NEUROPSYCHOLOGICAL INTERVENTIONS

NEUROPSYCHOLOGICAL INTERVENTIONS

Clinical Research and Practice

Edited by
PAUL J. ESLINGER

THE GUILFORD PRESS
New York   London

©2002 The Guilford Press
A Division of Guilford Publications, Inc.
72 Spring Street, New York, NY 10012
www.guilford.com

Printed in the United States of America

This book is printed on acid-free paper.

Last digit is print number: 9   8   7   6   5   4   3   2   1

Library of Congress Cataloging-in-Publication Data
available from the Publisher.

ISBN 1-57230-744-7

In memory of Rita and Frank

About the Editor

Paul J. Eslinger, PhD, is Professor of Neurology, Behavioral Science, and Pediatrics in the College of Medicine, Pennsylvania State University, and Director of Clinical Neuropsychology and Cognitive Neuroscience Programs in The Milton S. Hershey Medical Center and University Hospital Rehabilitation Center in Hershey, Pennsylvania. His research interests include functional organization of the frontal lobe, experimental analysis of neuropsychological interventions, developmental models of learning and executive functions, and functional brain imaging of emotional and cognitive processes. He presents workshops and lectures nationally and internationally, and serves on expert panels, review groups, and editorial boards in neuropsychology, aging, and disability.

Contributors

Steven W. Anderson, PhD, ABPP, Department of Neurology, University of Iowa College of Medicine, Iowa City, Iowa

Anna M. Barrett, MD, Departments of Medicine (Division of Neurology) and Behavioral Science, College of Medicine, Pennsylvania State University; The Milton S. Hershey Medical Center; and University Hospital Rehabilitation Center, Hershey, Pennsylvania

Thomas F. Bergquist, PhD, LP, ABPP, Department of Psychology, Mayo Medical School, Rochester, Minnesota

Keith D. Cicerone, PhD, Director of Neuropsychology, JFK–Johnson Rehabilitation Institute, Edison, New Jersey

Maureen M. Downey-Lamb, PhD, Department of Psychology, Temple University, Philadelphia, Pennsylvania

Paul J. Eslinger, PhD, Departments of Medicine (Division of Neurology), Behavioral Science, and Pediatrics, College of Medicine, Pennsylvania State University; The Milton S. Hershey Medical Center; and University Hospital Rehabilitation Center, Hershey, Pennsylvania

Claire V. Flaherty-Craig, PhD, Department of Medicine (Division of Neurology), College of Medicine, Pennsylvania State University; The Milton S. Hershey Medical Center; and University Hospital Rehabilitation Center, Hershey, Pennsylvania

Marjan Ghahramanlou, MA, Fairleigh Dickinson University, Teaneck, New Jersey

Lynn M. Grattan, PhD, Department of Neurology, University of Maryland Hospital and Medical School, Baltimore, Maryland

Elizabeth L. Glisky, PhD, Department of Psychology, The University of Arizona, Tucson, Arizona

Martha L. Glisky, PhD, private practice, Tucson, Arizona

Leslie J. Gonzalez-Rothi, PhD, Program Director, VA RR&D Brain Rehabilitation Research Center, Gainesville, Florida; Department of Neurology, University of Florida College of Medicine, Gainesville, Florida

Jacqueline J. Hinckley, PhD, Department of Communication Sciences and Disorders and Department of Psychology, University of South Florida, Tampa, Florida

Brian Levine, PhD, Rotman Research Institute, Baycrest Centre for Geriatric Care, Toronto, Ontario, Canada; Departments of Psychology and Medicine (Neurology), University of Toronto, Toronto, Ontario, Canada

James F. Malec, PhD, ABPP, Department of Psychology, Mayo Medical School, Rochester, Minnesota

Tom Manly, PhD, Medical Research Council Cognition and Brain Sciences Unit, Addenbrooke's Hospital, Cambridge, United Kingdom

Michael V. Oliveri, PhD, Department of Neuroscience, St. John's Mercy Medical Center, St. Louis, Missouri

Ian Robertson, PhD, Department of Psychology and Institute of Neuroscience, Trinity College, Dublin, Ireland

Caroline van Heugten, PhD, Institute for Rehabilitation Research, Hoensbroek, The Netherlands

Sarah Ward, BSc, Clinical Psychology Doctorate Programme, The University of Birmingham, Birmingham, United Kingdom

John Whyte, MD, PhD, Moss Rehabilitation Institute, Philadelphia, Pennsylvania

Preface

The scope of clinical practice and research concerned with neuropsychological disorders is rapidly expanding in many directions to meet increasing demands for accurate information and effective solutions. Approaches to diagnosis and management of brain-based behavioral impairments have always been multidisciplinary, bringing together the talents, skills, and knowledge of diverse psychologists, physicians, surgeons, therapists, and others to evaluate alterations in human behavior due to known and suspected ailments of the brain. These collaborations continue to grow and reach into many corners of society, from classrooms to medical centers, rehabilitation programs, medical offices, businesses, and retirement communities. The availability of expert diagnostic and rehabilitative care is a pressing need, with brain-based disorders of behavior a growing and leading cause of disability worldwide. While the provision of neuropsychological assessment services was sufficient at one time to facilitate the objective recognition and classification of brain-related behavioral impairments, the contemporary challenge is to link diagnostic and treatment procedures into pathways and protocols of effective service and adaptive outcome. Hence, advances in the scientific study of interventions for neuropsychological impairments provide the foundation and firm ground on which clinical services can be offered and patient disability can be reduced.

This book focuses on the linkage between clinical research and practice by addressing the ideas, methods, empirical data, conclusions, and models that drive interventions for neuropsychological disorders. Toward this goal, I am greatly appreciative of the efforts of the contributors, all very busy clinicians and researchers who care deeply about patients and their families and about the effectiveness of their craft. Their

comments and analyses are meant to be helpful for students, postgradu-
ate interns and residents, and practicing professionals from the clinical,
scientific, and educational arms of the psychology, medicine, and rehabilitation fields. The ideas and conclusions are meant to stimulate further research and implementation of interventions to reduce disability
and facilitate maximal adaptation of patients. I am also grateful to colleagues who carefully listened and counseled with regard to the aims of
this volume, particularly Arthur Benton, PhD, and Dan Tranel, PhD,
and to Rochelle Serwator, Sharon Panulla, and Seymour Weingarten of
The Guilford Press. Their encouragement and enthusiasm for advancing
neuropsychology and rehabilitation are admirable. My family and
friends have been unswerving sources of support. I am also indebted to
mentors, including Wayne Ludvigson, PhD, Ray Remley, PhD, Antonio
Damasio, MD, Gary van Hoesen, PhD, Hanna Damasio, MD, Richard
Tenser, MD, Marshall Jones, PhD, and Laszlo Geder, MD. It is my hope
that the findings presented in this volume will need revision in the near
future because of the scientific advances that will identify new interventions, revised interventions, combined medical–behavioral interventions,
as well as confirmed effective interventions to reduce the disability and
burden of neuropsychological impairments.

Contents

PART III   FUTURE DIRECTIONS

NEUROPSYCHOLOGICAL INTERVENTIONS

PART I

Foundations of
Neuropsychological Interventions

CHAPTER 1

Approaching Interventions Clinically and Scientifically

PAUL J. ESLINGER
MICHAEL V. OLIVERI

Health service delivery systems have adopted an increasing variety of neurological and neuropsychological interventions in the rehabilitation of patients with acquired brain damage. More recently, these activities have fallen under the rubric of neuropsychological rehabilitation, directed at remediating the behavioral, cognitive, and emotional deficits after brain injury and complementing the approaches of occupational, speech–language and physical therapies; therapeutic recreation; physiatry; social work; neuropsychiatry; and vocational rehabilitation. Hence, interventions are often multidimensional in nature and frequently are provided by a multidisciplinary team of rehabilitation professionals.

The magnitude of the problem for neurorehabilitation is a significant health concern. To cite only a few estimates, about 2 million people in the United States suffer stroke or traumatic brain injury each year, requiring medical evaluation and treatment (Guerrero, Thurman, & Sniezek, 2000; Thurman & Guerrero, 1999; Broderick, Brott, Kothari, et al., 1998; American Heart Association, 2000). Almost 10 million Americans are stroke survivors or are living with traumatic brain injury-related disability, causing an estimated economic burden approaching 90 billion dollars annually (American Heart Association, 2000; Goldstein, Adams, Becker, et al., 2001; Thurman, Alverson, Dunn, Guerrero, & Sniezek, 1999; Max, MacKenzie, & Rice, 1991). If one further considers the neurorehabilitation needs of those with neurodegenerative disorders (e.g., Alzheimer's disease), other cerebrovascular disease, cerebral neoplasms, hydrocephalus, and many other neurological causes of illness and disability, it should not be surprising that brain-based disorders are the leading cause of disability worldwide (World Health Organization, 2000). Therefore, the gravity of the human and economic burdens underscores the need for development and implementation of effective interventions that alleviate disability and hasten recovery of function.

Despite the multifaceted nature of brain injury rehabilitation, therapeutic interventions usually require innovative and individualized approaches (Wilson, 1991) due to the variable nature of deficits, personal background, and goals when comparing one patient to the next. In addition, the neurobehavioral consequences of any particular brain lesion are referable to variation in physiology and structure, momentum, etiology, and location, as well as to premorbid personality and cognitive factors, and postmorbid social and interpersonal issues (e.g., Lishman, 1978; Prigatano, 1999). Grimm and Bleiberg (1986, p. 499) recognized that the neurobehavioral sequelae of acquired brain injury may "defy any unified global description" due to the wide range of potential symptoms, syndromes, complicating factors, and recovery patterns. Despite the idiosyncratic nature of potential deficits, various themes consistently arise that pertain to the cognitive, behavioral, and emotional disturbances acquired after brain injury. Common neurobehavioral deficits include compromise to brain–behavior systems mediating self-awareness as well as attentional, memory, linguistic, sensory-perceptual, practic, executive, emotional, and social functions. In this volume, we emphasize that interventions for these diverse neuropsychological disorders need to be empirically and scientifically scrutinized for their effectiveness and linked to neuropsychological diagnoses.

Neuropsychological interventions are an evolving and growing enterprise. While at one time the fields of neuropsychology and behavioral neurology were comprised of "testers/diagnosticians" and "rehabilitators," this questionable dichotomy has never been tenable or advisable. Professionals who reported psychometric testing data in relationship to a particular lesion location or disease process were somehow perceived as more experimental and scientific, while rehabilitators were perceived as seeking a therapeutic effect from atheoretical and nonexperimental approaches (i.e., how can we make this person better?). Of course, these are stereotypical and extreme characterizations. Increasingly, the linkages between diagnosis and intervention are being probed and evaluated. It is reasonable to ask, "What are the clinical, professional, and scientific bases of service delivery?" This cuts across many aspects of neuropsychology, behavioral neurology, and rehabilitation, involving assessment, intervention, and management of cognitive, emotional, behavioral, and even vocational issues. Therefore, the chasm between assessment and rehabilitation/management is an artificial one, as the former is a critical foundation for the latter. By virtue of their multidisciplinary training, skills, and perspectives, specialists in neuropsychological rehabilitation are in position to bridge the continuum of care from acute to chronic stages of recovery. In addition to their providing descriptive and quantitative accounts of brain–behavior functioning from clinical evaluation and psychometric test results, they increasingly engage in providing real-time appraisals of the immediate functional implications of impairment, the types of rehabilitation interventions indicated for treatment, and anticipated outcomes, along with collaborating professionals.

In the 1987 text *Neuropsychological Rehabilitation*, Diller described an "uneasy" relationship between neuropsychology and rehabilitation and suggested the worthy goal of further integration between them. This gap is being filled admirably by recent texts that take a variety of approaches (e.g., Johnson & McCown, 1997; León-Carrión, 1997; Fraser & Clemmons, 2000; Sohlberg & Mateer, 2001; Wilson, 1999; Stuss, Winocur, & Robertson, 2000; Riddoch & Humphreys, 1994; Levin & Grafman, 2000) and by growing consensus about neuropsychological rehabilitation guidelines and goals (e.g., Harley et al., 1992; NIH Consensus Development Panel, 1999). The approaches are diverse, representing the growing needs for scientific data and clinical guidelines. While some investigators emphasize basic research, others focus on case-based therapeutic applications. Some are highly cognitive in their perspective, while others argue for a holistic, multidisciplinary program. This diversity is healthy and underscores the tremendous need for scientific scrutiny, evidence-based analysis, continuing publication of findings, multidisciplinary collaboration, and eventual linkage of detailed diagnoses with proven intervention protocols. In this volume, we emphasize in particular the clinical research that is driving current developments in neuropsychological interventions. More basic research lines (stem cells, trophic factors, etc.) are not covered, at least yet, because of the pressing need for clinical research that emphasizes scientific analysis, sound experimental designs with controlled studies, and application to clinically problematic areas that currently contribute to disability.

CLINICAL RATIONALE

It is the typical goal of clinical practice to determine which clinical interventions (short term and long term) are most likely to facilitate recovery of function. Within rehabilitation psychology and neuropsychology, it has been a long-term challenge to develop interventions directed at functional deficits that remain after acute medical management, in order to facilitate optimal adjustment (Diller & Gordon, 1981). Various approaches to neuropsychological rehabilitation and interventions have been developed, most often focusing on (1) restoration of function, to improve specific skill deficits, and/or (2) compensatory training in order to adapt to the presence of certain behavioral or cognitive problems.

In the 1980s, more comprehensive brain injury rehabilitation programs emerged, incorporating restorative and compensatory training, to address the cognitive, psychological, social, and vocational needs of patients with acquired brain injury (e.g., Ben-Yishay, 1982; Prigatano et al., 1986). Such programs have been viewed as holistic, due to multimodal interventions directed beyond specific cognitive deficits to include focus on emotional, interpersonal, and social areas. The goals of such programs have been to improve adaptive skills and to promote better psychological and vocational outcome. As a rule, brain injury rehabilitation programs have been predicated upon a clear and thorough delineation of the patients' underlying neurological, cognitive and social–emotional deficits. Beyond hospital-based acute rehabilitation management, clinical programming in outpatient follow-up has become quite comprehensive, including cognitive retraining, patient and family education, psychological adjustment counseling, and supervised prevocational and vocational placements. Treatment has been intensive, with frequency often on a daily basis, best represented by the emergence of day treatment brain injury programs, which have shown promise for improving outcomes of societal participation including vocational reintegration (e.g., Malec, 2001). At a basic level, brain injury rehabilitation management has been directed at improving patient self-awareness and promoting compensation strategies for residual deficits. Paramount among the goals for neuropsychological rehabilitation are (1) the need to focus on both the remediation of higher-level brain–behavior problems and their management in interpersonal situations, and (2) to help patients observe their behavior and thereby educate them about direct and indirect effects of their acquired brain injury (Prigatano, 1999).

FOUNDATIONS OF NEUROPSYCHOLOGICAL INTERVENTIONS

There are many patient, family, staff, and treatment setting variables that figure into building the foundations for neuropsychological interventions. A pivotal early component is to *demystify* as much as possible the medical diagnoses of brain disease and brain trauma, the resulting symptoms and disability, and the rehabilitation process. It is difficult for patients and families to focus on something they do not understand. Early programmatic services can address needed education in terminology, developing a common frame of reference with providers, delivering a view of where the patient and family are headed, and reinforcing a picture of recovery. A single form of management (e.g., medications) is rarely the solution. Instead, establishing collaborative relationships with patients and families underscores the necessity for a team approach and for multiple modalities of intervention.

Educational materials can be as creative and comprehensive as the rehabilitation team imagines. Schematics and metaphors can convey difficult concepts (e.g., recovery curve, half-life, multiple forms of attention/inattention). Profiles can provide comparative analyses. Emphasis on functional recovery and managing cognitive, behavioral, and emotional alterations can replace expectations of a "cure" after cerebral damage. Some of these interventions are critical in preventing pessimism, regret, loss of hope, and cascading decompensation in patients and family members. Identifying areas of strength is as important as identifying areas of impairment. The early stages of evaluation, therefore, not only begin to enumerate functional goals to emphasize, but also establish the attitudes with which rehabilitation services will be delivered and received.

Is insight on the part of patients necessary for demystifying their symptoms? For a complete understanding of their neurological conditions and symptoms, the answer is "Yes." However, partial insight or persistent lack of insight need not be a complete obstruction. Emphasis on specific behaviors, specific knowledge, and specific functional goals can still continue and be of observable benefit to patients. How the facts and events of their illness or trauma are packaged or reframed in behavioral, cognitive, vocational, or other terms in order to gain their awareness, understanding, and motivation may even influence the "insight" of the patient. Conversely, it is incumbent on providers to research their patients' frames of reference, common terminology, and expectations. Rooting out misperceptions, rigid beliefs, and false expectations may be the beginning of hopefulness and optimism.

As several authors in this volume discuss in detail, the World Health Organization (1980) has published the International Classification of Impairments, Disabilities and Handicaps. Three levels of trauma and disease consequences are suggested:

- *Impairments*: loss or abnormality of psychological, physiological or anatomical structures and functions.
- *Disabilities*: restrictions or lack of ability to perform activities in the manner or within the range considered normal.
- *Handicaps*: disadvantages for individuals that limit or prevent fulfillment of a role that is normal.

Pathology and impairment are located within body organs, such as the brain, and can be considered the neurobiological level of analysis. A fair amount of the literature of neuropsychology, behavioral neurology, and allied disciplines has focused on identifying and describing mechanisms and alterations of neurobiology. This is an important undertaking because impairments and pathology underlie disabilities and handicaps. Just as important, however, are the functional limitations (i.e., disabilities and handicaps) that are located within persons and their interface with the social and nonsocial environments. These are the levels at which disabilities and handicaps are expressed. The neuropsychology and allied literature have provided significant descriptive analysis and assessment methodology at these levels (e.g., Willmes & Deloche, 1997; Riddoch & Humphreys, 1994). However, these also need to be the focus of increasing efforts. Such broadening may be viewed as somehow "less scientific" if the goal is not to undercover mechanisms or anatomical–physiological correlates. This need not be the case. For example, while the primary actions of drugs are at the neurobiological level of pathology and impairment, the overriding interest in rehabilitation is on their effects at the disability and handicap levels, where functional limitations may be eased or worsened. There are strong conceptual challenges here, as Whyte describes in Chapter 4. While low-dose stimulant medication may improve inattentiveness after brain injury, its mechanism of action is on neurobiological transmitter systems that in turn influence the functional expression of numerous neural networks mediating attentional and other behaviors. Hence, expecting a drug cure for major functional impairments is scientifically and clinically naive and bypasses numerous levels of neurobiological action and pathophysiology. Similarly, most cognitive or functional neurobehavioral impairments remain minimally understood, be they nonfluent aphasia, memory retrieval inability, prosopagnosia, or intentional disorders of action. However, both neurobiological and neurobehavioral complexities continue to be unmasked a bit at a time, and it remains fair and reasonable to expect, as Levine and Downey-Lamb reinforce in Chapter 5, that efficacious interventions for functional impairments can be developed through empirical research.

AN APPROACH TO INTERVENTION RESEARCH

What treatment approaches are most efficacious for the remediation of neuropsychological impairments? Posing this question can lead to the following analysis:

Step 1	Step 2	Step 3	Step 4
Baseline assessment (variable X_1)	Assign subjects to treatment conditions	→ A → B → C	Reassess (variable X_2) and compare variables ($X_2–X_1$)

This analytical model represents only the initial planning steps for investigation of complex processes. For example, in remediation of attentional disorder, the following variables quickly surface:

- *Construct variables for attention*: verbal, initiate spatial, focus unimodal, sustain multimodal, shift divided/distraction.
- *Subject variables*: age, gender, etiology of brain injury, location(s) of lesion(s), focal–multifocal, early recovery phase, later recovery phase, comorbidity, medications.
- *Experimental design variables*: length of treatment, frequency of treatment, stimulus materials, measurement, control subjects/conditions, test–retest effects, randomization, frequency of assessment.

To design an informative Phase II-type treatment trial would entail not only hundreds of subjects across sites but also extensive facility, financial, and support staff resources, well beyond the capabilities of most centers and treatment facilities today. However, a more approachable question that each clinician and researcher can contribute to answering is, "What are the ideas, observations, and data that underlie interventions for neuropsychological disorders?" The need for innovative and informed research in remediation of brain-based cognitive, behavioral, and emotional impairments is widely acknowledged as pressing, important, and essential to the lives of many patients, to their families, to the continued improvement in health care quality and containment of costs, and to the leading causes of disability worldwide (e.g., Prigatano, 1999; World Health Organization, 2000).

Interventions for neuropsychological impairments cannot be accomplished as an isolated practice or limited to the acute and postacute phases of recovery after brain damage. Advances in effectiveness of interventions require insightful clinicians and therapists to detect and recognize deficits, formulate reasonable and attainable goals, implement innovative procedures, engage patients and their families in rehabilitation, and provide feedback and encouragement on progress toward those goals. Creative researchers and clinicians are also needed to frame empirical questions and hypotheses that can be addressed in clear, scientific, and measurable ways, encompassing both treatment effectiveness and real-world outcomes.

LINKING CLINICAL RESEARCH
AND PRACTICE THROUGH SCIENTIFIC
RESEARCH AND EVIDENCE-BASED ANALYSIS

Evidence-based analysis strives to complement individual clinical expertise with identification of the relative merit of particular patient care practices based on objective criteria. The focus of analysis is on clinically relevant research that bears directly on patient care practices such as sensitivity and specificity of diagnostic tests, efficacy of treatment protocols, and validity of prognostic indicators (e.g., Sackett, Richardson, Rosenberg, & Haynes, 1997).

In recent years, fiscal support for brain injury rehabilitation has been challenged by the broader erosion of economic support of health care. Despite this, rehabilitation programs focusing on remediation of neurocognitive deficits remain quite prevalent (Mazmanian, Kreutzer, Devany, & Martin, 1993). Even though there is a clear clinical need for management of these patients, the relative efficacy of both multimodal and modality-specific approaches to neuropsychological rehabilitation has been lacking. Without empirical support, it is easy for fiscal considerations to override established clinical needs in any individual case. There remains a pressing need to establish guidelines for neuropsychological interventions that are informed by both pragmatic clinical issues and sound scientific research.

There is ongoing debate about the utility of neuropsychological rehabilitation in rehabilitation medicine and in clinical neuropsychology. Evidence supporting the efficacy of such interventions is based on few studies (e.g., Prigatano et al., 1984; Ruff et al., 1989; Kay, Newman, Cavallo, Ezrachi, & Resnick, 1992; Rattock, et al, 1992). The research data base addressing the efficacy of cognitive rehabilitation has been criticized for lacking standardized treatment/remediation protocols, significant variability in subject selection, and problems with meaningful generalizability to functional activities (Ho & Bennett, 1997). With regard to neuropsychological rehabilitation, several lines of evidence are important to consider.

Within the purview of cognitive rehabilitation, some steps have been taken to establish guidelines for professional practice, even before efficacy has been established based on empirical evidence. In 1992, the

American Congress of Rehabilitation Medicine promulgated practice guidelines and recommendations, based on clinical expertise, for qualifications of specific providers (therapists) (Harley et al., 1992).

In 1998, a nonfederal panel of expert researchers and clinicians in various medical and rehabilitation fields came together to present findings to the National Institutes of Health regarding the scientific basis of the rehabilitation management of traumatic brain injury and related rehabilitation concerns (NIH Consensus Development Panel, 1999). The evidence was based on a review of the literature spanning January 1988 through August 1998, resulting in a bibliography of 2,563 references. Notwithstanding substantial methodological problems, a number of approaches were identified as having demonstrated efficacy. Cognitive interventions focusing on attention, memory, and executive skills have been supported by randomized controlled trials and case reports, based on intermediate outcome measures. Some support for computer-assisted exercises has been demonstrated through studies using global outcome measures. Some efficacy has been demonstrated for the use of compensatory devices such as memory books and electronic paging systems. Comprehensive interdisciplinary rehabilitation treatment, provided by a multidisciplinary team, received support for effectiveness. An extensive, evidence-based analysis of traumatic brain injury rehabilitation was sponsored by the Agency for Health Care Policy and Research and conducted by the Oregon Health Sciences University (Chesnut, Carney, Maynard, et al., 1999). A total of 3,098 abstracts addressing the efficacy of interventions from acute hospitalization to post-acute/longterm care were reviewed. Abstracts spanned 1976 to 1997 and were parsed down to 363 articles for review and abstraction. The review process identified significant fundamental problems in research design, so much so that most studies were not comparable. The primary problems included: insufficient description of cohorts, lack of uniformity in outcome measures, and inadequate description of interventions. It was concluded that some, albeit quite limited, support was discernable for:

1. psychiatrist-driven, multidisciplinary, acute rehabilitation with severe brain injury (one study),
2. direct transfer to formal inpatient rehabilitation that may improve outcome and decrease cost of care (one study),
3. cognitive rehabilitation, particularly involving compensation strategies, that showed positive effects on health outcome (3 studies), and
4. supportive employment (e.g., job placement, job site training, and coaching) that could improve rehabilitation outcome by increasing vocational success.

In a related systematic review of the literature pertaining to cognitive rehabilitation of persons with traumatic brain injury (Carney et al., 1999), 32 studies were ultimately abstracted. From these studies, two randomized controlled trials and one observational study suggested that specific forms of cognitive rehabilitation reduce memory failures and anxiety, and improve self-concept and interpersonal relationships.

Taken together, initial evidence-based review of contemporary neurorehabilitation argues for some support of comprehensive interdisciplinary rehabilitation treatment, provided by a multidisciplinary team, as well as modality-specific and directed interventions focusing on cognitive, psychosocial, and vocational issues. However, the optimal structure, content, timing, treatment, frequency, and implementation of such programs remains controversial (e.g., Salazar et al., 2000). Although this volume was not organized to undertake an evidence-based analysis of interventions for neuropsychological disorders, attention to evidence-based matters is extremely important and is presented in informal fashion throughout most chapters. This takes the form of consideration of subject variables, neurological variables (e.g., time since brain injury, location of brain lesions), reliability of treatment effects, generalization of treatment effects, measurement, appropriate control subjects and conditions, and the like. Even though some might argue that such analysis is premature for neuropsychological disorders, that concern has been answered. The Brain Injury–Interdisciplinary Special Interest Group of the American Congress of Rehabilitation Medicine recently published an initial evidence-based analysis of cognitive rehabilitation interventions (Cicerone et al., 2000). Their methods emphasized review of treatment efficacy and clinical effectiveness of interventions for disorders of attention, visual–perceptual and constructional abilities, language and communication, memory, problem solving, and executive functioning, as well as interventions that were multimodal and comprehensive–holistic. Results indicated a total bibliography of 655 articles, which were parsed to 171 studies meeting criteria and then classified according to experimental design characteristics (e.g., varying from prospective, randomized, controlled trials to single-subject designs). Results were further organized into three recommendation levels: practice standards, practice guidelines, and practice options. The results were encouraging indeed, with empirical support for neuropsychological interventions addressing language, attention, memory, and executive functions, among others, in patients with stroke and traumatic brain injury.

Though important for the evolving evidence-based support for neuropsychological interventions, the analysis and conclusions of Cicerone et al. (2000) clearly indicated where the field of interventions for neuropsychological disorders needs to go, and how it might achieve the objectives of reducing disabilities with sound scientific studies. Toward this end, this volume is organized to analyze the ideas, methods, and empirical data that currently underlie neuropsychological interventions and their scientific advancement.

AIMS AND SCOPE OF THIS BOOK

The aims of this book are rooted in two questions:

1. What are the ideas, models, and methods that are driving current research in interventions for neuropsychological deficits?
2. What are the results and current thinking from recent research in select areas of neuropsychological deficits—in particular, disorders of attention, learning and memory, language, praxis, visual perception, executive functions, emotional processing, and social behaviors?

While several excellent texts have been geared to the practical ("how-to") level of neurorehabilitation, to theoretical ideas, to animal models, to basic scientific findings, and to updates on progress and particular approaches to neurorehabilitation, we are hopeful that this volume combines several elements that are most sought by clinical practitioners, researchers, and students. Most importantly, we have aimed to provide the ideas, models, empirical data, and methodological frameworks that are guiding the scientific development, evaluation, and clinical application of new interventions for neuropsychological disorders.

The focusing question to the chapter authors concerned: "How is research in this area conceptualized, scientifically framed, and experimentally advancing?" Summarizing *what* studies have shown about rehabilitation focuses on where the field has been, but presenting *how* research is being formulated focuses on where it can go.

REFERENCES

American Heart Association (2000). *Stroke statistics*. Dallas, TX: American Heart Association.

American Heart Association (2000). *Economic cost of cardiovascular diseases*. Dallas, TX: American Heart Association.

Ben-Yishay, Y. (1982). *Working approaches to remediation of cognitive deficits in brain damage*. New York University Rehabilitation Monographs: No. 64. New York: New York University Medical Center Institute of Rehabilitation Medicine.

Broderick, J., Brott, T., Kothari, R., et al. (1998). The Greater Cincinnati/Northern

Kentucky Stroke Study: Preliminary first-ever and total incidence rates of stroke among blacks. *Stroke, 29*, 415–421.

Carney, N., Chesnut, R. M., Maynard, H., Mann, N. C., Patterson, P., & Helfand, M. (1999). Effect of cognitive rehabilitation on outcomes for persons with traumatic brain injury: A systematic review. *Journal of Head Trauma Rehabilitation, 14*(3), 277–307.

Chesnut, R. M., Carney, N., Maynard. H., et al. (1999). *Rehabilitation for traumatic brain injury: Evidence report no. 2.* Rockville, MD: Agency for Health Care Policy and Research. (http://www.ahcpr.gov/clinic/tbisumn.htm)

Cicerone, K. D., Dahlberg, C., Kalmar, K., Langenbahn, D. M., Malec, J. F., Berquist, T. F., Felicetti, T., Giacino, J. T., Harley, J. P., Harrington, D. E., Herzog, J., Kneipp, S., Laatsch, L., & Morse, P. A. (2000). Evidence-based cognitive rehabilitation: Recommendations for clinical practice. *Archives of Physical Medicine and Rehabilitation, 81*, 1596–1615.

Diller, L. (1987). Neuropsychological rehabilitation. In M. J. Meier, A. L. Benton, & L. Diller (Eds.), *Neuropsychological rehabilitation* (pp. 3–17). New York: Guilford Press.

Diller, L., & Gordon, W. A. (1981). Rehabilitation and clinical neuropsychology. In S. B. Filskov & T. J. Boll (Eds.), *Handbook of clinical neuropsychology.* New York: Wiley.

Fraser, R. T., & Clemmons, D. C. (2000). *Traumatic brain injury rehabilitation.* Boca Raton, FL: CRC Press.

Goldstein, L. B., Adams, R., Becker, K., et al. (2001). Primary prevention of ischemic stroke. AHA scientific statement. *Circulation, 103*, 163–182.

Grimm, B. H., & Bleiberg, J. (1986). Psychological rehabilitation in traumatic brain injury. In S. B. Filskov & T. J. Boll (Eds.), *Handbook of clinical neuropsychology* (Vol. 2). New York: Wiley.

Guerrero, J., Thurman, D. J., & Sniezek, J. E. (2000). Emergency department visits associated with traumatic brain injury: United States. *Brain Injury, 14*(2), 181–186.

Harley, J. P., Allen, C., Braciszeski, T. L., Cicerone, K. D., Dahlberg, C., et al. (1992). Guidelines for cognitive rehabilitation. *NeuroRehabilitation, 2*, 62–67.

Ho, M. R., & Bennett, T. L. (1997). Efficacy of neuropsychological rehabilitation for mild-moderate traumatic brain injury. *Archives of Clinical Neuropsychology, 12*(1), 1–11.

Johnson, J., & McCown, W. (1997). *Family therapy of neurobehavioral disorders.* New York: Haworth Press.

Kay, T., Newman, B., Cavallo, M., Ezrachi, O., & Resnick, M. (1992). Toward a neuropsychological model of functional disability after mild traumatic brain injury. *Neuropsychology, 6*(4), 371–384.

León-Carrión, J. (1997). *Neuropsychological rehabilitation.* Delray Beach, FL: GR/ St. Lucie Press.

Levin, H. S., & Grafman, J. (Eds.). (2000). *Cerebral reorganization of function after brain damage.* New York: Oxford University Press.

Lishman, W. A. (1978). *Organic psychiatry: The psychological consequences of cerebral disorder.* London: Blackwell Scientific.

Malec, J. F. (2001). Impact of comprehensive day treatment on societal participation for persons with acquired brain injury. *Archives of Physical Medicine and Rehabilitation, 82*, 885–895.

Max, W., MacKenzie, E. J., & Rice, D. P. (1991). Head injuries: Costs and consequences. *Journal of Head Trauma Rehabilitation, 6*(2), 76–91.

Mazmanian, P. E., Kreutzer, J. S., Devany, C. W., & Martin, K. O. (1993). A survey of accredited and other rehabilitation facilities: Education, training, and cognitive rehabilitation in brain-injury programmes. *Brain Injury, 7*, 319–331.

NIH Consensus Development Panel on Rehabilitation of Persons with Traumatic Brain Injury. (1999). Rehabilitation of persons with traumatic brain injury. *Journal of the American Medical Association, 282*(10), 974–983.

Prigatano, G. P. (1999). *Principles of neuropsychological rehabilitation.* New York: Oxford University Press.

Prigatano, G. P., Fordyce, D. J., Zeiner, H. K., Roueche, J. R., Pepping, M., & Wood, B. (1984). Neuropsychological rehabilitation after closed head injury in young adults. *Journal of Neurology, Neurosurgery, and Psychiatry, 47,* 505–513.

Prigatano, G. P., Fordyce, D. H., Zeiner, H. K., Roueche, J. R., Pepping, M., & Wood, B. C. (1986). *Neuropsychological rehabilitation after brain injury.* Baltimore: Johns Hopkins University Press.

Rattok, J., Ben-Yishay, Y., Ezrachi, O., Lakin, P., Piasesky, E., Ross, B., Silver, S., Vakil, E., Zide, E., & Diller, L. (1992). Outcome of different treatment mixes in a multidimensional neuropsychological rehabilitation program. *Neuropsychology, 6*(4), 395–415.

Riddoch, M. H., & Humphreys, G. W. (Eds.). (1994). *Cognitive neuropsychology and cognitive rehabilitation.* New York: Erlbaum.

Ruff, R. M., Baser, C. A., Johnston, J. W., Marshall, L. F., Klauber, S. K., Klauber, M. R., & Minteer, M. (1989). Neuropsychological rehabilitation: An experimental study with head-injured patients. *Journal of Head Trauma Rehabilitation, 4*(3), 20–36.

Sackett, D. L., Richardson, W. S., Rosenberg, W., & Haynes, R. B. (1997). *Evidence-based medicine.* New York: Churchill-Livingstone.

Salazar, A. M., Warden, D. L., Schwab, K., et al. (2000). Cognitive rehabilitation for traumatic brain injury. *Journal of the American Medical Association, 283,* 3075–3081.

Sohlberg, M., & Mateer, C. (2001). *Cognitive rehabilitation* (2nd ed.). New York: Guilford Press.

Stuss, D. T., Winocur, G., & Robertson, I. H. (Eds.). (2000). *Cognitive rehabilitation.* Cambridge, UK: Cambridge University Press.

Thurman, D. J., Alverson, C. A., Dunn, K. A., Guerrero, J., & Sniezek, J. E. (1999). Traumatic brain injury in the United States: A public health perspective. *Journal of Head Trauma Rehabilitation, 14*(6), 602–615.

Thurman, D. J., & Guerrero, J. (1999). Trends in hospitalization associated with traumatic brain injury. *Journal of the American Medical Association, 282*(10), 954–957.

Willmes, K., & Deloche, G. (1997). Editorial: Methodological issues in neuropsychological assessment and rehabilitation (Special Issue). *Neuropsychological Rehabilitation, 7,* 273–277.

Wilson, B. A. (1991). Theory, assessment, and treatment in neuropsychological rehabilitation. *Neuropsychology, 5*(4), 281–291.

Wilson, B. A. (1999). *Case studies in neuropsychological rehabilitation.* New York: Oxford University Press.

World Health Organization. (1980). *International classification of impairments, disabilities and handicaps: A manual of classification relating to the consequences of disease.* Geneva: Author.

World Health Organization. (2000). *The World Health Report 2000.* Geneva: Author.

CHAPTER 2

Theoretical Bases for Neuropsychological Interventions

ANNA M. BARRETT
LESLIE J. GONZALEZ-ROTHI

WHAT IS COGNITIVE REHABILITATION?

We recognize that the term "cognitive rehabilitation" is common usage. There is, however, little consensus as to its meaning. For example, some of us use the term to reflect rehabilitation programming directed at a certain population, that is, those with traumatic brain injuries (TBIs). In this context, "cognitive rehabilitation" defines that rehabilitation (exclusive of physical rehabilitation) provided to those with TBI. It may be done by a variety of professionals, including occupational therapists, neuropsychologists, speech pathologists, and so on. Another use of the term refers to a particular technology (specifically, highly structured, computerized programming) in the treatment of the cognitive deficits associated with neurological disease or injury. In addition to the professionals listed earlier, educational therapists in some rehabilitation units, for example, use this technological approach. We believe, however, that these uses of the term "cognitive rehabilitation" are far too restrictive, and we advocate a broader definition.

To expand the term, we could start by examining and defining its components. We define "cognition" as the ability to attend, to perceive, and to comprehend information; to manipulate, integrate, and maintain information; to intend to act or communicate; and/or to act or communicate. Thus, we would define a "cognitive disorder" as any impediment of these functions. In turn, what is rehabilitation? The Latin definition of "re + habilis" means "again + suitable"; that is, "re-" is applied in the instance of a loss of prior ability (as opposed to "habilitation"). With "habilis," in order to make something "suitable", one goal would be to maximize function via adaptation (through a focus on changing or accommodating the patient). A second goal would be to prevent or alleviate maladaptive behaviors. Thus, we suggest that "cognitive rehabilitation" is best defined as efforts to promote maximal adaptive cognitive functioning in patients with neurologically induced cognitive deficits. We do not believe that cognitive rehabilitation is defined by etiology; we believe that the potential methods available to this task are unrestricted (i.e., not limited to a particular method or technology). In fact, all neurorehabilitation efforts, whether focused on physical or cognitive deficits, may include experiential as well as physiological interventions. Physiological interventions may include drugs that render the system receptive to supporting functional recovery or minimize the impact or influence of maladaptive behaviors. We discuss some of these interventions later in this chapter. In contrast, experiential therapies cover a broad span of contextual enrichments, from applied therapies, such as strength training in the case of limb weakness, to modifications of the environment designed to accommodate dysfunction, such as the use of "beeping" watches to remind patients with memory problems of their appointments. Our definition of "cognitive rehabilitation" is open to treatments that involve physiological or experiential interventions, or combinations of both.

WHY TREAT COGNITIVE DISORDERS RESULTING FROM NEUROLOGICAL DISEASE OR INJURY?

We believe that, while not commonly treated, cognitive disorders resulting from neurological disease or injury require rehabilitation for the following reasons: First, cognitive impairments are common sequelae of neurological disease. Second, acquired cognitive deficits are thought to limit functional gains in rehabilitation. Third, the presence of these deficits may be used as a rationale to limit access to physical rehabilitation, because persons with cognitive deficits require more restrictive/costly living environments as a result of higher risk of injury due to decreased safety awareness and need for supervision. Most important, however, the presence of cognitive deficits after neurological disease or injury portends a poorer quality of life.

• *Cognitive deficits resulting from neurological disease or injury are common.* Acquired cognitive deficits can result from a variety of commonly occurring neurological causes, including traumatic brain injury (TBI), progressive neurological diseases, and vascular events. In the United States, an estimated 200–300 per 100,000 new cases are hospitalized with TBI each year (Jennett & MacMillan, 1981), and this figure does not include unhospitalized patients with mild head injuries, who we now know can manifest enduring and sometimes debilitating cognitive deficits. Combined figures for all types of head injury have been placed as high as 600 per 100,000 (Levin, Benton, & Grossman, 1982). The frequency of diseases of any kind that produce dementia doubles in 5-year age increments, from 7 per 1,000 in the 65- to 69-year age group to 118 per 1,000 in 85- to 89-year-olds (Bachman et al., 1993). Probable Alzheimer's disease alone has an incidence of 3.5 per 1,000 at 65 to 69 years, going up to 73 per 1,000 at 85 to 89 years (Bachman et al., 1993), and while the incidence of vascular dementia is lower than Alzheimer's disease, it is not an uncommon problem, with a prevalence estimated to be 15 per 1,000 in populations over the age of 65 years (Lindsay, Hebert, & Rockwood, 1997). By the mid-1990s, the incidence of stroke was 300–500 per 100,000 worldwide (Sudlow & Warlow, 1997), with a current prevalence of 2 to 3 million in the United States alone (Duncan, 1994; Lee, Huber, & Stason, 1996). It is noteworthy that all of these diseases/injuries are likely to yield a high proportion of enduring cognitive deficits. For example, in a prospective study of consecutive stroke admissions to a rehabilitation facility, 50% of patients displayed cognitive deficits (Paolucci et al., 1996). Thus, enduring cognitive deficits may result from a variety of causes, the incidences of which are indeed exceedingly high, thereby posing significant social and health concerns worldwide.

• *Those with cognitive deficits achieve less gain in rehabilitation.* While little is known about those with TBI or diseases that cause dementia, estimates of the number of patients placed in postacute rehabilitation settings after hospitalizations for acute stroke are surprisingly low, varying from 5% (Kuhlemeier & Stiens, 1991) to 16.5% (Lee et al., 1996). It is likely, however, that the number of patients receiving outpatient rehabilitation after stroke is higher. But most predominantly, the postacute rehabilitation services focus on physical rehabilitation despite the fact that cognitive dysfunction is known to be more enduring (Gresham et al., 1979) and to have a greater negative impact on quality of life (Ponsford, Olver, & Curran, 1995; Ponsford, Olver, Curran, & Ng, 1995). Importantly, many researchers have reported that the presence of cognitive disorders is a strongly negative predictor of rehabilitation outcome (Paolucci et al., 1966; Stineman, Maislin, Fiedler, & Granger,

1997). Standards of practice, as set in the U.S. Public Health Service's *Clinical Practice Guidelines for Post-Stroke Rehabilitation*, for referral to postacute (most predominantly, physical) rehabilitation include the establishment of "ability to learn," operationalized as a criterion score on one of two commonly used cognitive screens (Gresham et al., 1995). Thus, if a patient has a cognitive impairment that negatively impacts his or her performance on this general cognitive screen, he or she may be excluded from direct rehabilitation for physical limitations. This is an unfortunate recommendation considering that no data to date causally link (beyond correlation) ability to learn new motor skills with performance on these cognitive measures.

- *Persons with cognitive deficits resulting from neurological disease or injury require more restrictive/costly living environments and have a poorer quality of life.* While stroke more significantly relates to middle adulthood and dementia to late adulthood, TBI is a disorder associated with youth in that more than two-thirds of persons who sustain TBI are under 30 years of age (National Head Injury Foundation, 1984). Thus, those living each day with newly acquired functional deficits resulting from neurological disease or injury cover the adult lifespan. Additionally, the impact of TBI, stroke, or diseases that cause dementia, and their resultant functional deficits, makes the sufferer less independent and portends a poorer quality of life. For example, the impact of TBI on dependence of victims is significant, as evidenced by the fact that 33–75% of patients have to live with parents years after their injury (Kozloff, 1987; Tate, Lulham, Broe, Strettles, & Pfaff, 1989). Additionally, one study found that of those employed prior to their TBI, only 29% were employed 7 years after their brain injury (Brooks, McKinlay, Symington, Beattie, & Campsie, 1987).

Moreover, the functional impact of these neurological disorders very commonly includes cognitive deficits, with cognitive/neurobehavioral difficulties that are more disabling than physical impairments (Ponsford, Olver, & Curran, 1995; Ponsford, Olver, Curran, & Ng, 1995). For example, the prevalence of aphasia associated with stroke is 46–57% while the prevalence of memory impairment or disorientation is 47% (Bogouslavsky, Van Melle, & Regli, 1988; Scmidt, Smirnov, & Ryabova, 1988). Stroke is thought by some to be the most disabling chronic condition of all (Verbrugge, Lepkowski, & Imanada, 1989), possibly because so many stroke survivors have concomitant cognitive deficits. While 82% of first-time stroke patients are able to walk independently again, only 58% regain their independence in activities of daily living (ADLs) (Herman, 1981).

Evidence of the degree of disability associated with stroke is the finding in one study that only 59% of stroke sufferers under 65 years of age, employed before their stroke, were able to return to work in the poststroke years. A staggering 83% of stroke survivors reported that they had not returned to their prestroke quality of life (Niemi, Laaksonen, Kotila, & Waltimo, 1988). More practically, 6 months' poststroke onset, one-half to one-third of first-time stroke survivors require moderate to total assistance in carrying out basic ADLs (Allen, 1984; Andrews, Brocklehurst, Richards, & Laycock, 1984; Bamford, Sandercock, Dennis, Burn, & Warlow, 1990; Bonita & Beaglehole, 1988; Davaret, Castel, Dartigues, & Orgogozo, 1991; Dombovy, Basford, Whisnant, & Bergstralh, 1987; Kotila, Waltimo, Niemi, Laaksonen, & Lempinen, 1984; Wade & Hewer, 1987). It is frightening to consider this tremendously high level of dependence when one notes that only 47% of stroke survivors have a caregiver living with them at greater than 4.9-year postonset follow-up (Wilkinson et al., 1997); that is, a majority of stroke survivors either live alone or are institutionalized! Finally, dementia is defined by the presence of cognitive impairment, and the disabling nature of this problem is well known.

ARE COGNITIVE DEFICITS TREATABLE?

References to treatment of deficits in higher cortical functions (most predominately, spoken language) can be found in the literature as early as biblical times. Early efforts focused on methods such as herbal potions or placing stones in the mouth, and it was not until the world wars of the 20th century that behavioral manipulations were targeted for the management of these various deficits. Around the time of World War I, the majority of techniques used in aphasia rehabilitation were "borrowed" from the field of childhood education (Howard & Hatfield, 1987). In the years following World War I, aphasia treatment studies increased because of the large number of patients returning from the war with penetrating cranial injuries (Frazier & Ingham, 1920; Weisenburg & McBride, 1935). After World War II, the focus shifted specifically to treatment of aphasia associated with stroke. In the 1990s, we saw the emergence of interest in rehabilitation of a broader variety of cognitive disorders resulting from numerous causes (for reviews, see Prigatano, 1999; Riddoch & Humphreys, 1994; Stuss, Winocur, & Robertson, 1999).

The few anecdotal notes or experimental studies reported during the early 20th century extolled the benefits of treatment (Franz, 1906, 1924; Froeschels, 1914, 1916; Gutzmann, 1896, 1916; Mills, 1904). However, with the surge of interest in rehabilitation of cognitive deficits after the wars, controversy soon developed regarding the efficacy (or lack thereof) of these treatments (e.g., in the context of aphasia treatment, cf. Barton, Maruszewski, & Urrea, 1970; Sarno, Silverman, & Sands, 1970). This led Darley (1972) to suggest that research in aphasia treatment should focus on whether "language rehabilitation accomplish[es] measurable gains in language function beyond [that which] can be expected to occur as a result of spontaneous recovery" (p. 4). This is, of course, a reasonable question to ask with regard to treatments of all cognitive disorders.

In the last 25 years, we have witnessed an outpouring of investigations, many employing single-subject, multiple-baseline designs. These reports provide an opportunity to study the efficacy of cognitive treatment efforts. For example, in the area of aphasia rehabilitation, the issue of efficacy was addressed by Robey (1998), who reviewed 403 reports in the literature and found that 55 of them satisfied the strict, essential criteria for inclusion in a treatment outcome meta-analysis. Robey states that "on average, treatment for aphasic persons is effective" (p. 181; see also Hinckley, Chapter 9, this volume, for further discussion). Using within-subject method and experimental design offers a reasonable solution to experimental control problems found in several treatment studies (Kearns, 2000; Wilson, 1987; see also Levine and Downey-Lamb, Chapter 5, this volume, for further discussion). Thus meta-analysis of single-subject experiments may be used more extensively for studying the treatment outcomes for cognitive deficits other than aphasia. This likelihood is emphasized by work such as that reported by Malec and Basford (1996), supporting the suspected efficacy of broader-spectrum postacute brain injury rehabilitation when compared to natural recovery patterns. However, systematic meta-analysis of cognitive rehabilitation has not been done in areas other than aphasia treatment and remains a frontier of the future for neuropsychology and behavioral neurology research.

A RATIONALE FOR TREATMENTS OF COGNITIVE DEFICITS

We begin this section with a very basic assumption that on the surface seems painfully obvious. This assumption, shared by many neuroscientists (e.g., Kolb, 1995; Kandel, 2000), is that the action and interaction of neurons underlie behavior. If we accept this premise, then we must accept the notion that when behavior is pathologically deficient (e.g., aphasia), deficient behavior results from deficient action and interaction of the neuronal system underlying that behavior (e.g., language). Now we must take this logic to the next step, which is to assume that if recovery of this function occurs, it relates to the neurocellular, neurochemical, and neuropsychological events that define recovery of function after brain injury. Finally, if it is the interest of rehabilitation researchers to enable, encourage, and maximize recovery of function, then the rehabilitation process must be informed by what occurs at every level of brain function (cells, groups of cells, neuroanatomical, and neuropsychological systems). Therefore, it is our contention that rehabilitation efforts (prognosis and candidacy determination plus management) must be informed by what is believed to be happening not only at the functional level but also at cellular, neuronal network, and systemic levels. The purpose of this section is to review the cellular, network, and systemic changes that might inform our clinical decision making with regard to rehabilitation.

As others have objected (e.g., Kosslyn, 1996) when we study behaviors after brain damage, we cannot be certain whether improvement reflects evolution of restitutive activity in the injured brain or substitutive activity of intact systems, with *support of* deficient systems by intact systems (vicariation), or *replacement* of deficient systems by intact systems (compensation) (Rothi, 1995). For this reason, it is even more important to begin our overview of the physiological basis of recovery at the cellular level, where restitutive and substitutive changes are less ambiguous.

We begin with the precaution that applying results of bench research to human patients requires care. There are interspecies differences in brain morphology and neurochemistry, but human populations may also be relatively heterogeneous compared to normal animals or normal human tissue chosen for laboratory studies. With regard to the disorder being studied, environmental or genetic factors (e.g., sex) may differ between experimental animals or tissue and the typical human patient (cf. Barrett, 1999). Physiological studies may also be carried out with relatively small numbers of subjects or samples, and data may be examined using atypical procedures. Finally, the behavioral experiences of animals being studied are clearly different from the behavioral experiences of a typical neurorehabilitation patient (Kolb, 1995; Keefe, 1995), and we are not able to predict the variance that difference might contribute to each study's results. However, with these precautions in mind, there is still much to learn from the animal literature that might provide clues to a rationale for neurorehabilitation, and from this stance we proceed with caution.

Changes at the Synapse

Brain development may be a lifelong process, continuing throughout adulthood and into old age. This goes against the clinical teaching that there is a "critical period" of brain growth and learning from infancy to adolescence (for a review, see Finger & Stein, 1982). The classical dogma dictates that brain organization is completed in adulthood, and with aging, neurons degenerate and are not replaced: "In the adult brain, nervous pathways are fixed and immutable; everything may die, nothing may be regenerated" (Ramon y Cajal, 1928). While aged brains do show neuronal loss (Coleman & Flood, 1987), aged adults commonly demonstrate the integrity of their brain systems by performing complex cognitive tasks. Since the principal way in which the brain normally modifies itself is through change at the level of the synapse (Hebb, 1949), maintenance of performance as adults age means that new synapses (areas of electrical and chemical communication between neurons) develop as we age. Thus, neurons that remain continue to communicate and organize their activity, perhaps even more efficiently than before. Correlates of this activity involve changes in the axon, dendrite, or glia, and any of these changes would imply synaptic growth (Kolb, 1995). We, like others, define *synaptic plasticity* as enduring change at the synaptic level that leads to changes in the connections of cortical systems and, ultimately, to brain reorganization (Sanes & Donoghue, 1997).

Are our brains changing constantly beyond early adulthood? There is evidence that continuous, spontaneous neuronal remodeling normally occurs in the mature spinal cord (Purves & Voyvodic, 1987) and cortex (Coq & Xerri, 1998). Neuronal regeneration has also been noted to occur in the adult hippocampus (Kaplan & Hinds, 1977; Eriksson et al., 1998). Early reports (Konorski, 1948) described synaptic plasticity as a type of conditioned learning. Simply exposing an animal to a stimulating environment induces synaptic plasticity over hours to days (Hebb, 1948, 1949; Kolb, 1995). Adults, then, who continuously receive new environmental information, alter their attentional requirements by task demands, and engage in diverse cognitive activities, may undergo structural–dynamic brain changes on a staggering scale (Konorski, 1948). This conclusion endorses the desirability of maintaining exposure to enriched environments across the lifespan and, especially, well into late adulthood, when elderly persons are commonly relegated to less active lifestyles.

We observe that many adult subjects recover after brain injury, at least partially. If we accept our premise that changes in behavior reflect changes at physiological levels, and if we know that the mature brain is capable of synaptic plasticity, can we say that synaptic plasticity and neuronal remodeling underlie recovery of skills lost due to brain damage? Evidence suggests that they do (see Xerri, Merzenich, Peterson, & Jenkins, 1998; Seltzer, 1998), but whether synaptic plasticity restores normal function or assists the organism in compensating for lost function (again, restitutive vs. substitutive change) is still debated. Current thinking is that some changes, particularly in sensory maps, can occur in a matter of hours after injury (Kaas, 1991). Other changes may occur over weeks to months. In animals that have suffered ischemic brain damage, neurons that are temporarily nonfunctional but alive, located proximate to dead tissue, may demonstrate increased long-term potentiation (LTP), an activity-dependent change in synaptic transmission. This physiological alteration may mark slow functional recovery as it occurs for months to years poststroke (Hagemann, Redecker, Neumann-Haefelin, Freund, & Witte, 1998; Dobkin, 1998). Thus, might we question the time course over which therapies are typically planned? If plastic changes are still occurring in the brain months and years after brain injury, therapies may be usefully applied to the chronic as well as the acute patient, as currently typically practiced. Additionally, since rapid adaptation occurs in neurons, as well as slower recovery of function, some learning may be particularly strongly instantiated hours to days after a brain injury. We may wish to start some types of training as soon as possible, within hours. At the same time, because dysfunctional synaptic change can occur rapidly, we may also need to anticipate prevention of aberrant behaviors through control of patients' environment. This issue of the timing and nature of early enrichments remains to be determined in our human research, but there are clearly hints of its importance in the animal literature.

May we assume that if we can stimulate synaptic plasticity in mature brains, we can also do so after brain injury, with resulting functional recovery (e.g., Sanes & Jessell, 2000)? Unfortunately, plasticity may not be invariably beneficial. Massive cortical reorganization, similar to that correlated with synaptic remodeling (Pons et al., 1991), may occur with devastating or problematic results in patients who have chronic disease, for example, pain syndromes (Woolf & Salter, 2000), dystonia (Byl & Melnick, 1997; Elbert et al., 1998), or phantom limb sensations (Ramachandran & Rogers-Ramachandran, 2000). Additionally, aberrant synaptic plasticity has been associated with kindling (an animal model for epilepsy) (Sutula, He, Cavazos, & Scott, 1998), and may even be associated with worsening of the cellular pathology of Alzheimer's disease (Cotman, Cummings, & Pike, 1993). Finally, disuse can result in plastic changes and, in turn, loss of function (Nudo & Grenda, 1992). Do these pathological conditions represent deregulated, or dysfunctional, "learning"? The lesson to be learned from these instances of dysfunction related to plasticity may be that there is not a benefit-only outcome to all plasticity; that simply increasing the brain's propensity to change may not result in better performance (and in the case of postacute brain injury, functional recovery). Functional recovery as the result of synaptic remodeling must occur in the context of appropriate behavioral experiences. This is certainly the prediction of most connectionist models of cognition and learning (e.g., see Nadeau & Rothi,

1999), and it blends well with the current notions of errorless learning applied to cognitive rehabilitation (e.g., see Baddeley & Wilson, 1994).

Although postinjury brain adaptation may be more extensive for most adults than we previously hoped, it may still be limited in older subjects. For example, Corkin (1989) showed that as aging occurs in patients who have functionally recovered from a cerebral insult incurred in earlier years, there is evidence that they lose function more significantly than patients who did not have similar injuries. Thus, the aging brain may have less capability (decreased "reserve capacity") for plastic change (Finger & Stein, 1982; Bertoni-Freddari et al., 1996; Hatanpaa, Isaacs, Shirao, Brady, & Rapoport, 1999). Kolb (1995) proposes that the same mechanism that allows a patient to recover may allow compensation for neuronal loss with aging, and that at some point in the aging process, the two may compete, the net result being less efficient function; that is, eventually, synaptic plasticity may be maximally activated as the brain compensates for continued neuronal degeneration and adapts to new experiences. Synapses formed previously to compensate for brain injury may in this process be remodeled, "uncovering" old deficits (Kolb, 1995). By this reasoning, it is not surprising that older people show less recovery after brain injury (Teuber, 1975). However, paradoxically, aging may also benefit recovery in the injured region, depending upon how the injured region usually functions with aging (Stein & Finger, 1982). Normal, aged rats show impairments on behavioral tasks that rely on the frontal cortex, suggesting that frontal lobe function declines with aging. Aged animals with lesions in the frontal lobe cortex, however, return rapidly to their age-adjusted baseline, and their recovery can thus be more complete than that of younger animals with similar lesions. If our brains continuously remodel, vital cognitive functions may also become more localized or may be represented differently with age (Brown & Grober, 1983). Thus, some cortical lesions may be more devastating in older individuals, and others may have surprisingly little effect; some cortical lesions may respond better to one form of treatment than another in youth; some cortical lesions may respond well to one form of treatment in youth and not at all at a later age, and so on. We must become much better informed about the influence of age-related neural processes on treatment response in humans, and until this research is done, we must be wary of applying treatment strategies freely across the age span.

Changes in Neurotransmitter Systems

The extensive body of work on neurotransmitters in experimental models of brain injury has implications for rehabilitation (Flanagan, 2000;

Goldstein, 1998; Whyte, 1994). The scope of this chapter does not permit a comprehensive overview of these findings. Briefly, noradrenergic (NA) and dopaminergic (DA) stimulation may improve motoric function and orientation after brain injury (Feeney, 1997; Corwin et al., 1986). Enhancing acetylcholine activity, however, may also improve motor deficit (Ward & Kennard, 1942). Recent work suggests that acetylcholine release may also induce experience-dependent cortical remodeling, the assumed basis of neurological recovery after brain injury (Kilgard & Merzenich, 1998). Gamma-aminobutyric acid (GABA), an inhibitory neurotransmitter, may act against neurological recovery (Brailowsky et al., 1986).

Do medications acting upon neurotransmitter systems influence recovery? The answer is a qualified "yes." First, antihypertensives, antipsychotics, anxiolytics, and other medications that antagonize NA/DA and cholinergic systems, as well as GABAergic medications, may retard recovery after brain injury (Goldstein, Matchar, Morgenlander, & Davis, 1990). Second, although behavioral training alone aids motor recovery after brain injury, pharmacological treatments can work synergistically with conventional therapies to increase gains, even when only a one-time dose is given (Crisostomo, Duncan, Propst, Dawson, & Davis, 1988). NA/DA stimulants clearly have cognitive effects. They are helpful for patients with poststroke depression (Lazarus, Moberg, Langsley, & Lingam, 1994) and may improve distractibility and motivational deficit after brain injury (Powell, Al-Adawi, Morgan, & Greenwood, 1996; Whyte et al., 1997; Wroblewski & Glenn, 1994). Some investigators report that they improve recovery from aphasia (Wallesch, Mueller, & Hermann, 1997; Small, 1994). DA medication may improve spatial neglect, but patients may also experience paradoxical worsening (Heilman & Barrett, 1999). Cholinergic medication may have a beneficial effect on naming ability (Hughes, Jacobs, & Heilman, 2000; Jacobs et al., 1996; Tanaka, Miyazaki, & Albert, 1997).

How can we provide better treatment based on this information? First, although the effect of pharmacotherapy on cognitive rehabilitation is still being explored (see Whyte, Chapter 4, this volume, for further discussion), a trial of a DA, NA/DA, or cholinergic medication may be worthwhile for many patients. The choice among options depends upon the subject's specific deficits. Chronic patients, for whom there are few conventional rehabilitation options, may be excellent candidates for a trial of pharmacological therapy. Assessment of "target" and control behaviors before starting the drug, continuous monitoring while on the drug and again during periods of drug withdrawal are recommended (Barrett, Crucian, Schwartz, & Heilman, 1999). Finally, this literature again suggests the critical importance of applying these physiological treatments in conjunction with control of patients' experiences with targeted behaviors through therapy (Small, 2000). In Kilgard and Merzenich's (1998) study, cortical changes stimulated by electrically induced nucleus basalis activity in animals occurred only when associated with pure sensory experience. Additionally, their study underscores that an organism's environment can be constrained to enable errorless performance and this may permit optimal functional reorganization. When organisms respond incorrectly, the associated aberrant sensorimotor experiences may be strongly encoded and interfere with subsequent learning. Errorless rehabilitation strategies have been reported, with good clinical results for disorders of memory (Hunkin, Squires, Parkin, & Tidy, 1998; Clare et al., 2000). Others, however, suggest the possibility that "errorfull" and errorless techniques provide different learning advantages (Baddeley & Wilson, 1994), and optimal rehabilitation may integrate both techniques (Squires, Hunkin, & Parkin, 1997).

Functional Changes in Neuroanatomic Systems

Brain injury appears to disrupt the neural network of distributed, coordinated activity that occurs in many regions of the brain as we accomplish a behavioral task. One sign of this disruption is the remote deactivation of noncontiguous but functionally connected brain regions that occurs in the acute period after stroke, called *diaschisis*. A commonly recognized form of diaschisis is abnormal contralateral cerebellar function (which can be documented on functional imaging) after ischemic injury to the motor cortex, despite normal circulation to the cerebellum. It is likely that resolution of diaschisis plays a role in stroke recovery, and treatments to aid recovery may speed this process (Feeney, 1997). When a patient relearns a behavior after it has been lost due to brain injury, identifying the components of the newly functioning network can help us understand how recovery occurred and what facilitated it. When competence is not regained, we can look at the performance of other patients with similar brain lesions to learn if this type of brain damage may predict poor outcomes.

As functional networks subserving behavior reorganize after unilateral brain injury, we may ask whether the undamaged cerebral hemisphere now participates. In patients with motor deficits due to stroke, increased activity may occur in both hemispheres and in the perilesional region (Cramer, 1999; Weiller, Chollet, Friston, Wise, & Frackowiak, 1992). Some researchers have suggested that activation of motor and motor association areas in the damaged hemisphere (Picard, Hoffman, & Strick, 2000; Small et al., 1999; Small, 2000) or in both hemispheres (Seitz et al., 1998) may be associated with better recovery.

The contribution of different brain regions to recovery from aphasia after left-hemisphere brain injury is still being debated. Persons recovering from aphasia show increased activation in both the left and right hemisphere (e.g., Weiller et al., 1995) while attempting speech/language tasks. Some researchers have suggested that participation of the right hemisphere in speech/language tasks may be irrelevant or even detrimental to speech/language recovery. They posit instead that activation of spared left-hemisphere speech areas is crucial (Cao, Vikingstad, George, Johnson, & Welch, 1999; Samson et al., 1999; Heiss, Kessler, Thiel, Ghaemi, & Karbe, 1999; Karbe et al., 1998; Warburton, Price, Swinburn, & Wise, 1999). Others disagree (Musso et al., 1999; Thulborn, Carpenter, & Just, 1999; Weiller, 1998; Cappa et al., 1997). A possibility that has not been fully explored is whether right-hemispheric activity may be important during a limited phase of recovery. Although some therapies may be designed to activate a particular type of neural activity (e.g., using stimuli with emotional meaning may recruit right-hemisphere systems), it is unclear whether therapies definitely influence cortical functional networks. However, in two patients with dyslexia, tested more than 1-year poststroke, functional brain activity during reading changed after therapy improved their reading ability (Adair et al., 2000; Small, Flores, & Noll, 1998).

In patients with speech and language deficits, Dronkers (1996) investigated neuroanatomical correlates to recovery of function that differed from the classical localization of speech deficits. In her subjects, a lesion in the superior tip of the precentral insular gyrus, not in Broca's area, was associated with a persistent disorder of articulatory planning. Similarly, a lesion in the middle temporal gyrus and underlying white matter was associated with disruption of the lexical–semantic network (Dronkers, 2000). Careful use of neuroanatomical data to predict recovery of specific language function can, she suggests, allow for efficient speech therapy planning, concentrating on other deficits that can be expected to recover. However, further studies of the efficacy of targeted therapy are needed, since her anatomical–functional associations were based on patient groups in which all subjects received standard speech therapies.

These data also assume that neuroanatomical localization of functional networks subserving speech is relatively stable throughout life. It is possible that this is not true. Adult patients with fluent aphasias are significantly older as a group than persons with nonfluent aphasias (Obler, Albert, Goodglass, & Benson, 1978; Eslinger & Damasio, 1981; Brown & Grober, 1983). Brown and Grober (1983), noting a relationship among sex, aphasia type, and age, proposed that our brains reorganize normally over our middle-adult life: cognitive functions becoming increasingly localized and lateralized.

How can we design better therapies based on the implications of these changes in neuroanatomical–psychological systems after brain injury? First, because therapy may influence brain systems, we may ask again whether direct training of some behaviors should not begin earlier, during the acute period. Second, we may wish to reserve aphasia therapies that stimulate the right hemisphere for the postacute period, after recovery stabilizes, until more information is available about the right hemisphere's role in recovery of speech and language. Third, we may be able to determine whether a behavior is "lost" or only temporarily absent from the behavioral repertoire by using lesion data. As Dronkers (2000) suggests, patients who have new articulatory planning deficit but lack insular damage are likely to improve spontaneously. Treatment time may then be best invested in working on other language tasks. Finally, we may again ask about planning neurorehabilitation programs based upon a subject's age-related neural processes. If cognitive functions continuously reorganize as we age, and brain damage impedes this process, people under age 50 and suffering from brain injury may need periodic reevaluation and retreatment for emerging or "unmasked" deficits. In persons over age 50, whose cognitive functions may be differently localized, brain injury may have much less—or much more—impact on behavior. Subjects in the first category may benefit from intensive, early training over a shorter time period than their younger counterparts. Subjects in the second category, in whom a behavior may have been disrupted permanently by brain damage, may profit most from less intensive therapy geared toward compensatory changes by the caregiver or within the environment.

Although we primarily used language therapies for acquired aphasia when we discussed current issues in cognitive therapies, similar questions arise in the treatment of disorders of attention, memory, limb praxis, and visuospatial, social–emotional, and executive function. There is a need for outcome studies, particularly in the treatment of non-linguistic disorders, to investigate these questions.

CONCLUSION

In this chapter, we have defined what we mean by cognitive rehabilitation, described why cognitive rehabilitation should be part of the treatment of neurologically impaired patients, and have proposed a rationale for cognitive rehabilitation based on brain–behavior research. We suggest that the scope of cognitive therapies be widened beyond what the patient does with the therapist a few hours weekly, and that we categorize patients based upon both their disordered physiology (lesion location, neurotransmitter deficits, age) and the disordered behavior being treated. Comprehensive cognitive rehabilitation implies altering the patient's environment when outside therapy (limiting opportunities for dysfunctional learning or behavior), planning the time course of the therapy in relation to the brain injury (facilitating hyperacute administration of some therapies, as well as follow-up evaluation months and even years later for appropriate patients), coordinating behavioral training with pharmacological interventions, and tailoring therapeutic programs to the patient's age group. More systematic research is needed to help us define subgroups of patients who may differ in their natural recovery and response to therapies, so that we can offer effective treatments to individuals as well as to populations.

REFERENCES

Adair, J. C., Nadeau, S. E., Conway, T. W., Rothi, L. J. G., Heilman, P., Green, I. A., & Heilman, K. M. (2000). *Change in functional neuroanatomy after successful treatment of phonological alexia.* Paper presented at the Second National VA Rehabilitation, Research, and Development Conference, Washington, DC.

Allen, C. M. C. (1984). Predicting the outcome of acute stroke: A prognostic score. *Journal of Neurology, Neurosurgery and Psychiatry, 47,* 475–480.

Andrews, K., Brocklehurst, J. C., Richards, B., & Laycock, P. J. (1984). The influence of age on the clinical presentation and outcome of stroke. *International Rehabilitative Medicine, 6,* 49–53.

Bachman, D. L., Wolf, P. A., Linn, R. T., Knoefel, J. E., Cobb, J. L., Belanger, A. J., White, L. R., & D'Agostino, R. B. (1993). Incidence of dementia and probable AD in a general population: The Framingham study. *Neurology, 43,* 515–519.

Baddeley, A., & Wilson, B. A. (1994). When implicit learning fails: Amnesia and the problem of error elimination. *Neuropsychologia, 32,* 53–68.

Bamford, J., Sandercock, P., Dennis, M., Burn, J., & Warlow, C. (1990). A prospective study of acute cerebrovascular disease in the community: The Oxfordshire Community Stroke Project, 1981–86. 2. Incidence, case fatality rates and overall outcome at one year of cerebral infarction, primary intracerebral hemorrhage and subarachnoid haemorrhage. *Journal of Neurology, Neurosurgery, and Psychiatry, 53,* 16–22.

Barrett, A. (1999). Probable Alzheimer Disease: Gender-related issues. *Journal of Gender-Specific Medicine, 2,* 55–60.

Barrett, A. M., Crucian, G. P., Schwartz, R. L., & Heilman, K. M. (1999). Adverse effect of dopamine agonist therapy in a patient with motor–intentional neglect. *Archives of Physical Medicine and Rehabilitation, 80,* 600–603.

Barton, M., Maruszewski, M., & Urrea, D. (1970). Variation of stimulus context and its effect on word-finding ability of aphasics. *Cortex, 5,* 351–365.

Bertoni-Freddari, C., Fattoretti, P., Paoloni, R., Caselli, U., Galeazzi, L., & Meier-

Ruge, W. (1996). Synaptic structural dynamics and aging. *Gerontology, 42,* 170–180.

Bogousslavsky, J., Van Melle, G., & Regli, F. (1988). The Lausanne Stroke Registry: Analysis of 1,000 consecutive patients with first stroke. *Stroke, 19,* 1083–1092.

Bonita, R., & Beaglehole, R. (1988). Recovery of motor function after stroke. *Stroke, 19,* 1497–1500.

Brailowsky, S., Knight, R. T., Blood, K., & Scabini, D. (1986). Gamma-aminobutyric acid-induced potentiation of cortical hemiplegia. *Brain Research, 362,* 322–330.

Brooks, D. N., McKinlay, W., Symington, C., Beattie, A., & Campsie, L. (1987). Return to work within the first seven years of head injury. *Brain Injury, 1,* 5–19.

Brown, J. W., & Grober, E. (1983). Age, sex and aphasia type: Evidence for a regional cerebral growth process underlying lateralization. *Journal of Nervous and Mental Disease, 171,* 431–434.

Byl, N. N., & Melnick, M. (1997). The neural consequences of repetition: Clinical implications of a learning hypothesis. *Journal of Hand Therapy, 10,* 160–174.

Cao, Y., Vikingstad, E. M., George, K. P., Johnson, A. F., & Welch, K. M. (1999). Cortical language activation in stroke patients recovering from aphasia with functional MRI. *Stroke, 30,* 2331–2340.

Cappa, S. F., Perani, D., Grassi, F., Bressi, S., Alberoni, M., Franceschi, M., Bettinardi, V., Todde, S., & Fazio, F. (1997). A PET follow-up study of recovery after stroke in acute aphasics. *Brain and Language, 56,* 55–67.

Clare, L., Wilson, B. A., Carter, G., Breen, K., Gosses, A., & Hodges, J. R. (2000). Intervening with everyday memory problems in dementia of Alzheimer type: An errorless learning approach. *Journal of Clinical and Experimental Neuropsychology, 22,* 132–146.

Coleman, P., & Flood, D. G. (1987). Neuronal numbers and dendritic extent in normal aging and Alzheimer disease. *Neurobiology of Aging, 8,* 521–545.

Coq, J. O., & Xerri, C. (1998). Environmental enrichment alters organizational features of the forepaw representation in the primary somatosensory cortex of adult rats. *Experimental Brain Research, 121,* 191–204.

Corkin, S. (1989). Penetrating head injury in your adulthood exacerbates cognitive decline in later years. *Journal of Neuroscience, 9,* 3876–3883.

Corwin, J. V., Kanter, S., Watson, R. T., Heilman, K. M., Valenstein, E., & Hashimoto, A. (1986). Apomorphine has a therapeutic effect on neglect produced by unilateral dorsomedial prefrontal cortex lesions in rats. *Experimental Neurology, 94,* 683–698.

Cotman, C. W., Cummings, B. J., & Pike, C. J. (1993). Molecular cascades in adaptive versus pathological plasticity. In A. Gorio (Ed.), *Neuroregeneration* (pp. 217–240). New York: Raven Press.

Cramer, S. C. (1999). Stroke recovery: Lessons from functional MR imaging and other methods of human brain mapping. *Physical Medicine and Rehabilitation Clinics of North America, 10,* ix, 875–886.

Crisostomo, E. A., Duncan, P. W., Propst, M., Dawson, D. V., & Davis, J. N. (1988). Evidence that amphetamine with physical therapy promotes recovery of motor function in stroke patients. *Annals of Neurology, 23,* 94–97.

Darley, F. L. (1972). The efficacy of language rehabilitation in aphasia. *Journal of Speech and Hearing Disorders, 37,* 3–21.

Davaret, P., Castel, J., Dartigues, J. F., & Orgogozo, J. M. (1991). Death and functional outcome after spontaneous intracerebral hemorrhage: A prospective study of 166 cases using multivariate analysis. *Stroke, 22,* 1–6.

Dobkin, B. (1998). Activity-dependent learning contributes to motor recovery. *Annals of Neurology, 44*, 158–160.

Dombovy, M. L., Basford, J. R., Whisnant, J. P., & Bergstralh, E. J. (1987). Disability and use of rehabilitation services following stroke in Rochester, Minnesota, 1975–1979. *Stroke, 18*, 830–836.

Dronkers, N. F. (1996). A new brain region for coordinating speech articulation. *Nature, 384*, 159–161.

Dronkers, N. F. (2000). *Lesion site as a means of predicting recovery from aphasia.* Paper presented at the Seventh Annual Meeting of the American Society of Neurorehabilitation, San Diego, CA.

Duncan, P. W. (1994). Stroke disability. *Physical Therapy, 74*, 399–407.

Elbert, T., Candia, V., Altenmuller, E., Rau, H., Sterr, A., Rockstroh, B., Pantev, C., & Taub, E. (1998). Alteration of digital representations in somatosensory cortex in focal hand dystonia. *Neuroreport, 9*(16), 3571–3575.

Eriksson, P. S., Perfilieva, E., Bjork-Eriksson, T., Alborn, A. M., Nordborg, C., Peterson, D. A., & Gage, F. H. (1998). Neurogenesis in the adult human hippocampus. *Nature Medicine, 4*(11), 1313–1317.

Eslinger P. J., & Damasio, A. R. (1981). Age and type of aphasia in patients with stroke. *Journal of Neurology, Neurosurgery and Psychiatry, 44*(5), 377–381.

Feeney, D. M. (1997). From laboratory to clinic: Noradrenergic enhancement of physical therapy for stroke or trauma patients. *Advances in Neurology, 73*, 383–394.

Finger, S., & Stein, D. (1982). *Brain damage and recovery: Research and clinical perspectives.* New York: Academic Press.

Flanagan, S. R. (2000). Psychostimulant treatment of stroke and brain injury. *CNS Spectrums, 5*(3), 59–69.

Franz, S. I. (1906). The reeducation of an aphasic. *Journal of Philosophy, Psychiatry, and the Scientific Method, 2*, 589–597.

Franz, S. I. (1924). Studies in re-education: The aphasics. *Journal of Comparative Psychology, 4*, 349–429.

Frazier, C. H., & Ingham, D. (1920). A review of the effects of gun-shot wounds of the head. *Archives of Neurology and Psychiatry, 3*, 17–40.

Froeschels, E. (1914). Ueber die Behandlung der Aphasien. *Archiv für Psychiatrie und Nervenkrankheiten, 53*, 221–261.

Froeschels, E. (1916). Zur Behandlung der motorischen aphasie. *Archiv für Psychiatrie und Nervenkrankheiten, 56*, 1–19.

Goldstein, L. (1998). Pharmacologic effects on recovery of neurologic function. In R. Lazar (Ed.), *Principles of neurologic rehabilitation* (pp. 565–578). New York: McGraw-Hill.

Goldstein, L. B., Matchar, D. B., Morgenlander, J. C., & Davis, J. N. (1990). The influence of drugs on the recovery of sensorimotor function after stroke. *Journal of NeuroRehabilitation, 4*, 137–144.

Gresham, G. E., Duncan, P. W., Stason, W. B., et al. (1995, May). *Post-stroke rehabilitation: Assessment, referral and patient management. (Clinical Practice Guideline.* Quick Reference Guide for Clinicians, No. 16; AHCPR Publication No. 95-0663). Rockville, MD: U.S. Department of Health and Human Services, Public Health Service, Agency for Health Care Policy and Research.

Gresham, G. E., Phillips, T. F., Wolf, P. A., McNamara, P. M., Kannel, W. B., & Dawber, T. R. (1979). Epidemiologic profile of long-term stroke disability: The Framingham Study. *Archives of Physical Medicine and Rehabilitation, 60*, 487–491.

Gutzmann, H. (1896). Heilungsversuche bei centromotorischer und centrosensorischer aphasia. *Archiv für Psychiatrie und Nervenkrankheiten, 28*, 354–378.

Gutzmann, H. (1916). Stimm- und Sprachstörungen im Kriege und ihre Behandlung. *Berliner Klinische Wochenschrift, 53*, 154–158.

Hagemann, G., Redecker, C., Neumann-Haefelin, T., Freund, H. J., & Witte, O. W. (1998). Increased long-term potentiation in the surround of experimentally induced focal cortical infarction. *Annals of Neurology, 44*, 255–258.

Hatanpaa, K., Isaacs, K. R., Shirao, T., Brady, D. R., & Rapoport, S. I. (1999). Loss of proteins regulating synaptic plasticity in normal aging of the human brain and in Alzheimer disease. *Journal of Neuropathology and Experimental Neurology, 58*, 637–643.

Hebb, D. O. (1948). The effects of early experience on problem solving in maturity. *American Psychologist, 2*, 737–745.

Hebb, D. O. (1949). *The organization of behaviour.* New York: McGraw-Hill.

Heilman, K. M., & Barrett, A. M. (1999). Dopamine agonist treatment of neglect. *Neurology Network Commentary, 3*, 229–231.

Heiss, W. D., Kessler, J., Thiel, A., Ghaemi, M., & Karbe, H. (1999). Differential capacity of left and right hemispheric areas for compensation of poststroke aphasia. *Annals of Neurology, 45*, 430–438.

Herman, B. (1981). *Tilburg Epidemiological Study of Stroke—TESS.* Dutch Heart Foundation Final Report, Tilburg, The Netherlands.

Howard, D., & Hatfield, F. (1987). *Aphasia therapy: Historical and contemporary issues.* Hillsdale, NJ: Erlbaum.

Hughes, J. D., Jacobs, D. H., & Heilman, K. M. (2000). Neuropharmacology and linguistic neuroplasticity. *Brain and Language, 71*, 96–101.

Hunkin, N. M., Squires, E. J., Parkin, A. J., & Tidy, J. A. (1998). Are the benefits of errorless learning dependent on implicit memory? *Neuropsychologia, 36*, 25–36.

Jacobs, D. H., Shuren, J., Gold, M., Adair, J. C., Bowers, D., Williamson, D. J. G., & Heilman K. M. (1996). Physostigmine pharmacotherapy for aphasia. *Neurocase, 2*, 83–92.

Jennett, B., & MacMillan, R. (1981). Epidemiology of head injury. *British Medical Journal, 282*, 101–104.

Kaas, J. H. (1991). Plasticity of sensory and motor maps in adult mammals. *Annual Review of Neurosciences, 14*, 137–167.

Kandel, E. (2000). Cellular mechanisms of learning and the biological basis of individuality. In E. R. Kandel, J. H. Schwartz, & T. M. Jessell (Eds.), *Principles of neural science* (pp. 1247–1279). New York: McGraw-Hill.

Kaplan, M. S., & Hinds, J. W. (1977). Neurogenesis in the adult rat: Electron microscopic analysis of light radioautographs. *Science, 197*, 1092–1094.

Karbe, H., Thiel, A., Weber-Luxenburger, G., Herholz, K., Kessler, J., & Heiss, W. D. (1998). Brain plasticity in poststroke aphasia: What is the contribution of the right hemisphere? *Brain and Language, 64*, 215–230.

Kearns, K. P. (2000). Single-subject experimental designs in aphasia. In S. E. Nadeau, L. J. G. Rothi, & B. Crosson (Eds.), *Aphasia and language: Theory to practice* (pp. 421–441). New York: Guilford Press.

Keefe, K. A. (1995). Applying basic neuroscience to aphasia therapy: What the animals are telling us. *American Journal of Speech–Language Pathology, 4*, 88–93.

Kilgard, M., & Merzenich, M. M. (1998). Cortical map reorganization enabled by nucleus basalis activity. *Science, 279*, 1714–1718.

Kolb, B. (1995). *Brain plasticity and behavior.* Mahwah, NJ: Erlbaum.

Konorski, J. (1948). *Conditioned reflexes and neuron organization.* Cambridge, UK: Cambridge University Press.

Kosslyn, S. (1996). Carving a system at its joints. In *Image and brain* (pp. 42–45). Cambridge, MA: MIT Press.

Kotila, M., Waltimo, O., Niemi, M. L., Laaksonen, R., & Lempinen, M. (1984). The profile of recovery from stroke and factors influencing outcome. *Stroke, 15,* 1039–1044.

Kozloff, R. (1987). Networks of social support and the outcome from severe head injury. *Journal of Head Trauma Rehabilitation, 2,* 14–23.

Kuhlemeier, K. V., & Stiens, S. A. (1991). Rehabilitation admission after acute stroke hospitalization: Gender and racial disparities? *Archives of Physical Medicine and Rehabilitation, 72,* 840–841.

Lazarus, L. W., Moberg, P. J., Langsley, P. R., & Lingam, V. R. (1994). Methylphenidate and nortriptyline in the treatment of poststroke depression: A retrospective comparison. *Archives of Physical Medicine and Rehabilitation, 75,* 403–406.

Lee, A. J., Huber, J., & Stason, W. B. (1996). Poststroke rehabilitation in older Americans: The Medicare experience. *Medical Care, 34,* 811–825.

Levin, H. A., Benton, A. L., & Grossman, R. G. (1982). *Neurobehavioral consequence of head injury.* New York: Oxford University Press.

Lindsay, J., Hebert, R., & Rockwood, K. (1997). The Canadian study of health and aging: Risk factors for vascular dementia. *Stroke, 25,* 2343–2347.

Malec, J. F., & Basford, J. S. (1996). Postacute brain injury rehabilitation. *Archives of Physical Medicine and Rehabilitation, 77,* 198–207.

Mills, C. K. (1904). Treatment of aphasia by training. *Journal of the American Medical Association, 43,* 1940–1949.

Musso, M., Weiller, C., Kiebel, S., Muller, S. P., Bulau, P., & Rijntjes, M. (1999). Training-induced brain plasticity in aphasia. *Brain, 122*(9), 1781–1790.

Nadeau, S. E., & Rothi, L. J. G. (1999). Rehabilitation of subcortical aphasia. In R. Chapey (Ed.), *Language intervention strategies in adult aphasia* (pp. 457–471). Baltimore: Williams & Wilkins.

National Head Injury Foundation. (1984). *The silent epidemic.* Framingham, MA: Author.

Niemi, M. L., Laaksonen, R., Kotila, M., & Waltimo, O. (1988). Quality of life 4 years after stroke. *Stroke, 19,* 1101–1107.

Nudo, R., & Grenda, R. (1992). Reorganization of distal forelimb representation in primary motor cortex of adult squirrel monkeys following focal ischemic infarct. *Society for Neuroscience Abstracts, 18,* 216.

Obler, L. K., Albert, M. L., Goodglass, H., & Benson, D. F. (1978). Aphasia type and aging. *Brain and Language, 6,* 318–322.

Paolucci, S., Antonucci, G., Gialloreti, L. E., Traballesi, M., Lubich, S., Pratesi, L., & Palombi, L. (1966). Predicting stroke inpatient rehabilitation outcome: The prominent role of neuropsychological disorders. *European Neurology, 36,* 385–390.

Picard, N., Hoffman, D. S., & Strick, P. L. (2000). *Ipsilateral M1 is not involved in long-term recovery of distal arm movements after a contralateral M1 lesion.* Paper presented at the Second National VA Rehabilitation Research and Development Conference, Washington, DC.

Pons, T. P., Garraghty, P. E., Ommaya, A. K., Kaas, J. H., Taub, E., & Mishkin, M. (1991). Massive cortical reorganization after sensory deafferentation in adult macaques. *Science, 252,* 1857–1860.

Ponsford, J. L., Olver, J. H., & Curran, C. (1995). A profile of outcome two years following traumatic brain injury. *Brain Injury, 9,* 1–10.

Ponsford, J. L., Olver, J. H., Curran, C., & Ng, K. (1995). Prediction of employment status two years after traumatic injury. *Brain Injury, 9,* 11–20.

Powell, J. H., Al-Adawi, S., Morgan, J., & Greenwood, R. J. (1996). Motivational deficits after brain injury: Effects of bromocriptine in 11 patients. *Journal of Neurology, Neurosurgery and Psychiatry, 60,* 416–421.

Prigatano, G. P. (1999). *Principles of neuropsychological rehabilitation.* New York: Oxford University Press.

Purves, D., & Voyvodic, J. T. (1987). Imaging mammalian nerve cells and their connections over time in living animals. *Trends in Neurosciences, 10,* 398–404.

Ramachandran, V. S., & Rogers-Ramachandran, D. (2000). Phantom limbs and neural plasticity. *Archives of Neurology, 57,* 317–320.

Ramon y Cajal, S. (1928). *Degeneration and regeneration of the nervous system* (R. M. May, Trans.). London: Oxford University Press.

Riddoch, M. J., & Humphreys, G. W. (Eds.). (1994). *Cognitive neuropsychology and cognitive rehabilitation.* Hove, East Sussex, UK: Erlbaum.

Robey, R. R. (1998). A meta-analysis of clinical outcomes in the treatment of aphasia. *Journal of Speech, Language, and Hearing Research, 41,* 172–187.

Rothi, L. J. G. (1995). Behavioral compensation in the case of treatment of acquired language disorders resulting from brain damage. In R. A. Dixon & L. Backman (Eds.), *Compensating for psychological deficits and declines: Managing losses and promoting gains* (pp. 219–230). Mahwah, NJ: Erlbaum.

Samson, Y., Belin, P., Zilbovicius, M., Remy, P., Von Eeckhout, P., & Rancurel, G. (1999). Mechanisms of aphasia recovery and brain imaging. *Revue Neurologique, 155,* 725–730.

Sanes, J. N., & Donoghue, J. P. (1997). Static and dynamic organization of motor cortex. *Advances in Neurology, 73,* 277–296.

Sanes, J. R., & Jessell, T. M. (2000). The formation and regeneration of synapses. In E. R. Kandel, J. H. Schwartz, & T. M. Jessell (Eds.), *Principles of neural science* (pp. 1087–1114). New York: McGraw-Hill.

Sarno, M. T., Silverman, M., & Sands, E. S. (1970). Speech therapy and language recovery in severe aphasia. *Journal of Speech and Hearing Research, 13,* 607–623.

Scmidt, E. V., Smirnov, V. A., & Ryabova, V. S. (1988). Results of seven-year prospective study of stroke patients. *Stroke, 19,* 942–949.

Seitz, R. J., Hoflich, P., Binkofski, F., Tellmann, L., Herzog, H., & Freund, H. J. (1998). Role of the premotor cortex in recovery from middle cerebral artery infarction. *Archives of Neurology, 55,* 1081–1088.

Seltzer, M. (1998). Regeneration and plasticity in neurologic dysfunction. In R. Lazar (Ed.), *Principles of neurologic rehabilitation* (pp. 37–55). New York: McGraw-Hill.

Small, S. (2000). *Structure/function relationships in stroke recovery.* Paper presented at the Seventh Annual Meeting of the American Society of Neurorehabilitation, San Diego, CA.

Small, S. L. (1994). Pharmacotherapy of aphasia: A critical review. *Stroke, 25,* 1282–1289.

Small, S. L., Flores, D. K., & Noll, D. C. (1998). Different neural circuits subserve reading before and after therapy for acquired dyslexia. *Brain and Language, 62,* 298–308.

Small, S. L., Solodkin, A., Hlustik, P., Emge, D. K., Gullapalli, R. P., Genovese, C. R.,

& Noll, D. C. (1999). Cerebral cortical and cerebellar circuit reorganization after stroke [Abstract]. *Neurology, 52*(Suppl. 2), A14.

Squires, E. J., Hunkin, N. M., & Parkin, A. J. (1997). Errorless learning of novel associations in amnesia. *Neuropsychologia, 35,* 1103–1111.

Stineman, M. G., Maislin, G., Fiedler, R. C., & Granger, C. V. (1997). A prediction model for functional recovery in stroke. *Stroke, 28,* 550–556.

Stuss, D. T., Winocur, G., & Robertson, I. H. (Eds.). (1999). *Cognitive neurorehabilitation.* Cambridge, UK: Cambridge University Press.

Sudlow, C. L. M., & Warlow, C. P. (1997). Comparable studies of the incidence of stroke and its pathological types. *Stroke, 28,* 491–499.

Sutula, T., He, X. X., Cavazos, J., & Scott, G, (1988). Synaptic reorganization in the hippocampus induced by abnormal functional activity. *Science, 239,* 1147–1150.

Tanaka, Y., Miyazaki, M., & Albert, M. L. (1997). Effects of increased cholinergic activity on naming in aphasia. *Lancet, 350,* 116–117.

Tate, R. L., Lulham, J. M., Broe, G. A., Strettles, B., & Pfaff, A. (1989). Psychosocial outcomes for the survivors of severe blunt head injury. *Journal of Neurology, Neurosurgery and Psychiatry, 52,* 128–134.

Teuber, H. L. (1975). Recovery of function after brain injury in man. *Ciba Foundation Symposium, 34,* 159–190.

Thulborn, K. R., Carpenter, P. A., & Just, M. A. (1999). Plasticity of language-related brain function during recovery from stroke. *Stroke, 30,* 749–754.

Verbrugge, L. M., Lepkowski, J. M., & Imanada, Y. (1989). Comorbidity and its impact on disability. *Milbank Quarterly, 67,* 450–484.

Wade, D. T., & Hewer, R. L. (1987). Functional abilities after stroke: Measurement, natural history and prognosis. *Journal of Neurology, Neurosurgery and Psychiatry, 50,* 177–182.

Warburton, E., Price, C. J., Swinburn, K., & Wise, R. J. (1999). Mechanisms of recovery from aphasia: Evidence from positron emission tomography studies. *Journal of Neurology, Neurosurgery and Psychiatry, 66,* 155–161.

Ward, A. A., Jr., & Kenward, M. A. (1942). Effect of cholinergic drugs on recovery of function following lesions of the central nervous system in monkeys. *Yale Journal of Biology and Medicine, 15,* 189–228.

Weiller, C. (1998). Imaging recovery from stroke. *Experimental Brain Research, 123,* 13–17.

Weiller, C., Chollet, F., Friston, K. J., Wise, R. J., & Frackowiak, R. S. (1992). Functional reorganization of the brain in recovery from striatocapsular infarction in man. *Annals of Neurology, 31,* 463–472.

Weiller, C., Isensee, C., Rijntjes, M., Huber, W., Muller, S., Bier, D., Dutschka, K., Woods, R. P., Noth, J., & Diener, H. C. (1995). Recovery from Wernicke's aphasia: A positron emission tomographic study. *Annals of Neurology, 37,* 723–732.

Weisenburg, T., & McBride, K. E. (1935). *Aphasia: A clinical and psychological study.* New York: Commonwealth Fund.

Whyte, J. (1994). Toward rational psychopharmacological treatment: Integrating research and clinical practice. *Journal of Head Trauma Rehabilitation, 9,* 91–103.

Whyte, J., Hart, T., Schuster, K., Fleming, M., Polansky, M., & Coslett, H. B. (1997). Effects of methylphenidate on attentional function after traumatic brain injury: A randomized, placebo-controlled trial. *American Journal of Physical Medicine and Rehabilitation, 76,* 440–450.

Wilkinson, P. R., Wolfe, C. D. A., Warburton, F. G., Rudd, A. G., Howard, R. S.,

Ross-Russell, R. W., & Beech, R. R. (1997). A long-term follow-up of stroke patients. *Stroke, 28,* 507–512.

Wilson, B. (1987). Single-case experimental designs in neuropsychological rehabilitation. *Journal of Clinical and Experimental Neuropsychology, 9,* 527–544.

Woolf, C., & Salter, M. W. (2000). Neuronal plasticity: Increasing the gain in pain. *Science, 288,* 1765–1772.

Wroblewski, B. A., & Glenn, M. B. (1994). Pharmacological treatment of arousal and cognitive deficits. *Journal of Head Trauma Rehabilitation, 9,* 19–42.

Xerri, C., Merzenich, M. M., Peterson, B. E., & Jenkins, W. (1998). Plasticity of primary somatosensory cortex paralleling sensorimotor skill recovery from stroke in adult monkeys. *Journal of Neurophysiology, 79,* 2119–2148.

CHAPTER 3

Neuropsychological Assessment for Treatment Planning and Research

THOMAS F. BERGQUIST
JAMES F. MALEC

Neuropsychological evaluation has a relatively brief but impressive history as a diagnostic method to assess for the presence of brain dysfunction, as well as to assist in describing the nature of that dysfunction. Over the last 30 years, neuropsychological evaluations have played an increasingly important role with a variety of patient populations. These evaluations, for example, are still the principal means of diagnosing dementia, particularly in the early stages (McKhan et al., 1984). They are also a valuable and, in some cases, necessary means for diagnosing and describing the various cognitive and academic problems associated with developmental disorders such as learning disabilities (Rourke, 1989).

Neuropsychological evaluations have traditionally used a psychometric approach and determined the presence of brain impairment on the basis of deviation from the expected performance with reference to appropriate normative data. The determination of brain impairment is based on deviation of patients' performance on standardized psychometric tests from the expected level of performance for their particular demographic group. Clinical research in this area developed along these lines, with an emphasis on improving the normative base of psychometric testing. More recently, this has included developing a common normative base for various age and education cohorts (e.g., Halstead–Reitan Battery, Wechsler Adult Intelligence Scale—III (WAIS-III), Wechsler MEMORY Scale—III (WMS-III), Mayo Older Adult Normative Studies). The nature of possible brain dysfunction (e.g., cortical vs. subcortical dementia) can be further used to determine the underlying nature of the pathology. All of this work has helped to improve the efficacy of neuropsychological evaluations in determining the presence of brain dysfunction.

A NEW VENUE

With the rise of postacute brain injury rehabilitation in the 1970s and 1980s, a new venue was created for neuropsychologists to apply their testing acumen. In this setting, neuropsychological evaluations were used for different purposes. They were now required to determine an individual's pattern and level of *disability*, and not simply to comment upon *impairment* resulting from the brain damage. The emphasis of the evaluation in these settings was to identify realistic treatment goals and assess patients' capacity to benefit from treatment (Lezak, 1987). In order to accomplish this task, it was necessary to shift away from strictly diagnostically oriented neuropsychological assessment toward a more functional approach.

In our experience, it is very common for neuropsychologists to confuse level of *impairment* with level of *disability*. The International Classification of Impairments, Disabilities and Handicaps (ICIDH; World Health Organization, 1987) provides definitions of "impairment," "disability," and "handicap." The most recent edition (ICIDH-2) has exchanged the terms "activity" for "disability" and "participation" for "handicap" (World Health Organization, 1997):

- *Impairment* is an abnormality in a physical or mental function.
- *Disability/activity* is a limitation in performance of an activity because of impairment.
- *Handicap/participation* is a loss of social-role function because of a disability.

In postacute brain injury rehabilitation settings, neuropsychologists are asked to describe the effects of brain injury in terms of disability and handicap rather than impaired mental function alone. In these settings— which provide services primarily to persons with well-documented, moderate to severe brain injury—the diagnosis and neurological parameters of the injury itself have typically already been identified by other means (such as neuroimaging studies) and by other measures of injury severity (such as length of coma, length of posttraumatic amnesia, Glasgow Coma Scale score). In the postacute setting, using impaired test performance to characterize brain dysfunction adds information about the nature and severity of the injury but contributes little to the diagnostic evaluation.

The level of impairment in mental functions caused by brain injury is not the focus of treatment and intervention in these settings. Instead, the level of disability associated with brain injury is the focus of treatment. For example, a neuropsychological evaluation may identify memory impairment due to brain injury. Memory impairment itself may or may not justify further intervention. Some individuals accommodate to and learn to compensate for mild memory dysfunction easily, without professional assistance. The need for professional intervention depends on whether this impairment results in a change in valued activities in day-to-day life for individuals, in other words, whether or not their brain injury is associated with disability. The nature of that change (or disability) also determines the nature of those interventions.

SCOPE OF TESTING

Tests were developed based upon their ability to detect brain dysfunction within certain parameters. Neuropsychological evaluation conducted for the purpose of determining brain impairment typically includes assessment of several categories of mental functions. Generally accepted major categories of mental functions to be assessed are listed in Table 3.1 (Lezak, 1995).

In North America, neuropsychology has traditionally focused on psychometric testing used for diagnostic purposes. The emphasis has been on developing tests that can be demonstrated both to detect brain dysfunction (sensitivity) and describe the nature and scope of that dysfunction (specificity). Specificity has most often been assessed in terms of specific neurological diagnoses. However, patterns of cognitive impairment (e.g., learning disabilities) have also served as the basis for evaluat-

TABLE 3.1. Major Categories of Mental Function Included in Neuropsychological Evaluations (Lezak, 1995)

1. Orientation and attention	5. Construction
2. Perception	6. Concept formation and reasoning
3. Memory	7. Executive functions
4. Verbal and language functions	8. Motor/sensory abilities

ing the specificity of psychometric tests and test batteries. This approach, however, does not necessarily capture factors that have the most significant relationship to level of disability. The assessment of brain dysfunction depends on a test's ability to assess the integrity of brain structures. In contrast, assessment of disability focuses on the impact of a particular mental dysfunction on an individual's ability to perform an activity.

Self-awareness is an example of a mental function that typically is not included in diagnostic models of neuropsychological assessment. Since impaired self-awareness has recently been found to be present in approximately 25% of a normal adult population (Kruger & Dunning, 1999), the presence of impaired self-awareness following brain injury may not by itself be a valid indication of acquired brain dysfunction. Impaired self-awareness, however, is believed to result from brain injury (McGlynn & Schachter, 1989). Moreover, impaired self-awareness has been shown to be a major factor in determining the extent to which patients benefit from therapy (Prigatano & Fordyce, 1986) and a significant predictor of functional outcomes such as level of employment (Sherer et al., 1998).

Crosson and colleagues (1989) argued that clinical interventions in the postacute phase of brain injury rehabilitation are likely to be ineffective unless the level of self-awareness is accurately assessed. Specifically, level of self-awareness determines directly the degree to which patients are able to generalize gains made in treatment to other settings, and in so doing enables the therapist to determine the nature of interventions necessary to assist patients in achieving their highest level of functioning.

Sherer, Oden, Bergoff, Levin, and High (1998) describe several methods for assessing self-awareness, including (1) direct clinician ratings, (2) differences between patient and family ratings of abilities, (3) differences between patient and clinician ratings of abilities, and (4) differences between patient self-ratings and objective test performance. In instances in which differences between patient and staff or family ratings are to be used, scales have been developed that allow the clinician to assess accurately what constitutes a significant difference in ratings between patients and others (e.g., Malec, Machulda, & Moessner, 1997; Sherer et al., 1999).

Without attention to self-awareness, interventions may still result in improvements within the confines of the treatment setting and appear to be useful to the patient. Such improvements, however, will quite likely be ineffective in generalizing to behavior change that helps survivors of brain injury function better in day-to-day life (Gordon, 1987). Thus, while a neuropsychological assessment that does not assess self-awareness may be useful in detecting brain dysfunction and the pattern of cognitive dysfunction, it will be incomplete in assessing for level of disability and need for intervention following brain injury.

Although an appraisal of self-awareness may be critical to rehabilitation and intervention planning, differentiating between pre- and postmorbid disability is not necessary. In some situations, distinguishing the kind and level of disability that has resulted from a brain injury or illness is important, for instance, in legal consultations or consultations related to disability determination. However, in many cases, distinctions between pre- and postinjury cognitive, personality, emotional, and social functioning cannot be made confidently. In such cases, interventions based on an assessment of the patient's current psychological strengths and liabilities can proceed with a possibility of success. In still other cases, appraisal of preinjury functioning becomes confounded by impaired self-awareness. In these cases, when a patient's inaccurate attributions of the cause of his or her deficits interfere with treatment, identifying and clarifying the source of neuropsychological impairment with the patient may become critical for successful intervention. Some examples of such cases include patients who resist using compensation techniques for brain-injury-related memory problems because they inaccurately believe that their "memory has never been very good," or those who excuse preinjury, long-standing, maladaptive interpersonal behavior on the basis of their brain injury.

NEW SCOPE AND FOCUS

Evaluation of mood state, personality, motivation, and other psychological factors is often viewed as not essential to address many of the referrals for assessment of brain function. When assessed, these factors are often measured for the purpose of determining the degree to which they interfere with the validity of the evaluation. However, a lack of attention to other psychological factors in the neuropsychological evaluation may result in an inadequate assessment of disability. An approach that focuses solely on assessment of various cognitive domains has been criticized as leading to a lack of environmental validity and to difficulty in generalizing the results of testing to "real-world" situations (Sbordone, 1997). For example, significant behavioral disturbance often results from orbitofrontal injury and has a profound impact on an individual's ability to function independently in society. While this alteration in behavior is typically quite obvious in an unstructured and unsupervised environment, it is often underestimated in neuropsychological testing alone. This not only can lead to incorrectly describing the patient as having a lesser degree of brain impairment than is actually the case (false negative), but it also underestimates the level of disability following brain injury, leading to many unexpected problems in community, family, and vocational reintegration.

Similarly, neuropsychological assessment of someone who is highly anxious or has questionable motivation will likely not provide a valid measure of brain dysfunction. Since there is nothing neurologically wrong with this individual, a diagnostic neuropsychologist may feel limited to confirming the absence of brain dysfunction for the patient. At the extreme, using neuropsychological evaluations solely to determine the presence of brain dysfunction, while neglecting to address other psychological and emotional issues that are identified during the course of testing, has been described as unethical behavior (Binder & Thompson, 1995). For the neuropsychologist working in postacute brain injury rehabilitation settings, a comprehensive assessment of cognitive, emotional, personality, and interpersonal factors is an essential part of effective treatment planning.

Brain injury survivors may experience severe levels of anxiety and depression due to difficulties in coping with the often devastating effects of their injuries and illnesses. There is general consensus that in addition to the benefits of interventions targeting cognitive and behavioral impairments, supportive counseling and psychotherapy are very useful to assist patients and their families in improving mood, coping, and adjusting to significant changes in life circumstances (National Institutes of Health Consensus Development Panel, 1999). A neuropsychological evaluation can assist in assessment of these many factors and determine whether such interventions may be of benefit to the patient.

The malingering patient is not an appropriate candidate for neuropsychological treatment—and typically is not interested in such intervention. Perhaps because we work in a rehabilitative setting in which most patients are applying for treatment, our patients whose neuropsychological disability cannot be clearly attributed to brain dysfunction are rarely simple malingerers. It would be a gross oversimplification to define "malingering" as neuropsychological disability in the absence of a clear indication of neurocognitive impairment. Such disability most often results from a complex interaction of emotional, psychological, personality, and interpersonal factors, and—very possibly—higher order and executive cognitive functions that are not sensitively assessed by currently available psychometric procedures.

It is not surprising that models of functioning in individuals following brain injury, proposed by neuropsychologists working from a viewpoint of disability, are highly complex and include multiple, interacting variables to explain behavior following brain injury (Kay, Newman, Cavallo, Ezrachi, & Resnick, 1992; Ruff, Camenzuli, & Mueller, 1996). These models include not only cognitive status but also a variety of personality, emotional, and environmental factors. Together, these factors account for the wide variability in long-term patient outcome that is otherwise confusing when viewed simply in terms of whether brain dysfunction is present.

A neuropsychological evaluation is uniquely able to assess a wide variety of mental and psychological functions in medical and rehabilitative settings. Moreover, with their background in research design, methodology, and behavioral theory, neuropsychologists are uniquely positioned to conceptualize the multiple factors that interact to affect outcome in these cases (Johnston, Keith, & Hinderer, 1992). This is true whether or not the level of functioning the individual displays can be directly related to brain dysfunction.

Multiple factors beyond what can directly be attributed to brain dysfunction may affect test performance. The factors to be assessed, however, need to go beyond the categories of mental status typically included in the neuropsychological evaluations described earlier. Members of a consensus conference on neuropsychological rehabilitation discussed several topics related to these concerns, including use of neuropsychological evaluations to predict functional outcome such as employment (Bergquist et al., 1994). Unlike developers of the template for neuropsychological evaluations that focused on assessment of impairment (as shown in Table 3.1), this group attempted to develop a template that captures the information needed from a neuropsychological evaluation for assessment of level of functioning (Table 3.2).

The complete assessment of the impact of these factors on mental

---

TABLE 3.2. Major Areas to Be Assessed in a Neuropsychological Assessment When Planning for Intervention. (Bergquist et al., 1994)

1. Self-awareness of strengths and deficits
2. Compensation for cognitive, physical, and emotional deficits
3. Self-esteem and self-confidence
4. Extent of agreement between skill levels and personal/vocational goals
5. Constructive vocational and personal relationships
6. The need for environmental accommodations to achieve an effective match with the patient's specific cognitive, physical, and psychosocial needs

From Bergquist et al. (1994). Copyright 1994 by Aspen Publishers. Reprinted by permission.

function cannot be limited to neurocognitive testing. By changing the focus and the scope of how neuropsychological evaluations have traditionally been conducted, this evaluation can uniquely capture important information related to the effects of brain injury on day-to-day functioning and, in so doing, more completely describe the level of disability following brain injury.

Self-Awareness

We have already described methods to assess self-awareness. Assessment of most other areas described in Table 3.2 uses methods that require either observing the individual directly in real-life or simulated real-life environments, or obtaining such observational information from family, friends, or others who have the opportunity to observe the patient's functioning in real-life environments.

Disability

Several functional scales have been developed that measure disability due to a medical condition or illness. Hall (1992) provides a review of scales commonly used in inpatient settings to measure disability due to brain injury. However, these scales focus on more basic activities and physical status, and often do not capture the nature of disability present in ambulatory brain injured populations in the postacute phase.

   Crewe and Dijkers (1995) review a variety of scales used with disabled populations, including several suited to outpatient settings that assess functional changes due to brain injury. Of these, the Mayo–Portland Adaptability Inventory (MPAI; Malec et al., 1997), the Craig Handicap Assessment and Reporting Technique (CHART; Whiteneck, Charlifue, Gerhart, Overholser, & Richardson, 1992), and the Community Integration Questionnaire (CIQ; Willer, Rosenthal, Kreutzer, Gordon, & Rempel, 1993) seem to capture many of the activity and participation changes often present in individuals with brain injury in the postacute phase of recovery. These scales have demonstrated reliability and validity. The Web site of the Center for Outcome Measurement of Brain Injury (COMBI; *www.tbims.org/combi*) provides extensive information about psychometric and other properties of these and other scales that are useful in brain injury rehabilitation. Unfortunately, these scales are not familiar to most neuropsychologists and are most often used in rehabilitation settings as part of an overall team assessment. As we argue later, a team approach provides the best means of assessment in patients with this injury.

Compensation

Evaluating compensation for cognitive, physical, and emotional deficits, of course, requires identification of such deficits through neuropsychological, psychological, rehabilitation, or other types of formal assessments. However, evaluation in this functional domain also requires identifying methods that persons use to manage such impairments. Such compensation techniques for cognitive deficits may include calendars, notebooks, and personal digital assistants, as well as systems of prompts and cues that depend on other people. Emotional coping techniques may include both overlearned, internalized coping responses and systems such as "time out" that require assistance from other people. Physical compensation methods include orthoses, prostheses, and modifications of the physical environment.

Self-Esteem and Self-Confidence

These characteristics are best assessed as part of comprehensive clinical interview and observation of the patient. Limited self-awareness and defenses may interfere with accurate self-reporting of negative self-statements that nonetheless obviously interfere in actual behavioral performance settings. Congruence between goals and abilities, probably also best assessed behaviorally, is an aspect of self-awareness that goes beyond a verbal reporting of strengths and weaknesses to include the capacity to use information about strengths and weaknesses in selecting activities and making plans. Crosson and colleagues (1989) describe this as the *anticipatory* level of self-awareness.

Relationships and Environmental Accommodations

The last two items in Table 3.2 describe assessment at the level of handicap (participation). Relationships in home, community, and vocational settings can have dramatic effects on either minimizing or maximizing the translation of disability into handicap. Assessing environmental accommodations refers to the previously mentioned systems of prompts, cues, coaching, support, and physical modifications that increase the patient's ability to participate in home and community settings. Particularly in the area of handicap, it is difficult to obtain a complete and accurate assessment on the basis of a single interview or evaluation, even if information from multiple informants is obtained. Ongoing interaction, observation, and reporting that involve the patient, significant others, and involved professionals are usually required to develop an understanding of relationships and environmental factors that either reduce or enhance community participation.

ISSUES OF TRAINING

We have previously discussed the limitations in training of psychologists, including neuropsychologists, at both the doctoral and postdoctoral levels, to conduct interventions such as cognitive rehabilitation (Bergquist & Malec, 1997). Similarly, traditional training of neuropsychologists has not necessarily conferred either the skills or practical experience to conduct neuropsychological assessments in such a manner that they can be used to develop an appropriate treatment plan.

The recent Houston Conference on Specialty Education and Training in Clinical Neuropsychology arrived at a consensus on what training is necessary for the practice of clinical neuropsychology (Houston Conference, 1998). Tables 3.3 and 3.4 outline the knowledge base and skills, respectively, necessary for proficiency in this field. It is encouraging that skills related to treatment and intervention, as well as general knowledge of intervention techniques, are included in this document.

As formulated, however, these guidelines do not ensure that training includes developing competence in issues related to disability. As we have argued, a broader understanding of disability that includes not only impaired mental status but also other psychological and environmental factors is necessary in order to assess accurately the impact of brain injury on day-to-day functioning. In fact, there is little in the professional literature that describes specific procedures for disability assessment in neuropsychology or how to use neuropsychological assessments appropriately to design treatment programs to intervene with disability. Training in increasingly sophisticated methods of testing and measurement of impairments following brain injury is not a substitute for developing an understanding of issues related to adaptive functioning and disability following brain injury.

It appears to be a common aspiration of contemporary students in neuropsychology at the present time to identify new testing procedures with sufficient ecological validity to predict disability and handicap accurately. However, this assessment paradigm (i.e., laboratory testing) may simply be the wrong methodology for estimating disability and handicap. Other approaches to assessment may be more productive. Such assessment methodologies would focus on evaluation of the individuals undertaking activities in which they may experience disability as well as the introduction of methods or assistance that might be expected to minimize disability. A similar approach to the assessment of handicap

TABLE 3.3. Knowledge Base in Clinical Neuropsychology (Houston Conference, 1998)

A. Generic psychology core
    1. Statistics and methodology
    2. Learning, cognition, and perception
    3. Social psychology and personality
    4. Biological basis of behavior
    5. Lifespan development
    6. Cultural and individual differences and diversity

B. Generic clinical core
    1. Psychopathology
    2. Psychometric theory
    3. Interview and assessment techniques
    4. Intervention techniques
    5. Professional ethics

C. Foundations for the study of brain–behavior relationships
    1. Functional neuroanatomy
    2. Neurological and relative disorders, including their ideology, pathology, course, and treatment
    3. Non-neurological conditions affecting central nervous system functioning
    4. Neuroimaging and other neurodiagnostic techniques
    5. Neurochemistry of behavior (e.g., psychopharmacology)
    6. Neuropsychology of behavior

D. Foundations for the practice of clinical neuropsychology
    1. Specialized neuropsychological assessment techniques
    2. Specialized neuropsychological intervention techniques
    3. Research design and analysis in neuropsychology
    4. Professional issues and ethics in neuropsychology
    5. Practical implications of neuropsychological conditions

From Houston Conference (1998). Copyright 1998 by National Academy of Neuropsychology. Reprinted by permission.

would be to evaluate the individual in environments that both limit participation and maximize participation. Like classic behavioral assessment, these assessment methodologies for neuropsychology intertwine evaluation and treatment (Malec & Lemsky, 1995). As disabilities and handicaps are better identified, interventions can be implemented that test the validity of the assessment and whether the interventions diminish the identified disabilities and handicaps.

Many training programs continue to focus on developing skills in assessment of brain dysfunction. This is not surprising in a field whose origins and primary focus have been on assessment of brain–behavior relationships and detection of brain impairment. At the current state-of-the-art, training in disability issues probably needs to occur experientially rather than didactically. It is not possible, for instance, to provide a well-defined methodology or rulebook for such assessments. Potentially

TABLE 3.4. Skills in Clinical Neuropsychology (Houston Conference, 1998)

A. Assessment
1. Information gathering
2. History taking
3. Selection of tests and measures
4. Administration of tests and measures
5. Interpretations and diagnosis
6. Treatment planning
7. Report writing
8. Provision of feedback
9. Recognition of multicultural issues

B. Treatment and interventions
1. Identification of intervention targets
2. Specification of intervention needs
3. Formulation of an intervention plan
4. Implementation of the plan
5. Monitoring and adjustment to the plan as needed
6. Assessment of the outcome
7. Recognition of multicultural issues

C. Consultation
1. Effective basic communication
2. Determination and clarification of referral sources
3. Education of referral sources regarding Neuro Life Neuropsychological Services
4. Communication of evaluation results and recommendation
5. Education of patients and families regarding services and disorders

D. Research
1. Selection of appropriate research topics
2. Review of relevant literature
3. Design of research
4. Execution of research
5. Monitoring of progress
6. Evaluation of outcome
7. Communication of results

E. Teaching and supervision
1. Methods of effective teaching
2. Plan and design of courses and curricula
3. Use of effective educational technologies
4. Use of effective supervision methodologies

constructive approaches, based on principles described here, can be developed in working with individual cases. Thus, trainees will benefit most from greater experience in settings that conduct assessment and treatment to address disability following brain injury. As an example from another area of clinical practice, numerous psychologists are well skilled in assessment of personality and emotional function. Expertise in assessment without practical experience in conducting psychotherapy does not ensure that the practitioner will be an effective therapist. As mentioned previously, classic behavioral assessment may serve as a model for neuropsychological assessment in which both evaluation and therapy complement each other for the benefit of the patient.

Two case examples illustrate how knowledge, of testing procedures and clinical techniques alone are insufficient to ensure that a clinician is properly trained to conduct work in this area. These cases also illustrate the importance of behavioral observation and analysis in a disability assessment.

CASE 1

Joe, a 50-year-old male, underwent surgical resection of a right frontal area arterial venous malformation after developing seizures. The surgery was successful but involved resection of significant portions of frontal cortex. Joe underwent a course of inpatient rehabilitation followed by outpatient therapy for several weeks. Despite this therapy, he continued to have a variety of neurocognitive impairments, including impaired memory, poor attention span, and executive dysfunction, that affected his ability to function independently and return to his position in the health care field as an occupational therapist. Because of these continuing problems, he was referred to a specialized brain injury rehabilitation program and underwent a comprehensive team evaluation. The team recommended that Joe be enrolled in a postacute outpatient rehabilitation program, focusing on long-term goals of independent living, and return to work.

Joe started the rehabilitation program about 12 months after his initial neurosurgery. He was very compliant and cooperative in the program and, to the best of his ability, completed everything asked of him. He did not question the assessment of therapists in the program that he indeed had problems with memory and other cognitive functions, and that the various compensatory techniques he developed were helping him to function more independently. At the same time, it became increasingly clear that Joe was a very passive individual who avoided conflict at all costs and was hesitant to offer his opinion if it was in disagreement with others. Nonetheless, he was making progress, reflected in his reliably implementing compensation strategies and applying them in real-life settings.

After 6 months, Joe graduated from the treatment program and continued to receive intermittent follow-up. At that time, he discontinued using his compensation techniques, and his level of functioning quickly decreased. When he was seen for follow-up, Joe indicated that while he was receiving daily treatment in the program, his principal reason for working hard and being so compliant was to please the therapists he worked with and avoid any conflict. At the same time, Joe had never felt that he was as impaired as others had indicated. As a result, Joe did not believe he needed the various compensatory strategies he had been using. When away from the day-to-day structure of the treatment program, he no longer kept up with the routines he had developed and did not consistently apply the various compensatory strategies he had used effectively in the program.

This case illustrates how a patient's dependence on interpersonal cueing and reinforcement was a critical element in the maintenance of compensation techniques. It is unclear in this case to what degree Joe's dependent style predated or was created, or enhanced his brain injury. For treatment planning, determining the source of this habitual behavior was not nearly as consequential as the identification of this important source of motivation for the patient. His exquisite compliance during treatment might have been a clue to the team that approval from others was an important reinforcer for his behavior that should have been included in the long-term plan for maintenance of behaviors learned in the program. Without the benefit of hindsight, the patient's dependence was not identified until follow-up. It became clear that Joe needed environmental interventions and a clear support system to provide sufficient interpersonal cueing and support to use reliably techniques that he developed in the program to compensate for cognitive problems.

CASE 2

Sally is a 28-year-old female who suffered a severe traumatic brain injury, followed by a 2-week coma and a prolonged, acute hospital and rehabilitation stay. She eventually gained independence in activities of daily living. She was married at the time of her injury, and her husband was very supportive during her recovery. Their marriage remained relatively stable. Prior to her injury, she had been a nursing supervisor with a very good work history in an ICU in a major medical center. About 2 years after her injury, Sally and her husband had a child, for whose care she was primarily responsible during the daytime. Her husband helped with caring for their child on evenings and weekends. From reports of her family, she was a highly responsible and caring parent to her child. She had returned to school to take graduate-level classes in nursing. She had taken a total of three courses, one at a time, and received A's in all three. She desired to return to work as a nursing supervisor and was referred for a neuropsychological evaluation by the state vocational rehabilitation counselor who had been working with her for some time to help determine whether the vocational plan was appropriate.

The results of a neuropsychological evaluation identified average to high-average intelligence, good language skills, and low-average visuospatial and executive functions. Her attention span and speed of mentation were mildly impaired. While her complex attention was mildly impaired, her memory retention was impaired more severely. Based upon comparison of ratings of her level of functioning, made independently by Sally and her husband, she seemed to have an accurate appraisal of her own level of functioning and areas of impairment.

Based upon the results of testing alone, it seemed that Sally would likely have difficulty living independently, let alone caring for a toddler and doing well in graduate-level course work. Extensive discussions with her husband and the vocational counselor revealed that Sally had always been a very organized and driven individual, and that these basic character traits remained largely unchanged following her injury. By using a variety of compensatory techniques that she had developed through a course of outpatient therapy, Sally was able to function effectively well beyond what would be expected from her level of cognitive function alone.

These two case studies illustrate that while knowledge of testing procedures and clinical techniques is important to performing a useful assessment, this alone would not allow the clinician working on these two cases to make accurate predictions regarding individual levels of performance. Behavioral analysis of habitual traits that may or may not have been affected by brain injury assisted in developing a more accurate appreciation of these patients' strengths and disabilities.

The experience of following a patient about whom one has made specific predictions regarding long-term functioning and likely response to treatment can be quite humbling. It is this kind of experience, however, that produces an appreciation of the limitations of using test scores alone to predict functional outcome and of information that may be helpful in making such predictions more accurately. Observing how an assessed individual responds to various modes of treatment and actually functions over time in important daily activities is the most important teaching tool we know to gain competence in this area.

NEUROPSYCHOLOGICAL EVALUATION
AS PART OF A TEAM EVALUATION

If conducted appropriately, a neuropsychological evaluation provides a wide range of valuable information that can contribute to developing and implementing a treatment plan. A neuropsychological evaluation by itself, however, does not typically assess a patient's performance of specific, valued activities. For example, while impaired performance in one or more mental functions may affect a patient's ability to manage his or her checkbook, performing this activity is typically not assessed directly in such an evaluation. Moreover, in most rehabilitation settings, a neuropsychologist is not the most qualified professional to perform such an assessment.

Occupational therapists or other rehabilitation specialists who work in brain injury rehabilitation settings routinely assess such activities. Their training and expertise provide a framework to analyze various salient components of tasks. In order to develop an appropriate treatment plan for an individual who is experiencing difficulty with checkbook management following brain injury, for instance, there needs to be an understanding of both the difficulties with performing this activity and the impairments in mental status that contribute to this problem.

Impairments in one or more mental functions, including, for example, attention/concentration, visual scanning, arithmetic skills, memory, and reading, may result in problems with checkbook management. Impaired self-awareness determines the degree to which patients will independently generalize to everyday life what they have gained from the treatment setting. Determining whether inability to perform checkbook management is due to poor computational skill or poor scanning will lead to different approaches to intervention and result in the development of different compensatory skills. Describing the nature of a brain injury survivor's difficulties with managing a checkbook, along with detailing his or her neurocognitive, emotional, and motivational function, will provide the most comprehensive assessment of the problem and likely lead to the most effective treatment.

Working together, the neuropsychologist and other rehabilitation therapists can provide a more comprehensive assessment of problem areas. In our experience, an interdisciplinary team approach to rehabilitation of individuals disabled following brain injury results in the most effective rehabilitation plan and treatment (Malec, Schafer, & Jacket, 1992). This team approach is more than simply having several different rehabilitation professionals work on the individual problem areas in which each has the greatest expertise. Instead, this approach involves using a team of individuals working in concert toward achieving one or more of the patient's functional goals (e.g., returning to work), with the ultimate purpose of helping him or her achieve the highest level of functioning.

To be effective and complete, evaluation for possible treatment following brain injury needs to be done by a treatment team, with all parties working with the survivor of brain injury and the survivor him- or herself working as well. This task may seem daunting, but published general guidelines have outlined the areas that need to be assessed for

TABLE 3.5. Six Area Traumatic Brain Injury Assessment System (6A-TBIAS; American Congress of Rehabilitation Medicine, 1998; Revised 2001)

Area I: Etiology/pathology

A. Severity, specified by one or more of the following:
   1. Alteration or loss of consciousness
   2. Posttraumatic amnesia
   3. Glasgow Coma Scale
   4. Presence of injury-related intracranial abnormalities on neurodiagnostic studies
   5. Acute complications affecting cerebral functioning (e.g., hypotension, hypoxemia)
B. Chronicity (i.e., time since injury)
C. Treatment history/access to treatment

Area II: Preinjury status (Cushman & Sherer, 1995; Wade, 1992)

A. Preinjury medical diagnoses, including prior brain injury(ies), psychiatric disorders, substance abuse disorders, or developmental disorders (e.g., ADHD)
B. Functional status (e.g., mobility, activities of daily living)
C. Living independence (i.e., level of supervision or support)
D. Years of education
E. Employment status
   1. Professional/technical versus skilled versus semi- or unskilled
   2. Duration of episodes of unemployment
F. History of criminal convictions
G. History of physical or sexual abuse/trauma
H. Personality/coping style
I. Family roles
J. Social support system
   1. Extent
   2. Satisfaction
   3. Social roles
K. Gender
L. Age at injury

Area III: Injury/illness-related medical conditions

A. Systems
   1. Neurological, including autonomic
   2. Musculoskeletal
   3. Immunological
   4. Endocrinological
   5. Cardiovascular
   6. Other (e.g., vestibular)
B. Medication effects, therapeutic versus undesired side effects
C. Other conditions
   1. Sleep disorders
   2. Pain disorders
   3. Sexual dysfunction
   4. Psychiatric, including psychogenic conditions, malingering

(continued)

TABLE 3.5. (*continued*)

Area IV: Impairments

(any loss or abnormality of psychological, physiological, or anatomical structure or function [World Health Organization, 1987]) secondary to I, II, and III

A. Sensory–perceptual
B. Motor
C. Emotional
D. Behavioral
E. Cognitive, including language
F. Other somatic (as defined by *Guides to the Evaluation of Permanent Impairment*)

Area V: Disability

(any restriction or lack, resulting from an impairment, of ability to perform an activity in the manner or within the range considered normal for a human being [World Health Organization, 1987; Cushman & Sherer, 1995; Wade, 1992]) as assessed by:

A. Patient
B. Family/significant others
C. Professionals

Area VI: Handicap

(a disadvantage for a given individual, resulting from an impairment or a disability, that limits or prevents the fulfillment of a role that is normal, depending on age, sex, and social and cultural factors, for that individual [World Health Organization, 1987; Cushman & Sherer, 1995; Wade, 1992])

A. Indicators
   1. Living independence
   2. Vocational activity
   3. Avocational activity
   4. Psychosocial adjustment
   5. Quality of life
B. Influences
   1. Physical, environmental
   2. Social, attitudinal
   3. Financial
   4. Legal
   5. Social support
   6. Stress

From American Congress of Rehabilitation Medicine (1998). Copyright 1998 by American Congress of Rehabilitation Medicine. Reprinted by permission.

such an evaluation to be complete. The Brain Injury Interdisciplinary Special Interest Group of the American Congress of Rehabilitation Medicine (1998) has developed the Six Area Traumatic Brain Injury Assessment System (6A-TBIAS), which includes the major areas that need attention when conducting a comprehensive assessment (Table 3.5). Although 6A-TBIAS was developed specifically for the assessment of persons with traumatic brain injury, it can be applied with minimal modification to other types of acquired brain injury.

Note that even a thorough neuropsychological evaluation will not assess all six areas. Furthermore, a more traditional evaluation focused on assessment of brain dysfunction will cover only one of these six areas (Impairment). A larger, integrated team assessment, in contrast, can provide a more complete assessment of major aspects of all six areas related to functioning after brain injury. In this manner, a treatment plan with realistic and attainable treatment goals can be created that ultimately leads to the highest level of functioning for the survivor of brain injury.

SUMMARY

Neuropsychological evaluation is a tool with a long history of both diagnosing brain injury and describing the nature of brain dysfunction. With the rise of new forms of rehabilitation, there is the promise that the increasing number of individuals who survive severe brain injury will also be able to function at increasingly higher levels, as measured by independent living and returning to work. By documenting complex changes in brain function, neuropsychological evaluations are a very valuable tool in determining both the effects of brain injury and the needs of individuals following brain injury, and in contributing to the formulation of a comprehensive treatment plan. To accomplish this effectively, neuropsychological services need to expand beyond the impairment model of assessment to a model that also assesses level of disability. This will mean a broader conceptual and clinical view, both in the focus of the evaluation and the scope of the tests and other evaluation procedures employed by neuropsychologists. By using models of assessment that incorporate this broader focus, and by providing students as well as clinicians with appropriate training in these new models, clinical neuropsychology can make this shift. In so doing, it is more likely that our profession will best meet the needs of our patients and allow them to benefit from treatment and maximize their level of functioning and independence.

REFERENCES

Bergquist, T. F., Boll, T. J., Corrigan, J., Harley, J. P., Malec, J. F., Millis, S., & Schmidt, M. F. (1994). Neuropsychological rehabilitation: Proceedings of a consensus conference. *Journal of Head Trauma Rehabilitation, 9,* 27–38.
Bergquist, T. F., & Malec, J. F. (1997). The role of psychology in cognitive rehabilitation. *NeuroRehabilitation, 8,* 49–56.

Binder, L., & Thompson. L. (1995). The ethics code and neuropsychological assessment practices. *Archives of Clinical Neuropsychology, 10,* 27–46.

Brain Injury Interdisciplinary Special Interest Group of the American Congress of Rehabilitation Medicine. (1998). Six Area Traumatic Brain Injury Assessment System (6A-TBIAS). *Moving Ahead, 12*(1), 6.

Crewe, N., & Dijkers, M. (1995). Functional assessment. In L. Cushman & M. Scherer (Eds.), *Psychological assessment in medical rehabilitation* (pp. 101–144). Washington, DC: American Psychological Association.

Crosson, B., Barco, P., Velozo, C., Bolesta, M., Cooper, P., Werts, D., & Brobeck, T. (1989). Awareness and compensation in postacute head injury rehabilitation. *Journal of Head Trauma Rehabilitation, 4,* 46–54.

Cushman, L., & Sherer, M. (Eds.). (1995). *Psychological assessment in medical rehabilitation.* Washington, DC: American Psychological Association.

Gordon, W. (1987). Methodological considerations in cognitive rehabilitation. In M. J. Meier, A. L. Benton, & L. Diller (Eds.), *Neuropsychological rehabilitation* (pp. 111–131). New York: Guilford Press.

Hall, K. (1992). Overview of functional assessment scales in brain injury rehabilitation. *NeuroRehabilitation, 2,* 98–113.

Houston Conference on Specialty Education and Training in Clinical Neuropsychology. (1998). Policy statement. *Archives of Clinical Neuropsychology, 13,* 160–166.

Johnston, M., Keith, R., & Hinderer, S. (1992). Measurement standards for interdisciplinary medical rehabilitation. *Archives of Physical Medicine and Rehabilitation, 73,* S3–S23.

Kay, T., Newman, B., Cavallo, M., Ezrachi, O., & Resnick, M. (1992). Toward a neuropsychological model of functional disability after mild traumatic brain injury. *Neuropsychology, 4,* 371–384.

Kruger, J., & Dunning, D. (1999). Unskilled and unaware of it: How difficulties in recognizing one's own incompetence lead to inflated self-assessment. *Journal of Personality and Social Psychology, 77,* 1121–1134.

Lezak, M. D. (1987). Assessment for rehabilitation planning. In M. J. Meier, A. L. Benton, & L. Diller (Eds.), *Neuropsychological rehabilitation* (pp. 41–58). New York: Guilford Press.

Lezak, M. D. (Ed.). (1995). *Neuropsychological assessment* (3rd ed.). New York: Oxford University Press.

Malec, J. F., & Lemsky, C. (1995). Behavioral assessment in medical rehabilitation: Traditional and consensual approaches. In L. Cushman & M. Scherer (Ed.), *Psychological assessment in medical rehabilitation* (pp. 199–236). Washington, DC: American Psychological Association.

Malec, J. F., Machulda, M. M., & Moessner, A. M. (1997). Assessment of the differing problem, perceptions of staff, survivors, and significant others after brain injury. *Journal of Head Trauma Rehabilitation, 12*(3), 1–13.

Malec, J., Schafer, D., & Jacket, M. (1992). Comprehensive-integrated post-acute outpatient brain injury rehabilitation. *NeuroRehabilitation, 2,* 1–11.

McGlynn, S. M., & Schachter, D. L. (1989). Unawareness of deficits in neuropsychological disorders. *Journal of Clinical and Experimental Neuropsychology, 11*(2), 143–205.

McKhan, G., Drachman, D., Folstein, M., Katzman, R., Price, D., & Stadlin, E. (1984). Clinical diagnosis of Alzheimer's disease: Report of the NINCDS-ADADA work group 2 under the auspices of the Department of Health and Human Services Task Force on Alzheimer's Disease. *Neurology, 34,* 939–944.

National Institutes of Health Consensus Development Panel on Rehabilitation of Persons with Traumatic Brain Injury. (1999). Rehabilitation of persons with traumatic brain injury. *Journal of the American Medical Association, 282*, 974–983.

Prigatano, G., & Fordyce, D. (1986). Cognitive dysfunction and psychosocial adjustment after brain injury. In G. Prigatano (Ed.), *Neuropsychological rehabilitation after brain injury* (pp. 1–17). Baltimore: Johns Hopkins University Press.

Rourke, B. P. (1989). *Nonverbal learning disabilities: The syndrome and the model.* New York: Guilford Press.

Ruff, R. M., Camenzuli, L., & Mueller, J. (1996). Miserable minority: Emotional risk factors that influence the outcome of mild traumatic brain injury. *Brain Injury, 10*, 551–565.

Sbordone, R. (1997). The ecological validity of neuropsychological testing. In A. M. Horton, D. Wedding, & J. Webster (Eds.), *The neuropsychology handbook* (2nd ed., 365–392). New York: Springer.

Sherer, M., Bergloff, P., Levin, E., High, W., Oden, K., & Nick, T. (1998). Impaired awareness and employment outcome after traumatic brain injury. *Journal of Head Trauma Rehabilitation, 13*, 52–61.

Sherer, M., Oden, K., Bergloff, P., Levin, E., & High, W. (1998). Assessment and treatment of impaired awareness after brain injury: Implications for community re-integration. *NeuroRehabilitation, 10*, 25–37.

Sherer, M., Oden, K., Bergloff, P., Levin, E., High, W., Oden, K. E., & Nick, T. G. (1999). Impaired awareness and employment outcome after traumatic brain injury. *Journal of Head Trauma Rehabilitation, 13*(5), 52–61.

Wade, D. (1992). *Measurement in neurological rehabilitation.* New York: Oxford University Press.

Whiteneck, G. G., Charlifue, S. W., Gerhart, K. A., Overholser, J. D., & Richardson, G. N. (1992). Quantifying handicap: A new measure of long-term rehabilitation outcomes. *Archives of Physical Medicine and Rehabilitation, 73*, 519–526.

World Health Organization. (1987). *International classification of impairments, disabilities and handicaps.* Geneva: Author.

World Health Organization. (1997). *ICIDH-2: International classification of impairments, activities, and participation: A manual of dimensions of disablement and functioning (beta-1 draft for field trials).* Geneva: Author.

CHAPTER 4

Pharmacological Treatment of Cognitive Impairments

Conceptual and Methodological Considerations

JOHN WHYTE

Cognitive impairments result from a wide range of disease processes and traumatic events. Normal cognitive development may be compromised; mature adults may lose cognitive capacities, and elderly persons' capacities may undergo accelerated decline. Whereas these conditions were once accepted as immutable, increasing attention in recent decades has been devoted to understanding their origins and developing treatments to restore or slow the deterioration of cognitive abilities. Pharmacological treatments have been prominent in this treatment revolution, with considerable attention devoted to drug treatments for Alzheimer's disease, attention-deficit/hyperactivity disorder (ADHD), and Parkinson's disease, among others. Despite these advances, the role of pharmacological treatment remains unclear for many cognitively disabling conditions.

In light of the uncertain efficacy of many drug interventions for cognitive impairments, the purpose of this chapter is primarily conceptual and methodological. The conceptual framework underlying the enablement–disablement process is reviewed to demonstrate its importance as a framework for conducting high-quality research on pharmacological treatment of cognitive impairments. Various other methodological factors that constrain work in this area are addressed. Within this context, research models that potentially advance the understanding of pharmacotherapy are presented, with attention to the particular niche that each can fill in the ongoing development of the field. It is not my intent to review comprehensively evidence for the effectiveness of any specific drug treatment for any particular condition or impairment. However, I do present illustrative examples from the treatment literature, along with some of my personal experiences in research and clinical care.

Whereas this chapter emphasizes research and methodological issues, the perspective applies equally well to practicing clinicians. The same biases and confounds that impede research also hamper researchers' attempts to reach valid conclusions in the treatment of individual patients. While the formal researcher may have more tools available for circumventing these methodological obstacles, the clinician can also apply some of the available tools.

THE ENABLEMENT–DISABLEMENT MODEL

Disability has often been thought of as a property of a person—in psychological terms, a trait rather than a state. Through the combined influences of disability researchers and disability rights activists, however, it is increasingly recognized that disability is the product of an interaction between an individual and an environment. Individuals with hearing impairments are more disabled in a hearing culture than in a subculture where signing is the norm. Individuals in wheelchairs are more disabled in communities with multistory housing than in those with one-story ranch houses. Thus, we have increasingly come to understand that disability is a process that emerges from the interaction between traits of individuals and aspects of their environments. The process by which individuals become more disabled (either through deterioration of their own abilities or reduction in available environmental support) or less disabled (either through improved personal abilities or greater environmental support) is referred to as the enablement–disablement process (Institute of Medicine, 1997). Reconceptualizing disability as a process rather than an individual trait opens the door to a wide range of both individually and environmentally targeted interventions that influence the transition to lesser disability. Several different systems of nomenclature have been advocated to identify conceptual levels relevant to the enablement–disablement process. These systems differ in their details, but they share certain key points. In this chapter, I use the nomenclature recommended by the Institute of Medicine (1997).

"Pathology" or disease refers to loss of structure or function of biological tissue. For example, one may develop a brain infarction from cerebrovascular disease or neurofibrillary tangles from Alzheimer's disease. Pathology may or may not, however, lead to impairment, depending on its nature, location, and severity. "Impairment" refers to dysfunction of an organ or system. Thus, a brain infarction may lead to paralysis of the muscles in a limb. Dementia may lead to loss of bladder control. "Functional limitation" refers to difficulties in performing tasks. Thus, whereas pathology and impairment can be located in body organs, functional limitation is always located in a person. Paralysis may lead to difficulties in stair climbing. Memory impairment may lead to difficulty in shopping for groceries. Finally, "disability" refers to individuals' difficulty in fulfilling appropriate social roles. Disability is located at the interface of the individual and the environment. For example, an individual who cannot climb stairs may have employment problems (the role of "worker") if many job opportunities are to be found in buildings without elevators.

IMPLICATIONS OF THE ENABLEMENT–DISABLEMENT MODEL FOR TREATMENT OF COGNITIVE IMPAIRMENTS

Pharmacological agents are directed primarily at two levels in this conceptual hierarchy. Many drugs are used to prevent or treat pathology. For example, aspirin and drugs that lower cholesterol are intended to prevent brain infarction. Psychoactive drugs, however, are generally not used to prevent or cure a disease but to reduce the impairment that results from existing disease. Impairments in mood (Rush et al., 1998), attention (National Institutes of Health, 2000), memory (Mayeux & Sano, 1999), and impulse control (McElroy, 1989), due to a range of disease processes, may all be subject to modification by pharmacological agents.

The interrelationships among levels in this conceptual hierarchy present a key challenge to the use of drugs to enhance cognitive function and the performance of real-world tasks. Multiple, different diseases may produce the array of cognitive impairments that a patient displays. It is not uncommon, for example, to find a patient with mild dementia who suffers a stroke, or a child with a preexisting learning disability who experiences a traumatic brain injury. The relative contributions of different forms of neuropathology to the patient's cognitive impairments may be difficult to determine. Similarly, multiple cognitive impairments may underlie a patient's functional limitations. An individual may fail to complete doing the laundry as a result of a complex combination of attention, and anterograde and prospective memory impairments. Finally, an individual may fail to assume a social role, such as worker, due to a combination of functional limitations. The inability to drive, coupled with motor slowing and poor social skills, may work collectively to reduce employment options. This causal complexity is illustrated in Figure 4.1.

Within this context, the choice to treat a cognitive impairment invariably involves hypothesizing a relationship between the impairment and some functional limitation or disability that is the ultimate concern of the therapist and patient. If this hypothesized relationship is incorrect, then the treatment is unlikely to succeed.

This conceptual framework highlights some key problems in the use of drugs to improve cognitive function. The first problem has to do with the conceptualization of the impairment being treated. Physical impairments are generally defined rather concretely. Muscle weakness can be defined in measures of strength by using particular measurement devices. Range of motion of a limb can be defined by angular movements of joints, measured with a goniometer. But in the case of cognitive function, the impairments themselves are frequently hypothetical constructs. For example, controversy exists in terms of how precisely to define "attention," the number of subsidiary constructs contained in this larger domain, and the appropriate tools for measuring these constructs (Whyte, Polansky, Fleming, Coslett, & Cavallucci, 1995; Whyte et al., 1996). Similarly, should we refer to an impairment of "memory," of "anterograde declarative memory," or of "stimulus encoding"? One might question whether constructs such as attention exist at all as encapsulated mental faculties that can be measured independently of other faculties, or whether they are emergent properties of heterogeneous mental tasks.

The second problem pertains to the mismatch between the intended purpose of a psychoactive drug and the drug's mechanism of action. Psychoactive drugs are nearly always used to improve an impairment (e.g., to improve memory, attention, etc.), and sometimes even in the hope of improving a functional limitation (e.g., to improve reading abilities in children with ADHD). Yet the drugs' mechanisms of action are at the cellular or subcellular level, often through the manipulation of neurotransmitter systems. In reality, there is no "attention neurotransmitter." Neurotransmitters such as dopamine may be important for optimal attentional function, but other neurotransmitters are clearly also involved (Robbins, 1986). Moreover, dopamine is also implicated in a number of nonattentional systems (e.g., motor performance; Nutt & Holford, 1996). Invariably, when using a drug to improve a cognitive impairment, therefore, one risks inadvertently altering other brain systems and also failing to target adequately the range of neurochemicals relevant to the problem at hand. In this conceptual hierarchy, the mismatch between the level of drug action and the level of treatment goals is

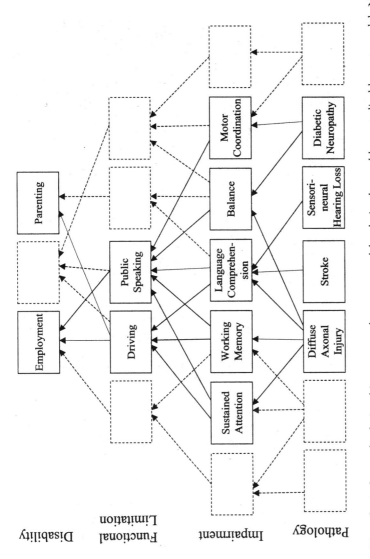

FIGURE 4.1. Hypothetical causal relationships among the conceptual levels in the enablement–disablement model. Note that an individual may have several distinct diseases (in this case, a diabetic individual with age-related hearing loss and a previous stroke suffers a traumatic brain injury in a motor vehicle accident) that result in multiple impairments, functional limitations, and disabilities. Adapted from Whyte (1994). Copyright 1994 by Lippincott Williams & Wilkins. Adapted by permission.

one of the most fundamental challenges to effective use of pharmacological treatments for cognitive disorders.

Because of the causal complexity, shown in Figure 4.1, and the complex relationship between neurotransmitters and functional behavior, the impact of even a successful drug intervention may be modest when measured in terms of functional behavior. The more causal "layers" separating the site of drug intervention (e.g., cells) and outcome assessment (e.g., return to work), the more intervening variables enter the causal chain. Thus, the proportion of variance in the outcome of interest that can be attributed to the intervention necessarily shrinks (Whyte, 1997). This phenomenon's important methodological implications are discussed later.

Both research on drug treatments of cognitive impairments and clinical management of individual patients require the same conceptual process on the part of the investigator or clinician: developing hypotheses that relate changes in the different levels of the conceptual hierarchy defined earlier and testing those hypotheses through the administration of a pharmacological "probe." A drug may fail to improve some aspect of function, then, for two different reasons. The drug may have failed to exert its intended psychopharmacological effect (e.g., psychostimulant drugs may fail to improve attentiveness), or the hypothesized relationship between the drug's pharmacological target and the therapeutic functional goal may have been incorrect (e.g., a child's poor reading skills may in fact not be related to attention impairments, but rather to a specific learning disability).

METHODOLOGICAL OBSTACLES TO DRUG TREATMENT OF COGNITIVE IMPAIRMENTS

In addition to the fundamental conceptual issues discussed earlier, a number of additional issues present obstacles to the systematic treatment of cognitive impairments with pharmacological agents. Most prominent among these is the presence of ongoing developmental change. When psychoactive agents are given to children, the associated cognitive changes must be disentangled from ongoing developmental maturation. When treating an individual with an acute onset of neuropathology (e.g., stroke or traumatic brain injury), spontaneous neurological recovery presents a similar confounding influence. Treatments for individuals with degenerative conditions present analogous challenges, because even successful drug treatments may merely decelerate deterioration rather than cause cognitive improvement. A more subtle confound of a similar nature is presented by all tasks that involve learning and practice. Thus, functional improvement may be attributed to a drug effect when, in reality, it is due merely to repeated performance of the task of interest. All of these examples require researchers and clinicians to sort out the cognitive effects of the drug of interest from a moving target of cognitive and functional performance. Some of the potential approaches to this problem are discussed later.

Drug treatment of cognitive impairments is also made more difficult by patient heterogeneity and by uncertainty about the level at which patients should be categorized for treatment. Within most neurological diseases and injuries, there can be considerable variation in the cognitive sequelae. Cognitive impairments experienced by individuals after stroke, for example, depend on the location, time course, and size of the resulting lesions, as well as on individual differences in the patients' premorbid brain organization. Similarly, traumatic brain injury produces a heterogeneous array of cognitive deficits depending on the severity of diffuse axonal injury, the presence and location of focal contusions, and the presence of secondary injury. This heterogeneity in neuoropathology makes it difficult to identify drug treatments for many neurological diseases or conditions. Therefore, one is more inclined to identify drug treatments for problems defined at the level of cognitive impairment rather than at the level of disease state.

Targeting patients for pharmacological treatment on the basis of cognitive impairment does not completely circumvent the problem of patient heterogeneity. Depending on the way in which a cognitive impairment is measured, it may be possible for two patients to demonstrate very similar behavioral deficits because of different underlying cognitive mechanisms. For example, a patient given a prospective memory task may fail to execute the required behaviors at the specified time. In principle, however, this might be due to an anterograde memory deficit (the patient remembers that something is to be done at a particular time, but forgets what), a prospective memory deficit (the patient fails to retain the goal over time but, with cuing, can report the required behavior), or an attention deficit (the patient becomes distracted by competing task demands at the time of the behavioral requirement). Each of these scenarios involves the failure to execute the required behavior, but the appropriate treatment might vary. If, then, one were trying to assemble a homogeneous group of patients for treatment with a given pharmacological agent, on what basis would one define this homogeneity?

Just as variations among individuals interfere with drug treatment assessment, cognitive and behavioral variability within an individual is also common after brain damage. In fact, some have argued that variability or inconsistency is one of the hallmarks of cognitive impairment, particularly after traumatic brain injury (TBI) (Stuss et al., 1989). However, verifying the impact of a drug treatment on cognitive performance, whether within an individual treatment context or in group psychophar-macological research, requires a comparison of performance on the drug of interest with performance in some other condition (e.g., no treatment, placebo, or an alternative drug). Greater performance variability im-pedes this comparison, by requiring either a larger sample size for group research or a larger volume of data from the individual whose treatment is being managed. Moreover, variability in performance from hour to hour or day to day challenges clinicians' ability to assess informally the impact of treatments. If a patient's performance is highly consistent, then a change induced by treatment is likely to be rather evident. However, if the treatment merely alters the proportion of good versus poor perfor-mance within a large and variable range, this alteration may be very dif-ficult to determine without careful collection of objective data that can be inspected for change. In addition to the inherent behavioral variabil-ity common among individuals with brain damage, variability can be af-fected by the reliability of the assessment measure being used: Unreliable assessment tools tend to magnify the natural behavioral variability.

All of this discussion assumes the availability of dependent mea-sures suitable for measuring the treatment-induced change. But this, too, can be challenging in the context of current theories of cognitive func-tion. In many cognitive domains, there are no generally agreed-upon measures of the constructs of interest, particularly if one is committed to measuring changes that have functional relevance. Although speed of in-formation processing, as measured in the laboratory, may respond to stimulant drug treatment, for example, we know little, as yet, about how this translates into the speed of performing useful work (Whyte et al., 1997). In the past, it has been particularly evident that "executive defi-cits" are difficult to measure with validated instruments, although recent developments appear to show progress in this area (Burgess, 1997; Norris & Tate, 2000).

The difficulty in selecting validated measures of drug effects relates both to remaining theoretical confusion about the constructs themselves and to the conceptual levels issue presented earlier. In the former realm, for example, one may wonder about the best way to operationalize an impairment in working memory. Is working memory a unitary cognitive process measured with a single assessment instrument? Does it involve an interaction between buffers and a central executive, such that its sep-arate components need to be measured? Are there different forms of working memory, depending on stimulus attributes (e.g., linguistic vs. nonlinguistic; Baddeley, 1992)? With regard to the conceptual levels is-sue, one must be concerned with the level at which to specify working memory—that is, whether to use highly controlled impairment-based laboratory tasks, functional limitation-based assessments in which working memory demands are salient, or both. It is quite conceivable that a laboratory measure of working memory might fail to correlate highly with the real-world demands on working memory, such that drug response, as measured by the former, might have little ecological validity.

The current managed health care environment presents additional methodological obstacles to the study of drug treatments for cognitive impairments. This is particularly true when one attempts clinical interventions rather than experimental research. To carefully study a patient's response to medication typically requires a considerable interval of time, particularly if the patient's performance is quite variable. In today's health care environment, although there may be time to provide the treatment, there is often insufficient time to judge its impact on the individual patient. Moreover, since many, if not most, psychoactive treatments for cognitive dysfunction can be classified as investigational (at least in the sense that a particular drug is not approved for the specific indication or patient population), there may be little insurance support for ongoing clinical contact to assess treatment impact.

POTENTIAL APPROACHES TO ASSESSMENT OF PHARMACOLOGICAL TREATMENTS OF COGNITIVE DYSFUNCTION

Despite the many challenges reviewed earlier in this chapter, progress can be made in delineating the useful roles of psychoactive drugs in cognitive rehabilitation. In the following sections, I review some of the most useful methods for addressing treatment efficacy questions, both in formal research and in clinical practice.

Research Approaches Using Parallel Group and Crossover Designs

Group research continues to be the most widely accepted method for documenting the efficacy of pharmacological interventions. Group studies of pharmacological intervention must consider three essential elements: subject selection, specifics of treatment, and measures of treatment impact.

SUBJECT SELECTION

Given the earlier discussion of subject heterogeneity, it is generally advisable that inclusion criteria specify both the disease state and the cognitive impairment. Thus, one might study treatment of patients' hemispatial neglect after stroke but not include individuals with neglect after

TBI, or individuals with stroke who lack hemispatial neglect. Such subject selection guarantees that all of the subjects will display the impairment of interest, and have room for treatment-induced improvement, and increases the chance of comparable underlying neurochemical mechanisms across the sample.

Whether further narrowing of inclusion criteria is warranted is generally controversial in the current state of knowledge. For example, should a study of stroke-related neglect enroll only individuals with cortical lesions? Or only those with right hemisphere lesions—in view of the fact that different neurochemical mechanisms may operate in these circumstances? If little is known about the relevant psychopharmacological differences, one may choose to enroll a relatively broad sample but plan for subgroup analyses dealing with pathoanatomical differences within the sample. If no such differences are found, one has the additional advantage of being able to generalize to a relatively broad clinical population. On the other hand, if there is strong a priori reason to expect different patterns of drug response by subgroup, one may choose to focus initial studies on the subgroup most likely to respond, and then, if positive results are found, begin to test the limits of the treatment on related samples.

It is also important to be able to characterize the prognosis of the sample being studied, in relation to the types of outcomes that will be used in the study. In acute neurological conditions, it is crucial to know not only how much cognitive recovery is likely in the absence of pharmacological intervention, but also what subject attributes best predict this recovery. Having this knowledge in advance of the clinical trial allows one to ensure balance in the predictive factors between study groups, helps one to know the sample size required to demonstrate that recovery is greater than expected, and helps one to determine the most appropriate time point at which to measure treatment response. Observational databases can be invaluable for this purpose. Standardizing time frames of clinical follow-up and measures of behavioral performance in such a database can provide pilot data that allow the investigator to examine natural history, number of potential subjects, and other important issues. In the absence of such a clinical database, a phase of pilot research in which the same inclusion and exclusion criteria are applied using the same outcome measures can be a useful prelude to a definitive clinical trial.

SPECIFYING THE TREATMENT

Specifying the treatment in drug studies is simpler than in studies of nonpharmacological cognitive interventions. Nevertheless, one must decide whether to deliver a standard dose of the study drug, a weight-adjusted dose, or a dose that can be titrated in relation to behavioral response. Because individual dosage adjustment within the trial complicates the design, this type of research should generally be reserved until the basic question of drug efficacy has been answered and more specific treatment refinements are pursued, unless the therapeutic window of the drug is so narrow and idiosyncratic that a positive effect may be missed altogether in a fixed-dose trial.

Parallel group designs (in which subjects are randomized to distinct treatment groups) are generally recommended over crossover designs (in which subjects spend part of the study receiving each treatment), because they do not contain the carryover problems of drug or practice effects. However, in parallel group designs, the two treatment groups must be well balanced with respect to prognostic factors to ensure comparability of outcome in the absence of a treatment effect. Simple randomization, particularly in a small study, cannot guarantee adequate prognostic balance. Crossover designs may be used if the drug's therapeutic effects are expected to occur relatively rapidly and to dissipate quickly after the drug is withdrawn. Drugs anticipated to alter permanently the course of the disease or recovery process are generally not suitable for crossover designs, because of large carryover effects in this context.

MEASURING THE TREATMENT EFFECT

Selecting the outcome measures for pharmacological trials is a complex task for many of the reasons discussed previously. The tradition in clinical trials designed for FDA approval is to select a single or very restricted set of primary outcomes as measures of treatment response. However, this is generally not appropriate in early stages of pharmacological research or in areas where considerable controversy surrounds the appropriate measures of the cognitive constructs of interest. Moreover, a single outcome located at the impairment level will not address questions of clinical significance, and a single outcome at the functional limitation or disability level will not be sensitive to subtle drug effects.

For these reasons, early stages of drug research ideally include several measures of treatment response addressing at least two conceptual levels. This reduces the chance of a negative trial due to an insensitive measure of treatment response. It also helps to clarify the relationship between impairment- and functional limitation-level changes. However, though casting the outcome net widely minimizes Type II error, it increases Type I error, because it increases the odds that at least one outcome measure will appear to show a treatment response. In recent research, we have addressed this problem by building a pilot and replication phase into the study; that is, we test a small sample of patients using a broad range of outcome measures and a liberal alpha-level cutoff. We then replicate the study on a larger sample, assessing only those outcomes that appeared promising in the pilot sample.

An alternative solution is to approach this problem sequentially rather than concurrently; that is, one can study several impairment-level outcomes in an initial study, hoping to determine the types of patients who show the most dramatic improvement in impairment with treatment. One can then conduct a subsequent study, enrolling only those subjects most likely to show improvement in impairment, and examine the impact of this improvement on their real-world functional limitations.

By either route, the range of variables to be studied should decrease over time as more is learned about which measures are most sensitive to drug response, and which measures are redundant with respect to specific psychological processes. While it might be ideal to have a fully developed model of the neural networks involved in various cognitive processes and their pharmacological control, it should be kept in mind that psychopharmacological interventions can be important probes with which to build such models; that is, to the extent that several cognitive measures routinely respond to a given agent (and several others routinely fail to respond), this suggests common mechanisms of neuropharmacological control of those processes that change together. This, in turn, may allow one to include just one measure for each cluster of processes in future studies of drug response.

A recent study of the effects of methylphenidate on attention deficits following TBI demonstrated this approach (Whyte et al., 1997). We administered methylphenidate, a short-acting psychostimulant, in a multiple crossover design to a group of 14 individuals with attentional complaints, while measuring a wide range of dependent variables, including several different computerized measures of attentional function, as well as videotaped records of independent work in a distracting environment. We found that a number of variables reflecting performance speed in several different tasks showed improvement in response to methylphenidate and could therefore be interpreted as overlapping measures of the same construct. In contrast, measures of patients' inappropriate orienting to extraneous environmental events were completely unaffected by the drug. This suggests that the pharmacological mechanisms underlying these two aspects of attentional performance are distinct and need to be measured separately.

Clinical Assessment Using Single-Subject Experimental Designs

Single-subject experimental designs can be used productively to understand the impact of pharmacological agents on cognitive function in individual patients. Single-subject designs (also called "N of 1" designs) are simply controlled experiments in which the universe of interest is the individual patient. Thus, these designs are particularly useful for answering patient-specific questions about treatment. However, if a series of patients is involved in such individual experiments, it may be possible to assemble patients into a larger test of the treatment question, with a correspondingly more general conclusion (Zucker et al., 1997). The process of assessing drug response in an individual is conceptually similar to the design of a group experiment. Reliable measures of the specific cognitive impairments and their task-related consequences, and knowledge of their practice effects, remain important issues. However, one does not have to deal with the problem of subject heterogeneity except implicitly, in the sense that one must have an idea about which patients are suitable for at least investigating a given treatment.

There are a number of advantages in using single-subject experimental designs. First, as mentioned, they allow the treating clinician to ask, no matter how unusual or idiosyncratic the patient's problems, whether a particular drug is effective in managing a patient's specific cognitive and behavioral problems. Second, such experiments may sometimes be carried out in the absence of time-consuming individual institutional review board (IRB) applications. For example, if the drug is already in clinical use with the patient population of interest for the impairments or symptoms of interest, and if the measures that will be used to judge its effect are also already in common use, then the IRB may conclude that the "experimental" intervention is simply the more rigorous and objective collection of data on treatment response—something that is surely no less ethical than dispensing the drug with more casual evaluation. Even when IRB review of individual treatments is not required, patients and caregivers should be fully aware that patients are receiving a drug for an unapproved indication and understand why the particular protocol is in place to judge the drug's effects, and this understanding should be documented in the patient's chart.

In single-subject experiments, the investigator must select one or more dependent variables for monitoring treatment response. This raises the measurement reliability and validity issues discussed earlier. Where possible, measures of response should be instruments whose reliability and validity have already been studied and found suitable for repeated administration. However, it may be necessary, or even desirable, to supplement these with measures that are individually tailored to the patient's presenting problems and therefore have high face validity. One must also consider the assessment protocol within which these measures will be collected; that is, the investigator may wish to standardize the time of day, the testing environment, and other factors, in order to minimize extraneous sources of performance variability.

In our applications of single-subject experiments to drug assessments, we have found it particularly useful to gather data at both the impairment and functional-limitation levels in order to test our hypotheses about the relationship between the two. For example, in the hope that a pharmacological intervention might improve their level of responsiveness, we have studied a number of patients who remain vegetative or minimally conscious after TBI. Here, the implicit hypothesis is that some level of arousal is needed in order to engage in meaningful behavior. Therefore, when treating with a drug known to influence central nervous system arousal, we record not only measures of arousal itself (e.g., amount of time spent with eyes open, amount of spontaneous movement) but also measures of meaningful responses (e.g., following commands, answering "yes"/"no" questions).

In principle, four different outcomes from such an experiment are possible, as shown in Table 4.1. If the drug produces more eye opening *and* more reliable command following, we can tentatively conclude that the drug is therapeutically useful and that its activity supports our hypothesized link between arousal and meaningful behavior. If the drug produces greater eye opening *without* more reliable command following, we know that the drug had the desired psychopharmacological effect on arousal, but we must question our hypothesized link with meaningful behavior. If the drug fails to alter either measure, we may question whether the drug was absorbed, whether the dose was adequate, and so on, but we have no data either to support or to refute the hypothesis. The least likely outcome, the finding that meaningful behavior improved without a change in eye opening, would suggest that the drug was therapeutically useful but for reasons other than those we hypothesized. Through the careful selection of hypotheses, drugs, and measures of the clinical effects, one can learn a great deal from both treatment successes and failures in this way.

In Table 4.2, we present data from 1 subject, who was in a vegetative state several years after TBI. The patient appeared drowsy much of

TABLE 4.1. Interpretation of Treatment Effects

Impairment outcome	Functional limitation outcome	
	Improved	No change
Improved	Therapeutic effect, hypothesis supported	No therapeutic effect on function, hypothesis refuted
No change	Therapeutic effect, not due to hypothesized mechanism	No therapeutic effect, hypothesis neither supported nor refuted

TABLE 4.2. Effect of Medication on Response Rate
and Accuracy in "Yes"/"No" Communication

Drug condition	Response rate[a]	Accuracy rate[b]
Baseline	18% (25/36)	52% (13/25)
Amantadine	37% (88/235)	45% (40/88)

[a]Finger movements/trials.
[b]Accurate finger movements/total finger movements.

the time, as evidenced by inconsistent eye opening. He demonstrated specific finger movements that his family interpreted as signals for "yes" and "no," but during a baseline assessment, we found these movements to be infrequent, and his responses were randomly related to "yes"/"no" questions with known answers. Thus, we performed a drug assessment with amantadine, a dopamine agonist, in an attempt to augment arousal, hoping that it would produce more accurate "yes"/"no" communication. As can be seen in Table 4.2, the drug produced a clear increase in arousal level, as measured by spontaneous finger movements, but it did not increase the patient's communication accuracy above chance.

Single-subject experiments require a considerable volume of data from each individual, particularly when performance is inconsistent. Moreover, inferring a drug effect is quite challenging when the patient's performance is improving rapidly due to spontaneous recovery. Thus, we find single-subject experiments for drug assessment to be most useful in the chronic recovery phase, when patient change is slow, or when the patient can be studied over a relatively long interval.

Many different specific experimental designs exist under the general rubric of single subject experiments. The simplest, but also the weakest, is an AB design, in which a particular behavior or aspect of performance is repeatedly measured prior to treatment (the A phase). The drug is then started and the same behavioral measure is continued. If performance during the A phase has a fairly flat slope with minimal variability, and if performance in the B phase either assumes a slope or remains flat but assumes a different intercept (see Figure 4.2), a drug effect can clearly be inferred. However, as mentioned earlier, some degree of slope is common during the A phase, as is considerable variability during both phases. Moreover, if the drug requires some time to reach a therapeutic dose or full behavioral effect, then there may be no abrupt transition between phases A and B. In the absence of an abrupt change in slope or intercept, it may be very difficult to distinguish a drug effect from practice or spontaneous recovery. In general, the greater the performance variability or slope in the A phase, the more data will be required in both phases to develop a firm conclusion.

A modification of the AB design that strengthens it is the ABA design. This is identical to the design mentioned earlier, except that the drug is withdrawn again and behavioral measurement continues. Because practice or recovery effects would be expected to continue into the second A phase, a deterioration in performance when the drug is withdrawn tends to disentangle these confounds. Of course, the use of an ABA design requires that the effect of the drug be reasonably rapidly reversible rather than "curative." While most psychoactive drugs are not expected to produce permanent "cures," the time frame over which their effects might dissipate varies considerably.

Perhaps the strongest single-subject design, though also the least commonly applicable, involves randomized reversal of drug phases (e.g., ABAABABBBA, where each letter might stand for a day, a week, etc.). We have found this design to be useful primarily in the assessment of psychostimulants, whose effects occur and dissipate rapidly. Collecting data in this way helps remove the observer bias if the many transitions are done blindly, and it controls powerfully for recovery and practice effects. Clearly, however, it cannot be used when the drug of interest requires a long interval to reach its full therapeutic potential or to wash out. Even short-acting stimulants typically require a dozen or so data points in each drug condition to evaluate the effect, unless it is extremely dramatic.

Analysis of the data from single-subject designs is a matter of some controversy. At a minimum, the data should be graphed sequentially, noting the point at which the drug of interest was introduced and/or withdrawn. Visual inspection, alone, however, is an inadequate analytic strategy unless the effects of the intervention are very dramatic (Kazdin, 1982). The celeration line approach can be used for AB designs. In this approach, a trend line is constructed through the baseline data and projected beyond into the intervention phase. According to the null hypothesis (no drug effect), approximately half of the intervention phase data points should fall above the trend line and half below (Ottenbacher, 1986). The binomial test can be used to determine whether the deviation from this 50/50 distribution is likely to have occurred by chance. However, this approach requires that the data trend be well represented by a straight line. If there is a curvilinear trend, projecting with confidence may be difficult. In addition, if measures such as percent correct are used, the natural ceiling (100%) may interfere with projecting an upward-sloping line.

Traditional inferential statistical tests cannot be applied validly to single-subject experimental data, because the observations are not inde-

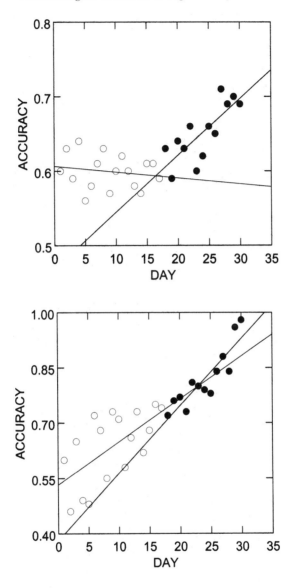

FIGURE 4.2. Top: The pattern of data that might be obtained in an AB single-subject experimental design, using a measure of a behavior anticipated to respond to the study drug (accuracy in responding to "yes"/"no" questions in a seriously impaired patient). Note that the slope during the baseline phase is relatively flat, with minimal variability, and there is a clear change in slope after the introduction of the drug. Bottom: In contrast to the top portion of the figure, variability and positive slope in the A phase result in a less clear drug effect.

pendent, as required by most statistical tests. Thus, the use of multiple regression or analysis of variance is questionable. Various bootstrap methods are increasingly available for such analyses. Readers interested in pursuing single-subject drug assessments will need to learn about the particular analytic strategies that are most appropriate given their experimental measures and experimental designs. Regardless of the analytic method chosen, however, it is useful to remember that merely graphing objective data in relation to time and drug dose is often a considerable step forward over more impressionistic methods of drawing treatment conclusions. We have also found that the clinical discussions that are required in order to agree on patient-relevant dependent measures, and to draw conclusions from the data, tend generally to promote a more analytic approach to patient care, one that extends well beyond the specific protocol.

THE CHRONOLOGY OF INVESTIGATION

In order to conduct high-quality, single-subject or group research on pharmacological treatment of cognitive impairments, many factors must be addressed: the selection of suitable patients, the selection of the candidate drugs and doses, and the identification of a range of reliable and valid dependent measures that can trace the drug effects from the cellular origins to meaningful behavioral impact. This large task requires a sustained effort over time. In order to be most productive, however, it is important to consider the order in which these research challenges might be approached (Whyte, 1997).

Single-subject experimental designs are often a useful starting point for exploration of drug effects on cognitive impairments. One can examine different drug doses and different measures of drug response in a detailed fashion, and solve some of the logistical problems associated with such trials (e.g., how to handle extraneous drug changes) at the same time.

At a similar, early phase, it is useful to begin constructing a descriptive database on the cognitive problem(s) of interest; that is, if one is treating a number of individuals with memory disorders, standardized data on the etiology, time since neurological event, initial memory test scores, follow-up memory test scores, and so on, can be obtained. This allows one to answer important questions, such as the number of such individuals available in the institution, the rate of spontaneous improvement, and other factors that predict outcome in terms of memory function. Recording the results of single-subject trials in this same database may help to demonstrate a pattern in terms of the profiles of patients who appear to improve with a given intervention.

One of the main questions in drug treatment of cognitive impairments is which patient should receive which drug. While it is often comforting, as clinicians, to think that we can select the "best" drug for a given patient, in the absence of research clearly demonstrating drug efficacy, such individual preferences may be little more than superstitions. Thus, a more productive approach may be to administer the same drug to all patients who demonstrate a given cognitive impairment (and who have no medical contraindications to it). This allows us to develop a volume of experience with the drug of interest and to begin to address whether subgroups of patients respond differently to the drug.

Needed testing of "hunches" that some patients may not respond as well to the drug can only occur if those patients are included in the study. Once a subgroup of patients has failed to respond, and that subgroup can be defined by some factor(s) other than a post hoc drug response, those patients can be selected for future studies using a different drug.

This kind of systematic clinical investigation of a specific patient population and a specific cognitive domain over time is necessary in order to make significant progress. This can be done in the context of formal research, in which the investigator builds from natural history studies to pilot treatment interventions, to large-scale clinical trials. It can also occur in the context of clinical specialization, in which the investigator assembles a clinical practice of patients with a common core of cognitive impairments, maintains a systematic clinical database, and implements specific treatment protocols tied to program evaluation and quality improvement efforts. In either case, the clinician/investigator who employs an empirical approach and sound methodology will develop increasing sophistication in the selection of treatment candidates, the management of the drug, and the measurement of drug effects.

CONCLUSION

Cognitive impairments are a source of significant disability after brain injury and illness. Many pharmacological agents are known to have effects on brain systems that subserve cognitive processes. Yet the number of cognitive impairments for which specific drugs are formally indicated remains small. Numerous factors have presented obstacles to progress in this area—conceptual, methodological, and practical in nature. In order to circumvent these obstacles, both clinicians and researchers can develop empirical and systematic approaches to a specific area of investigation and use a range of tools over time. The available tools are of use to both clinicians and researchers, and can help clinicians cope with uncertainty until formal drug recommendations are available.

Clinical intuitions followed by single-subject experiments can provide a useful starting point for a systematic approach to pharmacological interventions for cognitive impairments. Group studies are typically needed to arrive at formal "indications" for the use of specific medications to improve cognitive function. Only time will tell whether pharmacological treatments will best be selected by a patient's performance profile, his or her etiological diagnosis, or some combination of the two.

REFERENCES

Baddeley, A. (1992). Working memory. *Science, 255,* 556–559.

Burgess, P. W. (1997). Theory and methodology in executive function research. In P. Rabbitt (Ed.), *Methodology of frontal and executive function* (pp. 81–116). East Sussex, UK: Psychology Press.

Institute of Medicine. (1997). *Enabling America: Assessing the role of rehabilitation science and engineering* (E. N. Brandt & A. M. Pope, Eds.). Washington, DC: National Academy Press.

Kazdin, A. E. (1982). *Single-case research designs: Methods for clinical and applied settings.* New York: Oxford University Press.

Mayeux, R., & Sano, M. (1999). Treatment of Alzheimer's disease. *New England Journal of Medicine, 341*(22), 1670–1679.

McElroy, S. L., Keck, P. E., Jr., Pope, H. G., Jr., & Hudson, J. I. (1989). Pharmacological treatment of kleptomania and bulimia nervosa. *Journal of Clinical Psychopharmacology, 9*(5), 358–360.

National Institutes of Health. (2000). National Institutes of Health Consensus Development Conference Statement: Diagnosis and treatment of attention-deficit/hyperactivity disorder. *Journal of American Academy of Child Adolescent Psychiatry, 39*(2), 182–193.

Norris, G., & Tate, R. L. (2000). The behavioural assessment of the dysexecutive syndrome (BADS): Ecological, concurrent and construct validity. *Neuropsychological Rehabilitation, 10,* 33–45.

Nutt, J. G., & Holford, N. H. (1996). The response to levodopa in Parkinson's disease: Imposing pharmacological law and order. *Annals of Neurology, 39*(5), 561–573.

Ottenbacher, K. J. (1986). *Evaluating clinical change: Strategies for occupational and physical therapists.* Baltimore: Williams & Wilkins.

Robbins, T. W. (1986). Psychopharmacological and neurobiological aspects of the energetics of information processing. In G. R. J. Hockey, A. W. K. Gaillard, & M. G. H. Coles (Eds.), *Energetics and human information processing* (pp. 71–90). Dordrecht, The Netherlands: Martinus Nijhoff.

Rush, A. J., Crismon, M. L., Toprac, M. G., Trivedi, M. H., Rago, W. V., Shon, S., & Altshuler, K. Z. (1998). Consensus guidelines in the treatment of major depressive disorder. *Journal of Clinical Psychiatry, 59*(20), 73–84.

Stuss, D. T., Stethem, L. L., Hugenholtz, H., Picton, T., Pivik, J., & Richard, M. T. (1989). Reaction time after head injury: Fatigue, divided and focused attention, and consistency of performance. *Journal of Neurology, Neurosurgery and Psychiatry, 52*(6), 742–748.

Whyte, J. (1994). Toward a methodology for rehabilitation research. *American Journal of Physical Medicine and Rehabilitation, 73,* 428–435.

Whyte, J. (1997). Assessing medical rehabilitation practices: Distinctive methodologic challenges. In M. J. Fuhrer (Ed.), *The promise of outcomes research* (pp. 43–59). Baltimore: Brookes.

Whyte, J., Hart, T., Schuster, K., Fleming, M., Polansky, M., & Coslett, H. B. (1997). Effects of methylphenidate on attentional function after traumatic brain injury: A randomized placebo-controlled trial. *American Journal of Physical Medicine and Rehabilitation, 76*(6), 440–450.

Whyte, J., Polansky, M., Cavallucci, C., Fleming, M., Lhulier, J., & Coslett, H. B. (1996). Inattentive behavior after traumatic brain injury. *Journal of the International Neuropsychological Society, 2,* 274–281.

Whyte, J., Polansky, M., Fleming, M., Coslett, H. B., & Cavallucci, C. (1995). Sustained arousal and attention after traumatic brain injury. *Neuropsychologia, 33*(7), 797–813.

Zucker, D. R., Schmid, C. H., McIntosh, M. W., D'Agostino, R. B. D., Selker, H. P., & Lau, J. (1997). Combining single patient (N-of-1) trials to estimate population treatment effects and to evaluate individual patient responses to treatment. *Journal of Clinical Epidemiology, 50*(4), 401–410.

CHAPTER 5

Design and Evaluation
of Rehabilitation Experiments

BRIAN LEVINE
MAUREEN M. DOWNEY-LAMB

The brain injury epidemic has incurred massive societal costs from direct hospital care, loss of productivity, and emotional effects on the survivor and loved ones. These costs mandate effective, evidence-based strategies for improving quality-of-life outcomes. This need intensified in the cost-cutting climate of managed care. What is the evidence in support of neuropsychological interventions? A recent review covering more than 20 years of published research in cognitive rehabilitation for traumatic brain injury (TBI), the leading neurological cause of disablement in young adults (Max, MacKenzie, & Rice, 1991), revealed a total of 11 studies meeting criteria for properly designed randomized control trials (RCTs; Chesnut et al., 1999). Five of these studies addressed real-life outcome (as opposed to laboratory test performance); two of the five had positive results. A more comprehensive review of cognitive rehabilitation including both stroke and TBI, identified 29 RCTs, 20 of which showed clear, positive evidence (Cicerone et al., 2000). Although RCTs are not the only research design of value, it could nonetheless be argued that neuropsychological interventions have yet to meet the standards of practice typical of other health care services supported by an extensive history of efficacy and ongoing refinement through high-quality research.

What barriers affect progress in neuropsychological interventions?

Successful medical interventions reverse or compensate for the effects of specific diseases with a circumscribed, well-defined etiology and course. Such interventions are typically based on a thorough working knowledge of the affected organ systems. By comparison, the mechanisms of many neuropsychological disorders are less well understood. They are often nonspecific and highly interactive with external factors (e.g., the psychosocial milieu), and they involve both focal and diffuse damage to the least understood organ in the human body. In short, the problems addressed by neuropsychological interventions are among the most complex in biomedical science.

The status of neuropsychological interventions is thus comparable to that of other medical interventions 100 years ago. As with medical interventions, however, we believe that efficacious neuropsychological interventions can be developed through properly designed empirical research. In this chapter, we describe the ingredients that should be considered in the design of neuropsychological intervention research. We next briefly outline the advantages and disadvantages of different widely used research designs. We close with a section on novel methodologies from cognitive neuroscience research that can increase the yield for future rehabilitation research.

INGREDIENTS OF SUCCESSFUL
REHABILITATION STUDIES

Control groups, randomization, blindness, subject selection and description, selection and timing of outcome measures, treatment compliance, and theoretical relevance are research design issues that should be considered in the creation of neuropsychological interventions. Control groups, randomization, and blindness are explicitly addressed in the double-blind RCT, making it the fundamental design strategy necessary for establishment of evidence-based rehabilitation practice, as well as every other medical intervention (U.S. Preventive Services Task Force, 1996). As discussed in more detail later, the RCT's applicability is positively related to the specificity of the intervention. Specific treatments targeting circumscribed deficits are more easily studied within the RCT format.

Not surprisingly, the two distinguishing features of RCTs are the use of a *control group* and *random assignment* of subjects to control and treatment groups. These features are covered in every introductory experimental design and statistics class. Historically, the introduction of experimental control led to the elimination of ineffective or dangerous primitive medicinal treatments. In the present day, lack of appreciation for experimental control fosters superstitious belief in cause–effect relationships.

Although simple and known to us all, control groups and random assignment deserve some consideration, because their implementation can be far from straightforward in neuropsychological interventions. Due to the small effect sizes in behavioral research and the susceptibility of these effects to external confounds, they are the two most important (and perhaps neglected) aspects of design in neuropsychological intervention research.

Control Groups

When designing an intervention study, investigators seek to minimize or control extraneous factors that may influence results. In the case of brain trauma, for example, misinterpretation of natural recovery phenomena as treatment effects could result in the recommendation of expensive and unnecessary interventions. Conversely, when patients with a declining course (e.g., progressive dementia) fail to benefit from treatment, behavioral decline could be interpreted as a treatment failure, when, in fact, the treatment slowed the rate of decline. In both cases, a control group is necessary to observe the natural course of disease in the absence of treatment.

The benefits of experimental control are not limited to patients in a dynamic recovery phase. Control groups are necessary to assess practice effects of repeated testing. In their quantitative review of attention rehabilitation studies, Park and Ingles (2001) compared directly studies with and without control groups (i.e., with only pre- and postintervention assessments). Whereas studies without control groups showed significant improvement from pre- to posttesting, the effect size for studies with control groups was nonsignificant. This was also confirmed in studies that contained both pre- and posttesting and a control group. In other words, patients tended to improve on posttesting relative to pretesting due to the effects of repeated exposure to the outcome measures. This improvement could be mistakenly interpreted as a positive treatment effect.

Having decided on the inclusion of a control group, the investigator must next consider what aspects of the treatment should be controlled. In classic experimental design, the control group is matched to the experimental group in all aspects except for the variable of interest, as in a placebo-controlled drug trial. In neuropsychological intervention research, the variable of interest is a form of treatment whose precise therapeutic ingredients can be difficult to isolate. At a minimum, the control group should be matched to the experimental group for injury type and severity, stage of recovery, demographic/background characteristics, and amount of exposure to outcome assessments. Such a control group adequately covers cohort, natural recovery, and practice effects. However, this does not control for nonspecific effects, such as therapeutic attention and positive support, that accompany most interventions. To demonstrate that an intervention is specific and unique, members of both the control and the treatment group should have similar amounts of supportive contact with a member of the intervention team.

Randomization

The mere presence of a control group does not guarantee control, even when its demographics are closely matched to those of the experimental group. Systematic differences across the control and treatment groups may confound treatment effects if the two groups are drawn from separate populations. To protect against this bias, patients from the same population sample should be randomly assigned (*after* recruitment) to treatment or control groups such that confounding factors are distributed equally across both groups.

Randomization poses serious practical problems in real-world clinical settings. Randomization to a no-treatment control group is obviously unacceptable when treatment is available and sought by patients. This can be avoided by randomization to two alternative treatments (e.g., standard vs. experimental protocols), which is also an effective method of equating groups for nonspecific effects. Many patients, however, may decline to participate in an RCT if they believe they may receive a less effective intervention, even when the effectiveness of the standard intervention is unknown.

If a clinician believes that one intervention is superior to the other, he or she may still experience an ethical dilemma in randomizing patients to a treatment they perceive as less effective. Given the current status of neuropsychological interventions, there is often no empirical basis to support clinicians' feelings on treatment effectiveness, resulting in clinical debates stemming from intuition rather than data. In the absence of proven effectiveness, clinicians must also consider their ethical obligation to future patients to improve and validate their professional service. The RCT is the most widely accepted method of doing this. The knowledge that a specific intervention has been put to the test, and ultimately, we hope, disseminated to colleagues, benefiting a much larger pool of patients may compensate for the discomfort stemming from the temporary suspension of disbelief required by an RCT. Should it become clear during an RCT that one treatment is more effective than another, methods exist for terminating the RCT when statistical criteria have been met

(Fleming & DeMets, 1993; Simon, 1994). Furthermore, if the trial yields a significant effect, the patients in the less effective intervention can always be offered the more effective intervention. When an RCT is simply not an option, nonexperimental design strategies (discussed later) can still be considered.

Subject and Investigator Blindness

Double-blind studies, in which both the patients and the investigators are unaware of group membership, provide optimal protection against confounding expectancy effects. As humans are programmed to seek information and resolve discrepancies, double-blindness can require Herculean efforts. Patients' awareness of their membership in a group receiving a novel, cutting-edge treatment may inflate expectations or increase motivation, effort, and compliance. Investigators are no less subject to expectancies, especially given their high investment in finding a positive effect for their treatments. Accordingly, stroke rehabilitation effect sizes have been shown to be significantly higher in studies where raters were *not* blind to group membership (in direct comparison to blinded studies; Ottenbacher & Jannell, 1993). In other words, awareness of a patient's membership in the experimental group exerted a positive influence on the rater's assessment. This effect was attenuated in RCTs (as opposed to preexperimental or quasi-experimental designs; Ottenbacher & Jannell, 1993).

As with randomization, circumstances in rehabilitation settings can limit blindness. Patients on wait-list control groups are obviously not blind. Even when patients are initially blind to group membership, they may become aware of group membership through side effects or talking to other participants. Investigators may need to be aware of group membership for medical reasons. To maintain investigator blindness, it is often necessary to have outcome assessments performed by staff isolated from group membership information. Investigators should systematically document cases of unblinding in both patients and staff, and consider these cases separately when analyzing the data.

Selection and Description of Participants

Evaluation of neuropsychological interventions is critically dependent upon a thorough description of patient characteristics, including demographics (age, education, race, gender, socioeconomic status), injury characteristics (time since injury, lesion type and location, severity indicators), comorbidity, medical history, compensation seeking, mental status, neuropsychological test performance, and personality and psychosocial moderators. This information is necessary for future users of the intervention to determine its generalizability to their population. Additionally, these patient characteristics moderate outcome and can therefore be analyzed as independent variables.

Just as the study samples should be carefully documented, so also should the characteristics of those who declined to participate or dropped out of the study, along with the reasons for nonparticipation. Those who decide to participate in an intervention study may differ from nonparticipants in characteristics such as motivation, work status (e.g., unemployed patients have more time on their hands), or injury severity, affecting the representativeness of the study sample. Coding this information at the time of recruitment permits the later analysis of differences between participants and nonparticipants.

INJURY CHARACTERISTICS

The importance of documenting injury characteristics can be seen in the case of the RCT study of cognitive rehabilitation for military personnel with TBI, described by Salazar and colleagues (2000). Although there were no significant effects of inpatient cognitive rehabilitation compared to limited home rehabilitation, it was noted that 100% of the patients were gainfully employed (in the military) prior to the study, and 90% (inpatient group) or 94% (home group) returned to work following rehabilitation. These rates of employment are far higher than those typically reported for patients with TBI (Dikmen et al., 1994). It is therefore possible that the lack of significant differences were due to cohort effects specific to military personnel.

By carefully documenting injury characteristics, Salazar and colleagues' (2000) ability to identify subgroups with differential rates of response helped to refine their conclusions. Specifically, they found that individuals with more severe injuries (as defined by a loss of consciousness greater than 1 hour following TBI) in the inpatient group were more likely to be judged fit for duty at 1-year follow-up than those in the home-based group. Thus, the inpatient rehabilitation program, while not associated with improved employment outcome in the entire sample, showed promise for a subgroup of more severely injured patients (at least in comparison to the home study control group).

LESION LOCATION

Intervention studies of patients with focal brain damage should document lesion characteristics. Optimally, this would be done with chronic-phase magnetic resonance imaging (MRI) (as opposed to acute computed tomography). Careful documentation of lesion characteristics makes possible the identification of responders from nonresponders and to seek the reasons for these differences. For example, frontal lobe brain injuries can affect systems involved in arousal and self-regulation. Abulic patients with medial frontal damage are less likely to engage with rehabilitation initiatives and require a different approach than patients with damage confined to the dorsolateral frontal cortex affecting attentional or working memory processes (Eslinger, Grattan, & Geder, 1995).

NEUROPSYCHOLOGICAL TEST PERFORMANCE

Documentation of participants' neuropsychological test findings is necessary for external validity and useful for additional subgroup analyses. This should include standardized measures of attention, memory, language, visuospatial/visuoconstructive abilities, motor skills, executive functioning, and possibly personality and emotional functioning. Researchers performing population-specific interventions can use this information to assess the representativeness of the study sample (e.g., verifying that a sample of neglect patients has intact basic mnemonic functioning). These data can also be used in exploratory analyses of subgroup effects defined by divergent cognitive profiles. For example, it is possible that a group of nonresponders may have lower scores on memory measures, suggesting that memory deficits blunt an intervention's effectiveness or, alternatively, that memory-impaired patients require supplemental intervention (Ryan & Ruff, 1988).

Lesion- and performance-based triage can be used to target interventions at those most likely to benefit (Robertson & Murre, 1999). Patients with major tissue loss and minimal or no residual functional capacity are better candidates for compensation than for attempts at restitution or retraining. Those with minor brain damage and relatively preserved function are likely to recover spontaneously. A middle group with compromised (but partially preserved) functioning may derive the most benefit from guided intervention. For example, Heald, Bates, Cartlidge, French, and Miller (1993) used transcranial magnetic stimulation to assess central motor conduction in the hand following stroke. Individuals with partial response recovered to the same degree as those with normal response, whereas those individuals with no response showed significantly reduced recovery; that is, patients with residual sparing of connectivity showed the greatest potential for recovery.

PSYCHOSOCIAL MODERATORS

As discussed in more detail later, neuroplasticity research on individuals with brain damage has demonstrated remarkable effects on recovery due to environmental enrichment. It is therefore not surprising that the psychosocial context in which rehabilitation occurs can have significant effects on outcome that are independent of or interact with treatment decisions. Psychosocial moderators include living independence, coping skills, social support, and family involvement. Institutionalization is associated with impaired cognitive functioning in healthy older adults when compared to community-dwelling older adults, even when the two groups are carefully matched on intelligence and demographic characteristics (Winocur, Moscovitch, & Freedman, 1987). In further research with elderly persons, researchers noted that the cognitive changes were linked to psychosocial variables such as personal control, optimism, and well-being (Dawson, Winocur, & Moscovitch, 1999). As noted by Prigatano (1994), the family's working alliance with staff, as rated at discharge, was significantly related to productivity outcomes. Documentation of these moderators may prove fruitful at the data-analysis stage.

Selection of Outcome Measures

Outcome measurement is the final common pathway for intervention effectiveness. Poor selection and timing of outcome assessment can therefore render an effective intervention result inconclusive. A perpetual conflict facing investigators is that between sensitivity to the intervention and generalization to real life. Restricting outcome measurement to laboratory tasks that are specific to treatment may lead to the unsatisfying demonstration of a change in laboratory tasks, with unknown effects on day-to-day functioning. Alternatively, an ecologically valid measure may be too far removed from the intervention to be sensitive to intervention effects.

Neither specific nor general measures are expendable in a proper outcome battery. Specific measures should closely relate to the construct addressed by the intervention but with materials that do not overlap those used in the intervention. Including measures of processes unrelated to those targeted by the intervention can provide useful information concerning the intervention's specificity. Improvement on all measures reflects nonspecific effects, with any extra improvement in the targeted measure indicating specific treatment effects.

More broadly targeted interventions should be validated against functional outcomes such as productivity and quality of life. These include return to work/school, interpersonal relationships, and leisure activities (i.e., "work, love, and play"; Prigatano, 1989). These constructs are much harder to quantify than cognitive ones. Return to work or school is straightforward but should be accompanied by an assessment of changes in workload, responsibilities, and productivity. Other functional outcomes are generally assessed by questionnaires, which raises the issue of inaccurate self-appraisal in patients with compromised insight (Jennett, Snoek, Bond, & Brooks, 1981; Prigatano, 1991). In such cases, significant other ratings should also be collected. Several measures have parallel forms for patients and significant others (e.g., Burgess, Alderman, Evans, Wilson, & Emslie, 1996; Kay, Cavallo, Ezrachi, & Vavagiakis, 1995). It should be noted, however, that a significant other may also have distorted appraisal of a loved one's functioning due to inflation of perceived of preinjury function.

In summary, outcome batteries should be composed of carefully selected specific and general measures. When feasible, these should include assessment of productivity and quality of life as rated by both the patient and his or her significant other. Many investigators prefer to develop their own outcome measures. It is risky to rely on tasks without established psychometric properties. When homegrown measures are included, they should be accompanied by established measures.

Timing of Outcome Assessments: Baseline and Follow-Up

Prior to the start of any intervention study, baseline performance on measures of interest should be carefully documented, preferably with repeated assessments. As we noted later, this is a defining feature of well-designed case studies, in which changes from baseline indicate treatment effectiveness. In group studies, baseline assessments are necessary to ensure that the groups are equated on the dependent variables. Otherwise, preexisting differences cannot be ruled out as an explanation for group effects (see the later section on intervention experiments for an example of use of baseline group differences in interpretation of group effects).

Many intervention studies go no further than postintervention assessments of outcome, providing no information on the lasting effects of the intervention. For neuropsychological interventions, repeated follow-ups to at least 3 months postintervention are necessary to establish the durability of intervention effects. Even this level of follow-up, however, does not ensure lasting effects. In a well-controlled intervention study, Berg, Koning Haanstra, and Deelman (1991) found that memory strategy training improved memory test performance in TBI patients at 4 months, but these gains were not maintained when patients were reevaluated at 4 years (Milders, Berg, & Deelman, 1995). Several implications from these findings would not have been obvious from the 4-month trial alone, such as the need for intervening booster sessions to maintain treatment effects, the need for more sensitive outcome measures, or the possibility that patient groups tend to equalize over time in spite of short-term gains.

Treatment Compliance

Two forms of treatment compliance affect intervention studies. Most obviously, the participants' compliance and motivation need to be assessed during treatment. This may be accomplished through homework assignments, attendance, and group participation. Another form of compliance, addressed less frequently, is that of the trainer or therapist in the intervention protocol. The level of training required for therapists should be stated. Therapists' adherence to training protocols can be assessed through direct supervision, videotapes, and checklists. The best way to ensure consistency of an intervention's application is with a treatment manual, which is necessary for cross-center applications. An example from the psychotherapy literature can be found in the National Institute of Mental Health (NIMH) multicenter trial contrasting alternative depression therapies (Waskow, 1984).

Theoretical Grounding

In stroke patients, loss of neuronal input to the contralesional limb leads to learned nonuse and increased use of the less affected limb. Based on observations of this phenomenon in monkeys, Taub, Uswatte, and Pidikiti (1999) developed a novel technique for increasing function in the more affected limb: constraining the patient's less affected limb and training in use of the more affected limb, which resulted in substantial therapeutic gains in motor function in placebo-controlled trials. This research, which integrates behavioral theories of learned helplessness with neuroscience research on cortical reorganization, demonstrates the power of a specific theory to effect positive changes when operationalized in a novel intervention. Indeed, it shows that a therapeutic approach stressing increased use of the less affected limb would be harmful. Similarly, Wilson, Baddeley, Evans, and Shiel (1994) demonstrated that errorless learning (i.e., preventing patients' mistakes when teaching them new information) was significantly superior to effortful, error-prone learning in amnesics. This technique was also based on a synthesis from two previously unrelated literatures—implicit learning (Tulving & Schacter, 1990) and behavioral psychology (Terrance, 1963)—and directly contradicts alternative therapeutic techniques that encourage guessing.

There are, of course, numerous other examples of theory-driven neuropsychological intervention studies (Robertson, 1999). In practice, however, many rehabilitation techniques are based on clinical intuition. While certainly indispensable, clinical intuition cannot justify expensive interventions in the absence of empirically validated theoretical support.

As seen earlier, certain techniques can even be harmful when alternative, theory-driven approaches are not considered.

Like scripture, neuropsychological theory is subject to numerous interpretations and can be used to support a variety of practices. In some cases, rehabilitationists have assumed the mantle of neuropsychological theory, without carefully linking their interventions to the theory or testing their predictions against alternative theories. As in any medical science, the most successful interventions are more likely to emerge from a careful consideration of earlier research and a body of experimental evidence. In the next section, we discuss novel neuroscience methodologies that can be used to test specific predictions about intervention mechanisms at the level of neuronal systems.

DESIGN OPTIONS

Randomized Control Trial

As described in detail earlier, the RCT is the most widely accepted research design for intervention research and provides the best protection against threats to internal validity. Although it is considered a gold standard, the RCT is not without liabilities (Mohr & Brouwers, 1991). It is often difficult to recruit a sufficient number of participants to have an appropriate control group. Strict criteria for patient selection can make the ecological validity of the results questionable. A full-scale RCT study can be very costly in terms of financial resources and time commitment. Before undertaking such a large-scale study, it is desirable to have preliminary research results that demonstrate the effectiveness of the treatment on a smaller scale.

Moreover, many clinicians working in the trenches of real-life brain injury rehabilitation view the RCT as unrealistic. Clinicians in a rehabilitation setting are confronted with variable stages of recovery, complex and possibly conflicting interrelationships among staff and patients, family issues, a wide range of premorbid characteristics (e.g., substance abuse history), and the effects of litigation, to name just a few of the factors affecting treatment. Therapeutic changes may come only after sensitive and careful holistic assessment and management in a milieu-type setting, with therapeutic techniques and goals that vary from patient to patient. In such settings, intervention is an art as well as a science. Many authors object to the suggestion that the value of such interventions should be judged solely on impersonal empirical scientific criteria (Prigatano, 1999). Additionally, in large-scale trials, treatment effects that are specific to a select group of participants can be obscured (although careful selection and documentation of participant characteristics can guard against this, as discussed earlier).

Clearly, the previously described randomized control and other ingredients of intervention research are most easily applied to specific interventions, in which the treatment effects can be quantified using measures with known reliability and validity. Specific interventions validated in this manner may be integrated as components of evolving milieu-based programs. When a true intervention experiment is impractical, quasi-experimental or single-case studies can still provide valuable information. While these designs lack randomized control, other, previously described important design ingredients, such as the use of control groups and blind assessments, can be applied.

Quasi-Experimental Designs

New discoveries are often not predicted. When an interesting and novel observation is apparent in an intervention study, it can be quantified and analyzed so long as the treatment plan and operationalization of treatment effects are documented. If the observation and independent variable manipulations occur *a posteriori*, this would not be a true experiment. Rather, such studies are designated quasi-experimental (or *ex post facto*). In contrast to a true experiment, the investigator selects the independent variable from the natural environment and studies it "as if" it had been manipulated.

Teasdale, Hansen, Gade, and Christensen (1997) analyzed neuropsychological test data collected before and shortly after milieu-oriented treatment. Five years after treatment, preintervention test scores were superior to postintervention test scores in the prediction of return to work. In an experimental design controlling for other confounding variables, subjects might have been assigned to groups on the basis of their preintervention test scores. One such variable would be age, which in this study took up some of the variance in preintervention test scores, qualifying the conclusions. In spite of the design limitations, these findings are important in that they question the use of postintervention neuropsychological test scores as measures of treatment effectiveness. This study also shows how systematic quantification of baseline, outcome, and subject characteristics data in a clinical setting can be used to generate research.

Single-Case Designs

Single-case designs provide a cost-effective alternative for testing hypotheses about treatment effectiveness or for piloting for larger studies. They can be further useful in their own right when the research goals are oriented to the individual (without generalizing to the entire population; Franklin, Allison, & Gorman, 1997), when a single case can address a specific hypothesis or illustrate a novel syndrome (Shallice, 1988, Chapter 10). Indeed, many landmark advances in neuropsychology have been heralded by single cases.

Case studies need not be limited to qualitative reports. Use of within- and between-subject control in an appropriate single-case design can provide reasonable protection against internal validity threats. The two major classes of single-case designs, ABAB and multiple baseline, are described later. These designs have in common repeated assessments, with treatment effects expected to correlate in time with an intervention's onset. These can be extended to small groups of subjects (i.e., "small-N designs"). Although single-case research generally does not meet criteria necessary to make statistical inferences about the population, certain statistical analysis procedures can be applied to establish the reliability of the findings.

ABAB DESIGNS

In an ABAB design, a treatment is sequentially introduced and withdrawn. When treatment is withdrawn, performance is expected to return to baseline levels. ABAB designs can be useful for measuring direct effects of treatment; that is, increases in performances during treatment are clearly due to the treatment if removal of the treatment results in a return to baseline performance.

Although the ABAB design is useful for demonstrating direct effects of a treatment, it is only appropriate when lasting treatment effects (i.e., beyond cessation of treatment) are not expected, because these would prevent the return to baseline that is essential for this design (Mohr & Brouwers, 1991). For example, this design would be appropriate in case studies investigating the application of prosthetics, when the patient is not expected to internalize the therapy, such as a memory book in a severely amnesic patient. Withdrawing treatments in an ABAB design can also pose ethical issues for clinicians when the treatment benefits the patient (Kazdin, 1980).

MULTIPLE-BASELINE DESIGN

In a multiple-baseline design, several measures are taken before and after application of an intervention, with behavioral changes expected to relate to the timing and/or content of the intervention. In a multiple-baseline across-subjects design, the onset of the intervention varies across subjects. Thus, each subject has a different period of baseline assessment, with invariance in target behaviors expected until the intervention is applied. In a multiple-baseline across-behaviors design, multiple behaviors are assessed simultaneously, with change expected only in those behaviors targeted by the treatment. The specificity of treatment effects in multiple-baseline designs is supported by the *lack* of change when it is not expected (i.e., before intervention onset in the multiple-baseline across-subjects design, or on behaviors unrelated to the treatment in the multiple-baseline across-behaviors design). Unlike ABAB designs, multiple-baseline designs are appropriate when lasting treatment effects are expected.

The stability of baseline measurements is essential for a multiple-baseline design. A minimum of two baseline measurements should be assessed before treatment is introduced, but in situations where baselines are interrelated, more baseline assessments are desirable (Kazdin, 1980). When selecting baseline measures in a multiple-baseline-across-behaviors design, the interrelationship of measures should be carefully weighed if the goal is to demonstrate specificity of treatment effects. Although this design provides a strong test of an intervention's specificity, there is a risk of nonspecific findings should the treatment generalize to the "untreated" measures. A brief reversal phase can be useful to reinforce the causal relationships between the treatment and the targeted behavior (Kazdin, 1980).

ANALYSIS OF SINGLE-CASE DESIGNS

Although graphic display of data is useful (Kazdin, 1992), it is not sufficient to establish the reliability of treatment effects, which should be statistically assessed. When single-case designs do not meet the assumptions necessary for analyses with parametric tests (e.g., the assumption of random sampling), nonparametric tests are used. There are several tests that can be used depending on the type of design, number of participants, and the number of variables being assessed. For multiple-baseline designs, randomization tests are most appropriate (Marascuilo & Busk, 1988; Wampold & Worsham, 1986).

The Mann–Whitney U test can be used instead of a t test, for example, in a simple AB design in which a no-treatment condition is compared to the treatment condition on a single behavioral measure (Edgington, 1992). The chi-square test is useful for analyzing categorical data on two or more variables and provides a close approximation to F distribution. The Kruskal–Wallis test, a one-way analysis of variance by ranks, is used for analyzing data from a repeated behavioral measure.

The Rehabilitation Probe

As mentioned earlier, nonexperimental designs and single-case methodologies can be useful when a full treatment study as an initial foray into a rehabilitation technique is premature or infeasible. Alternatively, preliminary intervention experiments or rehabilitation probes (also known as analogue studies) can be used to support the efficacy of the proposed treatment.

The design and analysis of such studies are no different than a regular experiment. However, in the case of a rehabilitation probe, the experimental manipulation is meant to test a rehabilitation-related hypothesis. Thus, the manipulation involves an intervention, preferably applied in a mixed design, with pre- and posttesting, and a "handling" control group. As with any experiment, other conditions or groups can be added.

In our laboratories, a novel technique for treatment of executive dysfunction was applied to a group of TBI patients in the form of a rehabilitation probe (Levine et al., 2000). In its full form, this protocol (goal management training [GMT]; Robertson, 1996) can involve many hours of group and individual treatment. In brief, it targets attentional and intentional deficits in a staged approach, including "stop and think" strategies, defining the main task, breaking the task into subgoals, learning the subgoals, and monitoring to ensure that performance is concordant with the main task.

A case-study application of the expanded protocol with a postencephalitic patient was promising (Levine et al., 2000, Study 2). The rehabilitation probe was designed to examine the protocol's potential efficacy in patients with TBI before conducting an RCT. Patients were randomly assigned to two groups, GMT or motor skills training (MST). MST, involving standard procedural learning tasks (e.g., mirror tracing), was selected to equate experimenter contact across control groups and to act as a training task with effects independent from GMT. Patients in both groups were assessed pre- and posttraining on a battery of everyday attentional and executive tasks designed especially for this study.

A 2 × 2 mixed factorial design was used, with a between-subjects factor of group (GMT vs. MST) and a within-subjects factor of test session (pre- and posttraining). The effects of GMT were reflected in the interactions between group (GMT vs. MST) and test session (pre- vs. posttraining). However, this design also permitted the examination of main effects that influenced interpretation of the test scores, such as nonequivalence of pre- and posttest forms, fatigue, or practice effects, or group differences in speed and accuracy that inadvertently emerged from random assignment of subjects.

While less costly than a full randomized control study, the rehabilitation probe is nonetheless limited in that it is not a test of the full rehabilitation protocol. It is rather a miniature model that asks the question, "Could this intervention possibly have an effect?" in a controlled experimental setting. Many factors might promote or discourage an experimental effect when the treatment is expanded in a full-scale trial. In comparison to a case study, the rehabilitation probe has the advantage of generalization across individuals. Generalization to other conditions, however, is usually not assessed given the short-term nature of the intervention. One unique advantage of rehabilitation probes is the flexibility to test hypotheses with multiple groups, conditions, or both. In this study, for example, training modules containing different combinations of GMT components could have been used to isolate the components most associated with training effects.

Meta-Analytic Review

Meta-analysis, originally developed by Smith and Glass (1977) to quantify psychotherapy outcomes across studies, has since been used extensively across a wide range of disciplines (see Cooper & Hedges, 1994; Glass, McGaw, & Smith, 1981). A meta-analytic review offers all the advantages of a traditional literature review, but supplemented with standardized reporting of effect sizes.

Reporting effect sizes has been hampered by the scientific community's obsession with significance testing. Indeed, statistical significance (i.e., whether there is any effect at all; Cohen, 1988) is often misinterpreted as effect size (i.e., the magnitude of intervention effects in the population). Effect-size estimates can be derived from a given report's summary statistics, and these data can be tabled in a meta-analytic review.

The practical significance of effect size has further been pervasively underappreciated. One maxim among psychologists is that the correlation between dependent variable y and independent variable x is always around $r = .30$ (i.e., 9% of y variance is accounted for by x). What is the practical significance of such an effect size in an intervention study? Rosenthal and Rubin (1982) describe a method for displaying effect-size data in terms of how many people are likely to benefit from receiving treatment. As noted by Rosenthal (1987, pp. 114–115), an intervention with an effect size of $r = .30$ would increase the success rate from 35 to 65%. An effect size as small as $r = .20$ (accounting for 4% of the variance) would be associated with an increase in success rates, from 40 to 60%.

As the critical mass of neuropsychological intervention research accumulates, quantitative meta-analytic reviews will assume greater importance in treatment and health care policy decisions. It is notable that the influential review of cognitive rehabilitation by Chesnut and colleagues (1999) did not include quantitative data. By pooling data across a large number of studies, meta-analysis can reveal effects that are not judged as significant in individual studies due to low power (i.e., Type II error). In a rather dramatic demonstration of this problem and how it is addressed by meta-analysis, Antman, Lau, Kupelnick, Mosteller, and Chalmers (1992) documented that experts' recommendations for heart attack prevention in traditional literature reviews failed to consider more effective recommendations that had already been supported by cumulative, quantitative RCT evidence. This sort of error can arise from serial analysis of statistical significance in individual studies (as in a traditional literature review) that lack consideration of power and effect size.

Just as meta-analyses can reveal significant effects that were not apparent in individual studies, so can they indicate the lack of effect for certain interventions or research designs, as noted earlier in the Park and Ingles (2001) study.

NEUROSCIENCE APPLICATIONS IN NEUROPSYCHOLOGICAL INTERVENTIONS: NEURAL REORGANIZATION AND FUNCTIONAL NEUROIMAGING

Consider the following experiment (described in Kolb & Gibb, 1999): Rat pups were given frontal lesions at 4 days of age, followed by several days of stroking with a camel hair paint brush. These rats subsequently performed as well as controls on tasks known to be sensitive to frontal lesions. In other words, what should have been a profound behavioral disturbance in response to localized brain injury was reversed by a simple tactile stimulation maneuver.

The old maxim that central nervous system neurons do not regenerate no longer applies. In addition to hippocampal and localized neocortical neurogenesis (Gould, Reeves, Graziano, & Gross, 1999; Gould, Tanapat, Hastings, & Shors, 1999), massive regeneration and self-repair occur at the level of the synapse throughout the brain (Kolb & Gibb, 1999). Thus, the rats receiving tactile stimulation in the aforementioned study showed a reversal of atrophic neuronal changes and increased dendritic spine density, suggesting that this intervention reduced neuronal loss and increased synaptic connectivity among remaining neurons. At the systems level, recovery and rehabilitation effects are mediated through reconnection of damaged neural circuits (Robertson & Murre, 1999).

With the increasing availability of activation functional neuroimaging technologies, it is now possible to examine such reorganization *in vivo*. Activation studies (e.g., with $H_2{}^{15}O$ positron emission tomography [PET] or functional magnetic resonance imaging [fMRI]) are distinguished from clinical studies of resting metabolism (e.g., single-photon emission computed tomography [SPECT] or [^{18}F]fluorodeoxyglucose PET).

Activation studies measure brain activity in relation to specific mental tasks, revealing the brain's response to cognitive challenges that cannot be imaged in a study of resting metabolism.

Reliable PET and fMRI signatures of many cognitive activities have been established in healthy adults (Cabeza & Nyberg, 2000). Recent application of these techniques have delineated effects of normal aging (e.g., Reuter-Lorenz et al., 2000) and brain disease (e.g., Horwitz et al., 1995; Levine et al., 2001) on task-specific functional neuroanatomy. Most interesting to the rehabilitationist, these techniques have documented the changes in functional neuroanatomy in relation to behavioral recovery (Buckner, Corbetta, Schatz, Raichle, & Petersen, 1996; Chollet et al., 1991; Engelien et al., 1995; Weiller, Chollet, Friston, Wise, & Frackowiak, 1992; Weiller, Ramsay, Wise, Friston, & Frackowiak, 1993).

Weiller and colleagues (1995) studied the functional neuroanatomy of linguistic recovery in 6 patients recovered from Wernicke's aphasia following left posterior perisylvian language zone damage. On pseudoword repetition and verb generation tasks, healthy controls activated a left-lateralized network, including Wernicke's area (posterior superior and middle temporal gyri), Broca's area (inferior frontal gyrus), and lateral prefrontal cortex (with the latter two areas specific to the generation task), a pattern consistent with previously published findings on similar tasks (e.g., Petersen, Fox, Posner, Mintun, & Raichle, 1988). The patients showed more extensive right-lateralized activations, including the right homologues of the left temporal (Wernicke's area), lateral prefrontal, and inferior frontal gyrus regions activated in controls, as well as activation in the preserved left frontal regions similar to controls. The authors related the patients' additional activations to increased sustained attention and working memory.

These and other findings indicate reorganized functional neuroanatomy in relation to behavioral recovery (Grady & Kapur, 1999). The supplemental regional engagement by patients is not arbitrary; it includes regions known to be involved in healthy adults' performance of the same tasks. That is, recovery in these patients involves increasing reliance on regional pathways that are part of normal, task-specific networks.

It is tacitly assumed that neuropsychological rehabilitation changes the brain. If recovery-related regional neuronal engagement can be reliably imaged, nonrecovered patients could be trained to engage the same areas in the promotion of recovery, with changes studied before, during, and after treatment. It is, of course, also possible that task-related changes in brain activation reflect a response to greater task difficulty or brain injury effects (e.g., disinhibition of neuronal circuits) rather than functional reorganization. Rehabilitation experiments can discriminate among these hypotheses by tracking neuronal changes across repeated assessments in relation to manipulations that induce behavioral changes. In this way, rehabilitation research can contribute to theory. In the constraint-induced movement therapy discussed earlier (Taub et al., 1999), transcranial magnetic stimulation was used to map the cortical output area of a hand muscle in stroke patients before and after treatment. Results indicated a near-doubling of cortical hand area in the infarcted hemisphere in response to treatment; that is, treatment increased the number of neurons involved in movement. This plastic change in brain representation was associated with improved motor performance.

CONCLUSIONS

Neuropsychological intervention research has not enjoyed the same scientific status as other neuropsychological or biomedical research. This is attributable in part to the complexity of the questions asked by rehabilitationists and the obstacles to conducting research in clinical settings. Properly designed intervention research, however, improves efficacy of clinical care and contributes to neuropsychological theory. For the clinician/scientist, this means incorporating as many good design ingredients as possible into the applied research. Even in highly constrained clinical settings, control groups and theoretical grounding are not beyond the clinician's grasp. Intervention studies can also serve as powerful tests of theory, with fruitful opportunities for collaboration between clinicians and experimentalists. These opportunities are enhanced by recent technologies for documenting neural correlates of behavioral change.

ACKNOWLEDGMENTS

Work on this chapter was supported by the Canadian Institutes of Health Research, the Canadian Neurotrauma Research Program, and the Ontario Neurotrauma Foundation.

REFERENCES

Antman, E. M., Lau, J., Kupelnick, B., Mosteller, F., & Chalmers, T. C. (1992). A comparison of results of meta-analyses of randomized control trials and recommendations of clinical experts. *Journal of the American Medical Association, 268*, 240–248.

Berg, I. J., Koning Haanstra, M., & Deelman, B. G. (1991). Long-term effects of memory rehabilitation: A controlled study. *Neuropsychological Rehabilitation, 1*(2), 97–111.

Buckner, R. L., Corbetta, M., Schatz, J., Raichle, M. E., & Petersen, S. E. (1996). Preserved speech abilities and compensation following prefrontal damage. *Proceedings of the National Academy of Sciences of the United States of America, 93*(3), 1249–1253.

Burgess, P. W., Alderman, N., Evans, J. J., Wilson, B. A., & Emslie, H. (1996). The Dysexecutive Questionnaire. In B. A. Wilson, N. Alderman, P. W. Burgess, H. Emslie, & J. J. Evans (Eds.), *Behavioral assessment of the dysexecutive syndrome.* Bury St. Edmunds, UK: Thames Valley Test Company.

Cabeza, R., & Nyberg, L. (2000). Imaging cognition II: An empirical review of 275 PET and fMRI studies. *Journal of Cognitive Neuroscience, 12*(1), 1–47.

Chesnut, R., Carney, N., Maynard, H., Patterson, P., Mann, N., & Helfand, M. (1999). *Evidence report on rehabilitation of persons with traumatic brain injury* (99–E006). Rockville, MD: Agency for Health Care Policy and Research.

Chollet, F., DiPiero, V., Wise, R. S. J., Brooks, D. J., Dolan, R. J., & Frackowiak, R. S. J. (1991). The functional anatomy of motor recovery after stroke in humans: A study with positron emission tomography. *Annals of Neurology, 29*, 63–71.

Cicerone, K. D., Dahlberg, C., Kalmar, K., Langenbahn, D. M., Malec, J. F., Bergquist, T. F., Felicetti, T., Giacino, J. T., Harley, J. P., Harrington, D. E., Herzog, J., Kneipp, S., Laatsch, L., & Morse, P. A. (2000). Evidence-based cognitive rehabilitation: Recommendations for clinical practice. *Archives of Physical and Medical Rehabilitation, 81*(12), 1596–1615.

Cohen, J. (1988). *Statistical power analysis for the behavioral sciences* (2nd ed.). Hillsdale, NJ: Erlbaum.

Cooper, H., & Hedges, L. V. (Eds.). (1994). *The handbook of research synthesis* (Vol. 16). New York: Russell Sage Foundation.

Dawson, D., Winocur, G., & Moscovitch, M. (1999). The psychosocial environment and cognitive rehabilitation in the elderly. In D. T. Stuss, G. Winocur, & I. H. Robertson (Eds.), *Cognitive neurorehabilitation* (pp. 94–108). Cambridge, UK: Cambridge University Press.

Dikmen, S. S., Temkin, N. R., Machamer, J. E., Holubkov, A. L., Fraser, R. T., & Winn, R. (1994). Employment following traumatic head injuries. *Archives of Neurology, 51*, 177–186.

Edgington, E. S. (1992). Non-parametric tests for single-case experiments. In T. R. Kratochwill & J. R. Levin (Eds.), *Single-case research design and analysis: New directions for psychology and education* (pp. 133–157). Hillsdale, NJ: Erlbaum.

Engelien, A., Slibersweig, D., Stern, E., Huber, W., Döring, W., Frith, C., & Frackowiak, R. S. J. (1995). The functional anatomy of recovery from auditory agnosia: A PET study of sound categorization in a neurological patient and controls. *Brain, 118*, 1395–1409.

Eslinger, P. J., Grattan, L. M., & Geder, L. (1995). Impact of frontal lobe lesions on rehabilitation and recovery from acute brain injury. *NeuroRehabilitation, 5*, 161–182.

Fleming, T. R., & DeMets, D. L. (1993). Monitoring of clinical trials: Issues and recommendations. *Control Clinical Trials, 14*(3), 183–197.

Franklin, R. D., Allison, D. B., & Gorman, B. S. (Eds.). (1997). *Design and analysis of single-case research.* Mahwah, NJ: Erlbaum.

Glass, G. V., McGaw, B., & Smith, M. L. (1981). *Meta-analysis in social research.* Beverly Hills, CA: Sage.

Gould, E., Reeves, A. J., Graziano, M. S., & Gross, C. G. (1999). Neurogenesis in the neocortex of adult primates [see comments]. *Science, 286*(5439), 548–552.

Gould, E., Tanapat, P., Hastings, N. B., & Shors, T. J. (1999). Neurogenesis in adulthood: A possible role in learning. *Trends in Cognitive Science, 3*(5), 186–192.

Grady, C. L., & Kapur, S. (1999). The use of neuroimaging in neurorehabilitative research. In D. T. Stuss, G. Winocur, & I. H. Robertson (Eds.), *Cognitive neurorehabilitation* (pp. 47–58). Cambridge, UK: Cambridge University Press.

Heald, A., Bates, D., Cartlidge, N. E., French, J. M., & Miller, S. (1993). Longitudinal study of central motor conduction time following stroke: 2. Central motor conduction measured within 72 h after stroke as a predictor of functional outcome at 12 months. *Brain, 116*(6), 1371–1385.

Horwitz, B., McIntosh, A. R., Haxby, J. V., Furey, M., Rapoport, S. I., & Grady, C. L. (1995). Network analysis of PET-mapped visual pathways in Alzheimer type dementia. *Neuroreport, 6,* 2287–2292.

Jennett, B., Snoek, J., Bond, M. R., & Brooks, N. (1981). Disability after severe head injury: Observations on the use of the Glasgow Outcome Scale. *Journal of Neurology, Neurosurgery, and Psychiatry, 44*(4), 285–293.

Kay, T., Cavallo, M. M., Ezrachi, O., & Vavagiakis, P. (1995). The Head Injury Family Interview: A clinical and research tool. *Journal of Head Trauma Rehabilitation, 10,* 12–31.

Kazdin, A. E. (1980). *Research design in clinical psychology.* New York: Harper & Row.

Kazdin, A. E. (1992). *Research design in clinical psychology* (2nd ed.). Boston: Allyn & Bacon.

Kolb, B., & Gibb, R. (1999). Neuroplasticity and recovery of function after brain injury. In D. T. Stuss, G. Winocur, & I. H. Robertson (Eds.), *Cognitive neurorehabilitation* (pp. 9–25). Cambridge, UK: Cambridge University Press.

Levine, B., Cabeza, R., McIntosh, A. R., Black, S. E., Grady, C. L., & Stuss, D. T. (2001). *Functional reorganization of memory systems following traumatic brain injury: A study with H$_2^{15}$O PET.* Unpublished manuscript.

Levine, B., Robertson, I. H., Clare, L., Carter, G., Hong, J., Wilson, B. A., Duncan, J., & Stuss, D. T. (2000). Rehabilitation of executive functioning: An experimental–clinical validation of goal management training. *Journal of the International Neuropsychological Society, 6*(3), 299–312.

Marascuilo, L. A., & Busk, P. L. (1988). Combining statistics for multiple-baseline AB and replicated ABAB designs across subjects. *Behavioral Assessment, 10,* 1–28.

Max, W., MacKenzie, E. J., & Rice, D. P. (1991). Head injuries: Costs and consequences. *Journal of Head Trauma and Rehabilitation, 62*(2), 76–91.

Milders, M. V., Berg, I. J., & Deelman, B. G. (1995). Four-year follow-up of a controlled memory training study in closed head injured patients. *Neuropsychological Rehabilitation, 5*(3), 223–238.

Mohr, E., & Brouwers, P. (Eds.). (1991). *Handbook of clinical trials: The neurobehavioral approach.* Lisse, The Netherlands: Swets & Zeitlinger.

Ottenbacher, K. J., & Jannell, S. (1993). The results of clinical trials in stroke rehabilitation research [see comments]. *Archives of Neurology, 50*(1), 37–44.

Park, N. W., & Ingles, J. L. (2001). Effectiveness of attention rehabilitation after an acquired brain injury: A meta-analysis. *Neuropsychology, 15*(2), 199–210.

Petersen, S. E., Fox, P. T., Posner, M. I., Mintun, M., & Raichle, M. E. (1988). Positron emission tomographic studies of the cortical anatomy of single-word processing. *Nature, 331,* 585–589.

Prigatano, G. P. (1989). Work, love, and play after brain injury. *Bulletin of the Menninger Clinic, 53*(5), 414–431.

Prigatano, G. P. (1991). Disturbances of self-awareness of deficit after traumatic brain injury. In G. Prigatano & D. L. Schacter (Eds.), *Awareness of deficit after brain injury* (pp. 111–126). New York: Oxford University Press.

Prigatano, G. P. (1994). Productivity after neuropsychologically-oriented milieu rehabilitation. *Journal of Head Trauma Rehabilitation, 9,* 91–102.

Prigatano, G. P. (1999). Commentary: Beyond statistics and research design. *Journal of Head Trauma Rehabilitation, 14,* 308–311.

Reuter-Lorenz, P. A., Jonides, J., Smith, E. E., Hartley, A., Miller, A., Marshuetz, C., & Koeppe, R. A. (2000). Age differences in the frontal lateralization of verbal and spatial working memory revealed by PET. *Journal of Cognitive Neuroscience, 12*(1), 174–187.

Robertson, I. H. (1996). *Goal management training: A clinical manual.* Cambridge, UK: PsyConsult.

Robertson, I. H. (1999). Cognitive rehabilitation: Attention and neglect. *Trends in Cognitive Science, 3*(10), 385–393.

Robertson, I. H., & Murre, J. M. (1999). Rehabilitation of brain damage: Brain plasticity and principles of guided recovery. *Psychological Bulletin, 125*(5), 544–575.

Rosenthal, R. (1987). *The analysis of judgment studies.* Cambridge, UK: Cambridge University Press.

Rosenthal, R., & Rubin, D. B. (1982). A simple, general purpose display of magnitude of experimental effect. *Journal of Educational Psychology, 74,* 166–169.

Ryan, T. V., & Ruff, R. M. (1988). The efficacy of structured memory retraining in a group comparison of head trauma patients. *Archives of Clinical Neuropsychology, 3,* 165–179.

Salazar, A. M., Warden, D. L., Schwab, K., Spector, J., Braverman, S., Walter, J., Cole, R., Rosner, M. M., Martin, E. M., Ecklund, J., & Ellenbogen, R. G. (2000). Cognitive rehabilitation for traumatic brain injury: A randomized trial. Defense and Veterans Head Injury Program (DVHIP) Study Group [see comments]. *Journal of the American Medical Association, 283*(23), 3075–3081.

Shallice, T. (1988). *From neuropsychology to mental structure.* Cambridge, UK: Cambridge University Press.

Simon, R. (1994). Some practical aspects of the interim monitoring of clinical trials. *Statistical Medicine, 13*(13–14), 1401–1409.

Smith, M. L., & Glass, G. V. (1977). Meta-analysis of psychotherapy outcome studies. *American Psychologist, 32*(9), 752–760.

Taub, E., Uswatte, G., & Pidikiti, R. (1999). Constraint-induced movement therapy: A new family of techniques with broad application to physical rehabilitation—A clinical review [see comments]. *Journal of Rehabilitation Research and Development, 36*(3), 237–251.

Teasdale, T. W., Hansen, H. S., Gade, A., & Christensen, A.-L. (1997). Neuropsychological test scores before and after brain-injury rehabilitation in relation to return to employment. *Neuropsychological Rehabilitation, 7*(1), 23–42.

Terrance, H. S. (1963). Discrimination learning with and without "errors." *Journal of Experimental Analysis of Behavior, 6,* 1–27.

Tulving, E., & Schacter, D. L. (1990). Priming and human memory systems. *Science, 247,* 301–306.

U.S. Preventive Services Task Force. (1996). *Guide to clinical preventative services.* Baltimore: Williams & Wilkins.

Wampold, B. E., & Worsham, N. L. (1986). Randomization tests for multiple-baseline designs. *Behavioral Assessment, 8,* 135–143.

Waskow, I. E. (1984). Specification of the technique variable in the NIMH Treatment of Depression Collaborative Program. In J. B. W. Williams & R. L. Spitzer (Eds.), *Psychotherapy research: Where are we and where should we go* (pp. 150–159). New York: Guilford Press.

Weiller, C., Chollet, F., Friston, K. J., Wise, R. J. S., & Frackowiak, R. S. J. (1992). Functional reorganization of the brain in recovery from striatocapsular infarction in man. *Annals of Neurology, 31*(5), 463–472.

Weiller, C., Isensee, C., Rijntjes, M., Huber, W., Muller, S., Bier, D., Dutschka, K., Woods, R. P., Noth, J., & Diener, H. C. (1995). Recovery from Wernicke's aphasia: A positron emission tomographic study. *Annals of Neurology, 37*(6), 723–732.

Weiller, C., Ramsay, S. C., Wise, R. J., Friston, K. J., & Frackowiak, R. S. (1993). Individual patterns of functional reorganization in the human cerebral cortex after capsular infarction. *Annals of Neurology, 33*(2), 181–189.

Wilson, B. A., Baddeley, A., Evans, J., & Shiel, A. (1994). Errorless learning in the rehabilitation of memory impaired people. *Neuropsychological Rehabilitation, 4*(3), 307–326.

Winocur, G., Moscovitch, M., & Freedman, J. (1987). An investigation of cognitive function in relation to psychosocial variables in institutionalized old people. *Canadian Journal of Psychology, 41*(2), 257–269.

PART II

Models of Intervention for Neuropsychological Impairments

CHAPTER 6

The Rehabilitation of Attention

TOM MANLY
SARAH WARD
IAN ROBERTSON

The scientific analysis of attention disorders following brain damage is a relatively new and rapidly expanding field. Research increasingly indicates an important role for attention in recovery and in maximizing positive outcomes—as both a function in its own right and a facilitator to the expression of other abilities.

Attention should not, however, be regarded as a single entity. Growing evidence indicates that specific assessment of different attentional abilities is important in diagnosing, in predicting functional difficulties, and in informing rehabilitation.

In this chapter, we briefly review different forms of attention and address the question of whether they can be improved by systematic interventions. In particular we emphasize that rehabilitation can operate at a number of levels, including restoring basic function, compensatory strategies, and environmental support. The studies we consider suggest that cautious optimism is appropriate. However, more work is needed in assessing the impact of treatment on complex, everyday activities.

INTRODUCTION

The topic "attention" has become so broad that attempts at a concise, pithy definition seem increasingly futile. Describing the context that gives rise to this explanatory construct, however, remains relatively straightforward. As you read this book, you are being bombarded by competing information from other objects or events to which you might respond. Potential thoughts that you might think or memories that you might remember could intervene. Our ability to take up all these opportunities simultaneously is rather restricted—not least due to the finite number of sense organs and limbs at our disposal. This mismatch between opportunity and capacity means that *some* form of selection is inevitable.

One reasonably effective way to mediate this selection would be to rank all of the available options in terms of salience (defined by novelty, intensity, potential reinforcement, danger, etc.). A loud bang would be more likely to capture our resources than a small tap; a car speeding toward us would compel more response preparation than one speeding away. Such mechanisms are clearly present and may determine our behavior much of the time. A downside to such an arrangement—if unchecked by a degree of internal control—would be enormous difficulty in achieving some rather important goals. Eavesdropping on an interesting item of gossip being relayed on the other side of the room, for example, would be problematic, unless we are able to suppress the inputs from our current conversational partner. If we want to find our keys in an untidy office, it would be very useful to keep them in mind and resist having our actions "hijacked" by any other salient object we happen to see. To obtain the information contained in a not very gripping textbook, we may need to "internally" assist this stimulus in out-competing rivals for our attention.

An important reason to address these issues here, of course, is that many patients who have suffered neurological damage can experience profound problems in exercising such control. An example is Morris, a 56-year-old man who suffered a ruptured right middle cerebral artery aneurysm and had subsequent surgery to insert a right frontal shunt.

CASE EXAMPLE: MORRIS

Prior to his illness, Morris was the lone sales agent for a foreign manufacturer. He had to make and keep appointments, prioritize and complete paperwork, drive long distances, and keep on top of the details and needs of his clients. As far as we can tell, he was able to perform these high-level skills perfectly competently.

The right-sided brain damage left Morris with impaired vision in his left visual field (hemianopia) and tremendous difficulty in moving his left arm and leg. In addition, Morris suffered from a profound deficit in noticing, acting on, or even thinking about information from his left side that could not be accounted for solely on the basis of his visual difficulties. When asked to copy a drawing, he tended only to include information from the right side of the original. When asked to cross out particular stars, letters, or lines randomly distributed over a piece of paper, he was able to find targets on the right but missed many on the left. If he was asked to mark what he thought was the center of a horizontal line, his bisection was considerably to the right of the objective midpoint, suggestive of problems in detecting the left extent of the line. Examples of Morris's performance on tests are shown in Figure 6.1.

In the hospital ward, we asked Morris to describe his house for

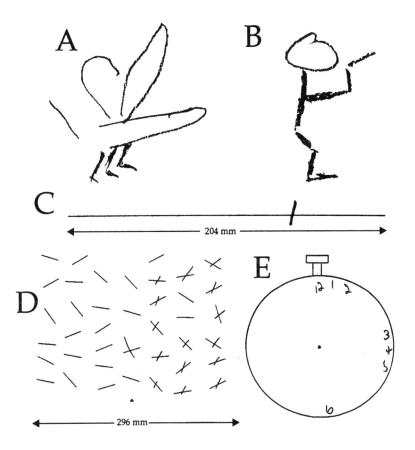

FIGURE 6.1. Morris's performance on standard tests of unilateral neglect. (A) Drawing a butterfly and (B) drawing a man from memory. (C) Marking the perceived center of a line. (D) Having been asked to cross out all of the lines shown on a page. (E) Drawing the numbers on the outline of a clock. Assessment procedures A–D are taken from Wilson, Cockburn, and Halligan (1987).

us—as if we were approaching from the front. His description was quite detailed except that he did not mention any of the rooms on the left-hand side. We then asked him to "walk in his mind" around to the back of the house, turn, and again tell us everything he would see. Now on the imagined right, information from the previously ignored side (including the lounge and two bedrooms) was suddenly available for Morris to report, demonstrating that his problems with the left were not restricted to the here-and-now but extended to details that he could remember from before his brain injury.

Morris's performance was consistent with one of the most striking manifestations of an acquired attentional disorder, termed unilateral or hemispatial neglect. Unilateral neglect has captured the interest of many scientists and clinicians because of the insights it offers into the nature of attention and awareness, and how they interact with perception and memory. It is also a pressing clinical problem associated with poor return to functional independence. We discuss further in this chapter how scientific insights have led to improved rehabilitation for the disorder.

Unfortunately, Morris's difficulties were not limited to the spatial domain. In common with many patients showing persistent neglect, he also had immense problems in keeping "on track" more generally (see a later section of the chapter for more discussion). During tests, his attention would wander so frequently that he needed prompts every few seconds to finish the simplest tasks. Similar difficulties affected his conversation, in which he tended to veer widely from the topic at hand or simply drift off midsentence.

Most of us do not show any bias in our awareness of space. However, many of us will occasionally experience something like Morris's problems in maintaining concentration, although almost certainly, to nowhere near the same degree. Although this familiarity may make such difficulties appear rather mundane in comparison with the dramatic spatial deficits of neglect, in many ways, they may actually pose a greater threat to Morris's functional recovery.

As our ability to assess attention improves, its role in mediating recovery becomes more apparent. Functional recovery from stroke, including motor ability, has been related to the integrity of attention systems (Denes, Semenza, Stoppa, & Lis, 1982; Fullerton, McSherry, & Stout, 1986; Ben-Yishay, Diller, Gerstman, & Haas, 1968; Blanc-Garin, 1994; Robertson, Ridgeway, Greenfield, & Parr, 1997; Robertson, Manly, et al., 1997). Increasingly, research into social and occupational outcomes highlights attention as an important predictive variable (Brooks & McKinlay, 1987; McPherson, Berry, & Pentland, 1997; Woischneck et al., 1997). Whether as functions in their own right or as adjuncts to the recovery of other systems, developing effective interventions for attentional disorders is therefore a key issue for professionals working with people with brain damage.

This chapter is primarily concerned with sharing recent developments in therapy for adult neurological patients and the models that guide new interventions. Although the role of attention deficits in a range of developmental and psychiatric conditions has received increasing emphasis, we cannot do justice to these substantial topics in this chapter.

In the first sections of this chapter, we consider some of the theoretical advances in the study of attention that have been very influential for clinical approaches. Although the focus of this chapter is intervention, we briefly highlight some important questions in assessment that are relevant to our subsequent discussion. We then turn to the relatively few—but rather promising—rehabilitation studies of attention that have emerged in recent years. Research in this area is at an early stage. The examples we use are not designed to represent a "how to" manual of attention rehabilitation but rather to illustrate current issues and approaches. Much more work and careful evaluation are required in this area to promote effective rehabilitative change.

CONTEMPORARY MODELS OF ATTENTION FUNCTION

Attention is at once everywhere and nowhere. This is a fundamental difficulty faced by both clinicians and researchers in trying to assess or characterize "it." We cannot look at attention without asking people to do *something*. That *something* will inevitably involve other perceptual, cognitive, and motor factors. At the same time, we cannot examine these other factors in isolation—without taking attention into account as a potentially important modulating variable.

The application of experimental methods to this field has provided one way out of this entanglement, by operationalizing attention as *the consistent variability in performance of some "other" task*. If we can hold constant as many as possible of the perceptual, cognitive, and motor aspects of an activity, while systematically manipulating attention, we may be able to see and measure its effects more clearly.

Perhaps the simplest example of this approach, and certainly one of the most influential, is a computerized task that has become known as the Posner Cueing Paradigm. In the task, volunteers are asked to look at a computer screen and not move their eyes from a central (fixation) cross. They are told that a visual target will be presented on either the left or the right side of the screen, and that they should press a button as quickly as possible after they have detected it. Under normal conditions, response times to left- and right-sided targets are robustly equivalent. If, however, people are given an accurate hint as to the side of the screen on which a target is more likely to occur, their responses will be quicker than normal. If the hint is wrong and the target appears on the opposite side, response times are slower than in the uncued condition (Posner & Snyder, 1975). Because there are no eye movements, the objective information from the target in each case is effectively identical. This applies also to the aim of pressing the button as quickly as possible, and the basic perceptual and motor processes required to perform the task. The small but reliable differences in reaction times can therefore be attributed to the action of a "hidden" system that is influenced by task instructions—attention.

The use of such measures has promoted a considerable resurgence of scientific interest in attention over the past few decades. It has also allowed the patient deficits that clinicians had long reported to be examined and quantified more precisely. Most recently, the patterns of activation within the brains of healthy volunteers as they perform attentional tasks have been considered using new functional imaging technology. Reviewing these areas in 1990, Posner and Petersen proposed a model outlining three key principles of attentional function

> First . . . the attention system of the brain is anatomically separate from the data processing systems that perform operations on specific inputs even when attention is oriented elsewhere. In this sense, the attention system is like other sensory and motor systems. It interacts with other parts of the brain but maintains its own identity. Second, attention is carried out by a network of anatomical areas. It is neither the property of a single centre, nor a general function of the brain operating as a whole. . . . Third, the areas involved in attention carry out different functions and these specific computations can be specified in cognitive terms. (p. 26)

For clinicians working with brain-injured patients, these principles have important implications. An anatomical and functional separation between attention systems and other sensory, motor, or cognitive systems means that damage to that area can produce a deficit that is *exclusively or predominantly attentional in nature*.

The differentiation of attentional functions within different regions, again depending on the location of any damage, means that an impairment *can occur to one attention function while another may be relatively intact*. In order to assess a patient adequately, therefore, we need to use tasks that place differential demands on different forms of attention. Furthermore, we need to take into account the nature of the impairment in making predictions about difficulties in everyday life and in informing rehabilitative interventions.

In their 1990 review, Posner and Petersen proposed a broad, three-way division of voluntary attention based on this functional and anatomical separation.

The first, *orienting* or *spatial attention*, referred to the capacity to move attention within space. The second, termed *target selection*, but also frequently referred to as *selective* or *focused attention*, concerns the ability to use stored information (such as memory for something you are looking for) efficiently to sort out relevant from irrelevant information. The third attention system has been variously characterized as *alerting*, *vigilance*, or *sustained attention*, that is, the self-maintenance of an alert, "ready-to-respond" state.

These broad divisions, and those proposed in other taxonomies (see Van Zomeren, Brouwer, & Deelman, 1984; Mirsky, Anthony, Duncan, Ahearn, & Kellam, 1991; Cohen & Kaplan, 1993) are, of course, provisional. Work carried out since the Posner and Petersen review has clarified the nature of some of these systems and challenged other aspects of this approach. Additional separations, for example, of the ability to divide attention between two tasks or to switch attention smoothly from one activity to another, certainly appear to have clinical merit. Nevertheless, the basic premise of separability has informed—and indeed been further supported by—subsequent clinical work.

ANATOMICAL AND ETIOLOGICAL FACTORS

There is good evidence that the right hemisphere of the brain subserves a particular role in supporting attention. Unilateral neglect is a strong example. Conventionally, unilateral neglect has been seen as arising primarily from damage to the parietal lobe of the right hemisphere, particularly the inferior parietal lobule (Heilman & Watson, 1977; Vallar & Perani, 1986). Neglect has also been observed, however, following damage to other regions, including the right prefrontal cortex, basal ganglia, and brainstem structures (Mesulam, 1981). A recent analysis of 53 patients indicated that the key area of lesion overlap predicting persistent neglect lay in middle temporal gyrus and/or the temporoparietal paraventricular white matter of the right hemisphere (Samuelsson, Jensen, Ekholm, Naver, & Blomstrand, 1997). Such findings have led a number of authors to conclude that neglect can arise following damage to a widely distributed right-hemisphere-dominant network supporting spatial orientation (Mesulam, 1981; Heilman & Valenstein, 1979; Heilman, Watson, Valenstein, & Goldberg, 1987; Posner & Petersen, 1990).

Right-hemisphere dominance is also observed in some nonspatial attention functions. Neuropsychological studies have consistently shown that right-hemisphere lesions disproportionately impair a cluster of related abilities, including the following:

- *Alertness*—measured in most cases by the maintenance of a readiness to respond in simple reaction time tasks (De Renzi & Fagliono, 1965; Benson & Barton, 1970; Boller, Howes, & Patten, 1970; Howes & Boller, 1975; Posner, Inhoff, & Friedrich, 1987; Ladavas, Pesce, & Provinviali, 1989; Sturm, Reul, & Willmes, 1989).
- *Arousal*—as defined by the overall responsivity of the nervous system to external stimuli (Gainotti, 1972; Heilman, Schwartz, & Watson, 1978).
- *Sustained attention*—as defined by self-maintaining performance on tasks with low or intermittent demand (Wilkins, Shallice, & McCarthy, 1987; Rueckert & Grafman, 1996; Knight, Hillyard, Woods, & Neville, 1981).

These findings have been further supported by recent functional imaging studies (Cohen et al., 1988; Cohen, Semple, Gross, King, & Nordahl, 1992; Pardo, Fox, & Raichle, 1991; Lewin et al., 1996; Sturm et al., 1999) that highlight the particular importance of the right prefrontal cortex in these abilities.

The frontal lobes make up approximately one-third of the total cortical areas of the brain. Lesions to these anatomically heterogeneous areas have been observed to cause a very wide variety of symptoms. At least some of these have fueled a persuasive view of the frontal lobes as being somewhat akin to a conductor leading an orchestra. While the conductor does not contribute any sound, he or she plays a vital role in coordinating the efforts of the individual musicians to produce harmonious results. In the same way, the prefrontal cortex has a role in regulating the functions of more specialized processing units in order to produce coherent output and to free the system from "slavish" response to immediate environmental contingency (Luria, 1966; Stuss & Benson, 1984; Shallice, 1988; Shallice & Burgess, 1991; Foster, Eskes, & Stuss, 1994; Duncan, 1995).

Distractibility, one consequence of such poor control, has certainly long been noted as a common symptom of prefrontal damage (e.g., Hecaen & Albert, 1978; Luria, 1966). As we have seen, there is evidence linking the capacity to sustain attention to the activity of the right prefrontal region (particularly the dorsolateral cortex). In addition, a number of neuropsychological and functional imaging studies have linked selective attention performance to prefrontal and underlying anterior cingulate areas (e.g., Pardo, Pardo, Janer, & Raichle, 1990; Corbetta, Miezin, Dobmeyer, Shulman, & Petersen, 1991; Janer & Pardo, 1991; Bench et al., 1993).

As would be expected given the distributed nature of networks supporting attention, deficits have been described in almost all commonly seen neurological conditions including head injury, cerebrovascular disease, tumor, and progressive degenerative disease (e.g., De Renzi & Fagliono, 1965; Howes & Boller, 1975; Van Zomeren & Deelman, 1976, 1978; Vallar & Perani, 1986; Robertson & Marshall, 1993; Whyte, Polansky, Fleming, Branch-Coslett, & Cavallucci, 1995; Loken, Thornton, Otto, & Long, 1995; Bak & Hodges, 1998). Deficits in the first two of these, head injury and stroke, have formed the major focus for the work we describe here.

As many clinicians can attest, the neat linkage between symptoms and lesion location presented in the textbooks can sometimes bear little resemblance to the picture that is apparent in day-to-day practice. In addition, for every patient we see with a discrete, focal lesion, we see many more with distributed damage encroaching on many systems. In this context, rules of thumb on anatomy can be useful, but the primary aim lies in the assessment and treatment of *function*, that is, what a particular individual can and cannot do when presented with the challenges of assessment materials and—most importantly—real-life situations.

THE ASSESSMENT OF ATTENTION

As we mentioned earlier, there are fundamental problems in assessing a postulated "central" function such as attention. In order to get at "it," we must go through any number of input and output stages, each of which can add their own "noise" to our measurement. There are three main options available to the clinician to get around this difficulty.

The first is to use rating scales and questionnaires to capture the patients', their relatives', or care-staff's understanding of the attentional contribution to patients' difficulties. The advantage of such measures is that they, in principle, distill this experience, over long periods of time and across many contexts, into a useable form. Often, this is also the only practical way to assess the achievement of complex functional goals or instances of particular errors in real-world settings.

There are, however, many difficulties with this approach. Patients, particularly those with attentional/executive impairments, may not always be ideally placed to report problems (Heaton & Pendleton, 1981; Wilson, Alderman, Burgess, Emslie, & Evans, 1997; Burgess, Alderman,

Evans, Emslie, & Wilson, 1998). The reports of others may suffer from positive or negative halo effects, from low interrater reliability and insensitivity to small changes in function. There may also be a considerable gulf between an author's theoretically driven perspective and lay understandings of cognitive cause.

Despite these problems, the use of such measures remains crucial to the evaluation of rehabilitation effects in everyday life. Where possible, the use of published measures with known validity and reliability, rather than untested "in-house" scales, is a considerable advantage. In this respect, we have found measures by Broadbent, Cooper, FitzGerald, and Parkes (1982), Ponsford and Pinsella, (1992), Burgess, Alderman, Wilson, Evans, and Emslie (1996), and a scale designed for the assessment of attention-deficit/hyperactivity disorder (ADHD) in adults (Brown, 1996), to be particularly useful for attention, although many others may be of equal value.

The second option in assessing attention, as with many experimental approaches, is to examine a single task under two conditions and interpret the *difference* between them. The color–word Stroop Test (Trenerry, Crosson, DeBoe, & Leber, 1989), for example, looks at the additional interference caused by the incompability between the color of ink in which a word is written and the color name that it spells. The Robertson et al. Telephone Search test in the Test of Everyday Attention (Robertson, Ward, Ridgeway, & Nimmo-Smith, 1996), compares visual search performance under single- and dual-task conditions, interpreting the decrement as the cost of dividing attention. Many tests of neglect compare performance on the left- and right-hand side of the *same* task. In these ways, factors that are common to both conditions or sides of space are relatively well controlled. A difficulty for this approach in clinical practice lies in the inherent volatility of difference scores. The final result is vulnerable to a change on either the control or test task, and small changes in either can produce large and somewhat difficult-to-interpret fluctuations.

The final option places greater reliance on the clinician to use a range of measures in ruling out nonattentive causes for failure. One of the best validated measures of sustained attention, for example, is to ask patients to keep a count of the number of slowly presented tones they hear within a set period (Wilkins et al., 1987; Broks, Preston, Traub, Poppleton, Ward, & Stahl, 1988; Pardo et al., 1991; Robertson, Ward, Ridgeway, & Nimmo-Smith, 1996; Robertson, Manly, et al., 1997; Manly, Robertson, Anderson, & Nimmo-Smith, 1999). Although inefficient attention to task is the most likely reason for an individual to perform poorly, it is clearly necessary to rule out sensory impairment and task comprehension as "contaminating" factors.

One major advantage of performance test measures over rating scales is that the upper limit of performance becomes a matter of fact rather than opinion. They can allow a much finer analysis of theoretically specified abilities and can form more objective measures of change. However, as with all tests there are limitations. At best, they represent a "snapshot" of abilities taken under one-to-one conditions, usually over a rather brief period. Their use as a predictor of performance under the complexities and distractions of everyday life remains a topic of current debate.

For rehabilitationists, both in research and clinical practice, careful evaluation of the effectiveness of interventions is crucial. If we are to claim a specific effect of a specific strategy, we need to exclude the influence of "spontaneous recovery" or more general effects of the rehabilitation environment. As with any treatment, the gold standard is the blind randomized trial in which patients who share the same levels of disability, age, time since injury, and so forth, are randomly allocated either to a treatment or control group—the group status of each patient being unknown to those assessing the treatment. Because many standardized measures do not have parallel forms or known repeat administration reliability, this design also has a major advantage in the range of measures that can be used. Because both control and treatment groups share common exposure to the assessments, disproportionate change can be reasonably assessed. Even in this case, the use of measures such as the Test of Everyday Attention (Robertson et al., 1996), which has parallel forms and normative data on retest effects, can offer interpretive advantages.

There are, however, often practical drawbacks to random allocation designs. First, there may be an insufficient number of patients with common difficulties—or patients who are matched on sufficient relevant characteristics—to form the necessary groups. Second, there are potential ethical issues in allocating people, who may be at a critical stage in their recovery, to activities that are designed *not* to help them (although relatively benign control conditions are often used, such as general education on the effects of brain injury or the training of another function).

For single-case or small-group studies, further methods have been developed that allow statistical interpretation of the treatment effects. In particular, these are necessary when the treatment is hypothesized to cause a lasting change (as is usually desirable). One design that has particular relevance for measure selection involves an interrupted time series analysis (e.g., Gottman & Glass, 1978). Here, single patients or groups will generally complete the same measures every day over the period of the study. The aim is to establish that the introduction of treatment causes a significant change in performance, over and above the variability that is observed during a baseline period. While the design can cope with a progressive improvement in performance over the baseline that is attributable to practice effects (assuming that the treatment effect is marked by a much steeper increase), factors such as the sensitivity of the measures (e.g., vulnerability to ceiling effects, how much change is required in order to score an additional point, and so forth) become crucial. As we discuss in a later section, we have found the structured observation of the frequency of real-life behaviors (rather than rating scales) to be a particularly useful measure in this respect.

The use of these designs in attention rehabilitation, together with the measures that have been adopted, are discussed in more detail in a later section.

A Note on Attention and Executive Function

There is considerable overlap between the concepts of attention and executive (sometimes also termed "frontal") function. The distinction is often one of terminological preference rather than substance. Attention can be viewed as one of the functions of a broader executive system; conversely, executive functions may be attributed to the working of attention. Both can imply the notion of a central system that acts to coordinate or orchestrate the actions of more basic perceptual, cognitive, and output processes, and both are thought to be particularly reliant on the prefrontal cortex.

In practice, the term "executive" is more frequently applied to complex activities involving multiple processes (such as formulating, carrying out, and evaluating a plan, or remembering the consequences of previous responses and using this adaptively in the generation of new ones). This emphasis is reflected in clinical assessments that tend to be more open-ended, and require strategy and the generation of novel responses. Attention tests, on the other hand, generally use very explicit instructions about what the individual needs to do, may take multiple trials of the same activity, and often involve a timed component.

(An excellent discussion on executive disorders is presented by Cicerone, Chapter 11, this volume.)

REHABILITATION

In the last 20 years, we have seen a considerable shift in the perceived goals of clinical interventions across a range of disciplines. Rather than focusing exclusively on the restitution of damaged function (e.g., an impairment in walking), it is argued, we should focus on more generally specified goals relating to an individual's "quality of life" (such as being independently mobile or having access to community opportunities; World Health Organization, 1980, 1986). Although restitution of basic function remains an important component within this—walking, for example, being an exceptionally useful means of being independently mobile, it is not the only approach. These are important issues for cognitive rehabilitation: Our ability to restore function in damaged brain circuits remains questionable, and the relationship between particular impairments and functional outcome is more often assumed than tested.

There is little doubt that functional, *goal-based* approaches tailored to an individual patient's disabilities and aims are currently the most promising route to effective rehabilitation. In other words, if a patient wishes to get to the store to buy food, then it is better that he or she be trained in this particular activity—or modify the activity such that it can be achieved—rather than abstractly trained in the cognitive functions thought to support the activity (for further discussion, see McLellan, 1991; Wilson, 1996). These are the early days of research, however, and further investigation of factors that can modulate underlying capacities remains crucial. In this chapter, we therefore adopt a broad definition of "rehabilitation" that encompasses interventions at a number of levels: restitution or enhancement of basic function, prosthetic aids to attention, and specific goal-based training. The review is restricted to studies that have used appropriate research designs, allowing substantiated conclusions on efficacy. While there is growing interest in a potential role for pharmacological therapies in acquired disorders of attention, our discussion here is restricted to behavioral/psychological interventions.

UNILATERAL NEGLECT

Scanning Training

Most patients who show unilateral neglect immediately after a stroke spontaneously recover from the most striking spatial symptoms within a few weeks (Hier, Mondlock, & Caplan, 1983; Stone et al., 1991; Stone, Patel, Greenwood, & Halligan, 1992). For those that do not, the impaired awareness of objects and events on the left side of space would be expected to cause problems in almost all everyday activities, including independent mobility, self-care, and reading. Chronic unilateral neglect therefore represents one of the clearest example in which improvement in underlying capacity could most efficiently improve outcome across many domains. There is also evidence, for example, from the observation that patients may become more aware of left-sided information if cued to do so (e.g., Riddoch & Humphreys, 1983; Mattingley, Pierson, Bradshaw, Phillips, & Bradshaw, 1993), that there may be considerable residual function that is not *expressed* in everyday activities. Interventions aimed at increasing this expression could therefore produce valuable functional results.

Unilateral neglect patients can be curiously unaware of their deficits, including the denial of left-sided hemiplegia (Critchley, 1949; McGlynn & Schacter, 1989; Gialanella & Mattioli, 1992; Berti, Làdavas, & Corte, 1996). It is certainly the case that, by definition, these patients do not appear to "expect" left-sided information or view their performance on tasks as incomplete. There is also evidence that "spontaneous" recovery from unilateral neglect involves increasing compensatory visual scans into left space (Goodale, Milner, Jakobson, & Carey, 1990; Robertson et al., 1994; Mattingley, Bradshaw, Bradshaw, & Nettleton, 1994) and that these may be mediated by more "voluntary" frontal circuits (Henik, Rafal, & Rhodes, 1994). Encouraging patients to make such scans, therefore, seems a useful place to begin rehabilitation.

Early attempts at this approach tended to show improvements in spatial awareness on the trained materials but little generalization to other activities (Seron, Deloche, & Coyette, 1989; Robertson, 1990; Wagenaar, Wieringen, Netelenbos, Meijer, & Kuik, 1992). Sometimes the specificity of these effects can be striking. Lawson (1962), for example, describes how a nun, who had learned to read her own Bible effectively, returned to a lateralized pattern of errors when a different typeface was used. Such failure to generalize does not mean that this approach has no value for rehabilitation. It simply suggests that training should take place on materials/tasks relevant to the patient's life. If careful training is required for each and every important activity that a patient performs, however, such rehabilitation may well exceed available clinical resources.

More encouraging results on generalization from scanning training have emerged over recent years. Pizzamiglio et al. (1992) provided scanning training to 13 patients between 3 and 34 months poststroke. The training took place over 40 sessions and included a scanning task in which patients were asked to identify computer-projected digits on a large screen. Cues, such as the presentation of a warning tone, the flashing of relevant parts of the display, and the therapist's encouraging the patient to look for targets, were systematically faded over the course of the training. Other tasks included reading, copying line drawings, and describing complex scenes. Significant improvements were observed on nontrained cancellation tasks and, importantly, in semistructured behavioral observation of untrained, real-life like activities.

The AB design of this initial study means that attribution of improvements to the training must be advanced with caution. However, a subsequent evaluation (Antonucci et al., 1995) using a randomized control group confirmed the improvements and the generalization to activities of daily living. The authors attribute the success of their training relative to previous studies principally to the increased duration of training rather than to particular differences in method.

Right parietal damage is known to compromise "covert" visual attention—that is, moving attention without moving the eyes (Posner, Walker, Fredrich, & Rafal, 1984). Ladavas, Menghini, and Umilta (1994) compared 30 hours of training on tasks that required overt eye movements with 30 hours of training in moving attention without accompanying eye movements. Both produced significant improvements in cancellation task performance relative to a general therapy control. While generalization of the effects to everyday activity was not examined, the results are useful in that they suggest that the movement of attention—rather than eye movements per se—may be an important component in achieving the previously reported therapeutic effects.

Limb Activation

An alternative approach to the amelioration of unilateral neglect emerged from the observation that spatial bias can be modulated by task and action context. Robertson, Nico, and Hood (1995, 1997) for example, demonstrated that when unilateral neglect patients reached as if to pick up a metal rod, they were significantly nearer to the center of the rod than if they were asked to point at the center. Halligan and Marshall (1989) showed how, in a single case, a patient's use of the left hand to perform a cancellation task significantly reduced lateralized error. Later, Halligan, Manning, and Marshall (1991) further demonstrated how these effects were modulated by the position of the left hand relative to a patient's midline. The intentions, limb of action, and the spatial locations of actions all, therefore, appear to allow access to different representations of space that may be more or less vulnerable to unilateral neglect.

These effects were systematically analyzed by Robertson and colleagues (Robertson & North, 1992, 1993, 1994; Robertson, North, & Geggie, 1992). They found reliable effects of reduced spatial bias when patients moved their left hand as they performed spatial tasks—even minor movements, in the case of partial hemiplegia. Moving the right hand within left space did not produce these dramatic improvements, and if both hands were moved simultaneously, the improvements were abolished or even reversed. The main findings of these studies are summarized in Figure 6.2.

These experimental findings have been extended to show improve-

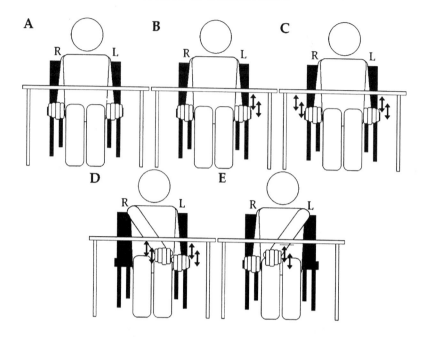

FIGURE 6.2. Principal findings from Robertson and colleagues' studies of limb activation effects in unilateral neglect. Compared with a no-movement condition (A), movements of the left hand in left space (B) produced significant reductions in neglect. Moving both hands in left and right space (C) or in left space alone (D) reduced or abolished the benefits of left-hand use. Moving the left hand within right space (E) also reduced the benefits.

ments on everyday activities (Robertson et al., 1992; Robertson, Hogg, & McMillan, 1998). A portable "neglect alert device" was developed to substitute for the therapist in cueing left-sided movements during task performance. The device consisted of a variable timer, a buzzer, and a switch. If the switch was not pressed within a predetermined interval, then the buzzer would sound, reminding the patient to make the action. Significant improvements in a number of everyday spatial activities (including combing the hair and navigating around a hospital route) coincided with the onset of the movement cueing.

The experimental findings suggest a rather immediate and direct effect of limb activation on spatial bias. If the limb is in use, the bias is reduced. If the use stops, the bias returns. If patients do not spontaneously remember to use their hand, the continued environmental cues provide one route for generalizing the rehabilitation effect across many contexts. For some patients in the study, however, the end of external cueing was not accompanied by a decline to previous levels of performance (Robertson, Hogg, et al., 1998), suggesting that the approach may have a training as well as an immediate effect.

We recently found similar results in using limb activation with a patient to improve his self-care skills (Wilson, Manly, Coyle, & Robertson, 2000). CL, a 62-year-old man, had suffered a right cerebral artery infarct that left him with a strong neglect for left-sided stimuli, including an underuse of his left hand and arm despite residual function (that is, he could use this hand if he was cued to do so by the therapist). Importantly, his neglect was affecting his ability to care for himself and therefore jeopardizing his return to a degree of independence in living.

By dividing up the patient's self-care program into discrete steps (washing upper body on both sides; washing lower body on both sides, and so on) and taking as the measure the number of verbal prompts needed to complete each stage, we were able to quantify the functional effects of his lateralized bias over a 10-day baseline. Using an interrupted time series design, as with previous studies, the onset of "limb activation" saw a significant and rather dramatic improvement. After the end of the training the improvements were well maintained (see Figure 6.3).

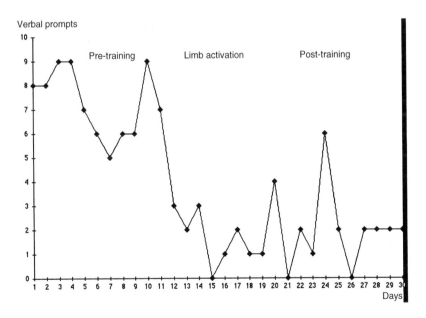

FIGURE 6.3. Improvements in self-care with the onset of limb activation training for a male neglect patient. Improvements were relatively well maintained following the end of the explicit training period.

Because the patient was observed to make more spontaneous use of his hand after training, it is possible to speculate that the increased awareness of left space (including the body), *caused* by using the left hand, itself leads to increased use of the left hand. By this means, a rather positive feedback loop could be established that maintains and enhances the effect.

Sustained Attention Training

Another area in which immediately observed improvements in spatial attention can become consolidated into stable beneficial effects follows from a common clinical observation: Neglect patients can find it very difficult to remain engaged in a task, regardless of its spatial content.

As we discussed earlier, both spatial attention and sustained attention have been related to predominantly right-hemisphere cortical networks. On this basis alone, we would expect that damage to the right hemisphere could produce coexisting deficits in both capacities. Evidence has emerged, however, that suggests a more intimate, functional relationship between the two.

Robertson, Manly, et al. (1997) examined the performance of stroke patients on a nonspatial tone-counting paradigm. Keeping a count of simple tones, especially when the tones are separated by long intervals, is a particularly tedious activity. Wilkins et al. (1987) have previously shown that patients with right prefrontal lesions perform disproportionately poorly at voluntarily maintaining their attention on this dull task. Not surprisingly, Robertson et al. found that right-hemisphere stroke patients were poorer at performing the tone-counting measure[1] than *left*-hemisphere stroke patients. *Within* the right-hemisphere group, however, patients with visual neglect had significantly greater difficulty than patients without—indeed, this nonspatial tone-counting test was a better predictor of neglect than some spatial measures. Samuelsson, Hjelmquist, Jensen, Ekholm, and Blomstrand (1988) have similarly shown that, within a right-hemisphere group, neglect patients are more impaired in self-maintaining a "readiness to respond" on variable interval, nonspatial reaction time tasks.

Although these associations are suggestive of a relationship between the capacities, a more compelling method for demonstrating this link is through experimental manipulation. If patients with neglect are asked to judge which of two lateralized events happened first, they show a spatial

---

[1]The "Elevator Counting" subtest of the Test of Everyday Attention (Robertson, Ward, Ridgeway, & Nimmo-Smith, 1996).

bias. Left-side objects need to appear about 200 ms before right-side objects in order for the two to be seen as happening simultaneously (Rorden, Mattingley, Karnarth, & Driver, 1997). Robertson, Mattingley, Rorden, and Driver (1998b) showed that playing a loud, alerting tone for neglect patients just before occasional trials in this computerized test abolished or even reversed this bias. The results suggest that increasing arousal/alertness using external stimuli can compensate for a deficit in the self-maintenance of such a state in patients, and that this has direct effects on spatial awareness.

Robertson, Tegnér, Tham, Lo, and Nimmo-Smith (1995) addressed the question of whether training neglect patients in self-maintenance of an alert state would improve spatial attention. Along lines first described by Meichenbaum and Cameron (1973), patients were encouraged to use conscious verbal manipulation to enhance impaired attentive function. Initially, they were provided with an inherently "alerting" external stimulus (the therapist banging on the desk) and asked to tell themselves out loud to "*pay attention!*". Over time, the external component was systematically faded, and patients were only cued to use the self-instruction. Eventually, patients were asked to use covert or "inner speech" to give themselves the cue.

Eight neglect patients were trained in this manner, and the rehabilitative effects were examined in two related designs. The first, multiple-baseline by function, tests for the specificity of improvements to targeted symptoms. Improvements in lateralized spatial tasks, but *not* in impaired memory, for example, at least suggest that generalized spontaneous recovery has not taken place (this relies on an assumption of parallel spontaneous recovery rates within different functions). In the second approach, multiple-baseline by subjects, patients were randomly allocated different baseline lengths, the expectation being that improvements related to the training would follow the order of training onset. Both methods significantly supported the impact of the sustained attention training—both on sustained attention function and, importantly, on lateralized spatial function.

At least three very different approaches have therefore produced significant rehabilitative results with unilateral neglect. Unilateral neglect is a general term that covers a now highly fractionated set of symptoms (Robertson & Marshall, 1993). More research is needed to clarify the applicability of these methods to different manifestations of spatial bias—and, indeed, to determine whether the effects may be additive in some cases.

As we shall see, rehabilitation research is considerably more advanced for neglect than for nonspatial attentional disorders. There are two, somewhat related factors that may underpin this relative progression. The first factor is that neglect has been extensively studied from a theoretical perspective. Views of processes underlying neglect have led to effective rehabilitation strategies that are unlikely to have emerged from focusing only on the surface symptoms. The second factor is that the assessment of neglect is relatively easy and unambiguous. Frank, spatial biases are not generally seen in the healthy population (Wilson et al., 1987) and abstract test performance (e.g., on a cancellation task) bears a clear functional relationship to everyday difficulties (such as eating food from one side of the plate). As we look for a pattern of differential performance *within* an individual, many extraneous factors (task comprehension, motivation, etc.) can be effectively excluded.

For *non*spatial attention disorders, there is much less agreement on classification and paradigmatic definitions. The relationships between tasks developed within experimental psychology—where most of the constructs emerged—and everyday difficulties are also often less straightforward or are untested. Under these conditions, it is perhaps not surprising that the rehabilitation of nonspatial attention is at a very early stage in its development.

NONSPATIAL ATTENTION

A Behavioral, Goal-Based Approach

One way around some of the conceptual difficulties that we have highlighted is to target an important goal activity rather than the inattention that is thought to affect it. Wilson and Robertson (1992), for example, focused on the reading difficulties experienced by a man who had sustained a severe head injury. Although the injury had left many of his cognitive abilities relatively intact (e.g., including *above*-average performance on memory tasks), he showed impairments on tests of attention. Similarly, while all his basic processes of reading were preserved, he had great difficulty in "keeping his mind" on the text—often having to reread the same paragraph a number of times to get its meaning.

A baseline was established with the patient, indicating each attentional slip as he experienced it. At the outset of training, he was asked to read a novel for only very brief periods, the aim being to maximize his experience of "nonslip" reading. If he completed three trials without a slip, the duration of reading time was increased by 10%. In this way, over 160 sessions in 40 days, he attained the goal of reliably reading for 5 minutes without a slip. Most importantly, the number of slips reported when he read material relevant to his job—although not directly trained—had also been significantly reduced.

This systematic, shaping approach does not tell us a great deal about the underlying nature of the difficulties experienced by the patient. It does show, however, that appropriate reinforcement and learning can modulate the consequences of poor attention—at least in this context.

Behavioral Shaping of Attention as a Stage in Achieving Complex Goals

Behavioral approaches have also been used to clarify the contribution of attentional deficits to complex difficulties. Alderman, Fry, and Youngson (1995) worked with a patient (SK) who, following herpes simplex encephalitis, was left with behavioral disturbance, dysexecutive deficits and difficulty in monitoring her own performance and staying "on task." Aspects of her behavior, particularly, a very high frequency of stereotyped repetitive speech, seriously affected her access to rehabilitation and community opportunities. Initial treatment using "response cost" (the patient needed to give away a token for each incident) was successful in reducing the behavior during therapy sessions. However, very little generalization was observed.

The authors felt that some of the difficulty experienced by SK in gaining control over this behavior may have resulted from her relative inattention to its occurrence. They tested this by asking her to record instances of her own predefined problematic verbal behavior using a counter, while a therapist kept an independent record. Initially, the agreement levels were very low—around 9%. Training began with SK being rewarded if her record of instances approximated that of the therapist. The margins were systematically reduced—shaping the *detection* behavior. At no point during this stage of the training was any attempt made to reduce the frequency of her inappropriate verbal output.

Only when SK's self-monitoring achieved high levels of accuracy was reinforcement for reducing the behavior introduced. This resulted in statistically and clinically significant reductions in her behavioral problems to a level that was socially appropriate and that generalized across contexts. These gains were well maintained at 5-month follow-up.

This example is interesting in that targeting the potential attentional component was, in some ways, a move *away* from the desired functional goal. However, the observed success of the intervention confirms the authors' view that inattention was a major component in the problem, and it provides further evidence that attention can be shaped by cueing and rewards.

Improving Attention through General Training

The acquisition of a new skill—such as driving a car, playing a musical instrument, or learning a foreign language—takes many, many hours of practice. While adults may envy the speed and flexibility of children's learning, they can nevertheless achieve these goals. It seems reasonable to assume that relearning a cognitive skill, or learning new ways to achieve similar ends, would not occur within a few hours of training. We have already discussed evidence from Pizzamiglio et al. (1992) and Antonucci et al. (1995) that the long duration of their scanning training in visual neglect may have been the crucial factor in their positive results.

The revolution in computer technology and price over the last two decades has increasingly made possible long periods of systematic and reflexive training. For researchers, the use of computers to "deliver" therapy also means that exposure to treatment can be highly standardized, improving the interpretation of particular factors that can promote performance change.

Gray, Robertson, Pentland, and Anderson (1992) performed a randomized, controlled study of computerized attentional retraining. Thirty-one patients with reported attention difficulties were randomly allocated to one of two conditions, approximately 15 hours of either computerized training or recreational computing. This relatively short training comprised (1) a reaction-time task with feedback on speed, (2) identification of two identical-digit strings from a briefly presented array of four digits, (3) a digit–symbol translation task, and (4) a color–word Stroop task.

Immediately following the 3- to 9-week training, the experimental group showed significant improvements on two *nontrained* tasks relative to the controls: the Wechsler Adult Intelligence Scale—Revised (WAIS-R) Picture Completion subtest, which requires visual search and reasoning, and the Paced Auditory Serial Addition Task (PASAT), widely considered to be primarily a measure of processing speed (Gronwall & Sampson, 1974; Deary, Langan, Hepburn, & Frier, 1991). At a 6-month follow-up, the benefits on these measures had been maintained and, in addition, further untrained measures showed training benefit (backward digit span, mental arithmetic, and the WAIS-R Block Design).

Because the groups were well-matched on task performance prior to training, the results suggested both that the training produced generalized improvements and that a "sleeper effect" led to continued improvement beyond the training period. While little evidence exists for this, it is possible to speculate that such "sleeper effects" emerge through both consolidation of the learning and increased exposure to attentionally demanding situations consequent to initial improvements.

The results persuasively suggest a specific effect that, thanks to the well-matched control group, cannot be interpreted in terms of generalized recovery. The generalization to *functional activities* of everyday life was not, however, examined in this study.

Training Specific Functions

Sturm, Willmes, et al. (1997) have also reported encouraging results from computerized training of a much longer duration. Unlike their previous work with a rather general computer training program (Sturm & Willmes, 1991, using a program by Brickenkamp, 1986), they developed computerized tasks designed to train *specific* and putatively separable attention systems. In an elegant design, 38 stroke patients (selected on the basis of attentional impairments) were randomly allocated to a particular *order* of training. Whereas one patient would begin the treatment period using the sustained attention training program, another would not encounter this until the end of the examination period. The logic of this design is that distinct forms of attention should show specific training effects. Improvements in, say, sustained attention should be significantly greater following sustained attention training than following training on the selective attention task.

There are a number of advantages to this approach. First, it can provide further supportive evidence for the functional separability of attention. Second, all patients are engaged in training and not assigned to a control condition that is hypothesised *not* to help them—while spontaneous improvements are still controlled. Third, unlike ABAB style designs, this approach does not require return to baseline in order to support the effect. This makes it suitable for interventions that are hypothesized—indeed, hoped—to be lasting.

A criticism that can be leveled at some psychologists is a tendency to view the types of tasks that are used in psychological tests or experiments (where simplicity is desirable) as ideal materials for training. All over the world, people voluntarily spend vast amounts of their own time engaged in visuospatial and reaction-time tasks that are the stock-in-trade of the computer games industry. This is because they look good, make noises when a point is won, and contain a plot (or, at the very least, a high death toll). Neurological patients in rehabilitation, on the other hand, may be encouraged repeatedly to judge which of two lines is longer or to respond to red squares but not green triangles, which may be rather less than engaging.

Sturm and Willmes (1991) creditably set their computer training tasks within a game context. Alertness, for example, was trained by controlling an on-screen motorbike. Aspects of selective attention were trained by patients' having to shoot some, but not other, objects flying across the display. As patients improved their performance on the tasks, the difficulty level was increased. In all, each patient completed some 56 hours of training (14 hours for each component).

The results supported the hypothesis, with generally the greatest improvements in a particular capacity being seen after that capacity was trained. The detection rate for targets in the untrained test battery vigilance task, for example, was significantly improved only after vigilance training and not following training in selective or divided attention. Similarly, reaction times in the selective attention test were improved following selective, but not sustained, attention training. As might be expected, some crossover effects were also observed. Performance on the divided attention task, for example, was significantly enhanced following training in selective, as well as divided, forms of attention.

Although these important findings are of theoretical as well as clinical interest, it is important to note again that the improvements were measured on another, albeit *non*trained, computerized battery (Zimmermann, North, & Fimm, 1993). Important questions of spontaneous generalization outside the computer training context therefore remain. Although it strains credulity to believe that the brain has capacities untouched by daily life and reserved only for neuropsychological tasks, issues such as context-dependent expression of ability remain crucial to evaluating the effectiveness of interventions.

Environmental Support for Attention during Complex Tasks

We have argued that impairments in attention can prevent the adequate expression of other abilities. Recently, we (Manly, Hawkins, Evans, & Robertson) have examined whether providing environmental support to one aspect of attention can improve performance on a complex, life-like task.

The Six Elements test was originally devised by Shallice and Burgess (1991) to test complex "executive" functions such as planning and strategy application in patients with prefrontal lesions. In the test, patients are asked to attempt each of six tasks within a 15-minute period. The crucial aspect is that fully completing each of the tasks would take much longer than is available for the test as a whole. The emphasis is therefore on being able to plan and switch strategically between the tasks. A common type of error is for patients to get so caught up in performing one component activity that they neglect this most important, overall goal.

We asked patients with traumatic brain injuries to perform a modification of the task under two conditions. In the "environmental support" condition, a relatively salient tone was presented at random points. We simply asked patients to "try and be aware of what they were doing" when they heard the tone. Our view was that attention to current activity is in competition with attention to the overall goal in the task. By briefly disrupting the ongoing activity, we predicted that the representation of the main goal would stand a better chance of expression.

The results were consistent with this view. The patients significantly improved both the number of tasks they attempted and the amount of time they spent on each task. The findings suggest that the patients had not forgotten the overall goal, but that without the periodic environmental cue, they were less likely to attend to it spontaneously. The findings also suggest that providing this environmental support to the attentive aspects of the task allowed the more *useful* expression of the other, required abilities.

Tasks such as the Six Elements test have the advantage of allowing reliable measurement of complex, life-like activities. As such, they can provide a useful "test-bed" for rehabilitative strategies that may have applications across different tasks and settings.

There is, therefore, growing evidence that nonspatial attention is amenable to shaping by reward contingencies, general training effects, and enhancement through environmental support. In each of these areas, whether using a desktop PC in the clinic or taking rehabilitation into the patient's day-to-day activities using "palm-top" technologies, there is considerable scope for productive relationships between clinicians and computer programmers. The potential additive value of combining structured rehabilitation with pharmacological treatments is another barely explored area. In each of these areas, however, it is important to keep an eye on the main goal of rehabilitation, namely, to demonstrate that improvements on tests generalize to improvements in patients' independence, capacity, and quality of life.

SUMMARY

1. The scientific study of functions that are *specifically* attentional is a relatively recent development. These ideas have begun to inform both assessment and rehabilitation practice.

2. Attention is not just one thing. Contemporary research suggests that the attention functions of the brain are subserved by distinct networks—separate from basic perceptual functions and from one another. This means that damage to the brain can produce specifically attentional dysfunction, and that where that damage occurs will influence the type of attentional impairment observed.

3. Increasingly, there is evidence that attention deficits can interfere

with good recovery from brain damage. While they are a pressing problem in their own right, attention deficits may also act to prevent the adequate expression of other abilities, the relearning of lost skills, and the flexible adaptation to disability.

4. Clinicians have tried in a number of ways to work with adult neurological patients to improve attention by teaching them the functional goals that require attention, by changing the environment or other aspects of function that support attention, and through teaching the practice of attentionally demanding tasks.

5. The spatial biases of unilateral neglect have been successfully ameliorated in three distinct ways. The training of leftward scanning has not always produced generalized improvements, but there is evidence that the duration of training may be an important factor. Experimental observations of interactions between use of the left limb in left space have led to "limb activation" training that has reliably improved spatial function across a number of contexts. Training patients in self-maintenance of an alert, ready-to-respond state has also reduced spatial bias in test and functional settings.

6. The rehabilitation of nonspatial attention is at an early stage in its development. Results show that training patients in a specific goal activity that is limited by poor attention can produce positive results. There is also evidence that the much greater exposure to training activities made possible by computers can produce measurable improvements. This work further supports the need for careful assessment in targeting training at the particular attention system that is compromised.

7. Demonstrating improvements in everyday function that are related to improved attention is extremely difficult. Evidence of such generalization will, however, be very important if the techniques described here are to be more widely adopted.

REFERENCES

Alderman, N., Fry, R. K., & Youngson, H. A. (1995). Improvement in self-monitoring skills, reduction of behaviour disturbance and the dysexecutive syndrome: Comparison of response cost and a new programme of self-monitoring training. *Neuropsychological Rehabilitation, 5,* 193–221.

Antonucci, G., Guariglia, C., Judica, A., Magnotti, L., Paoloucci, S., Pizzamiglio, L., & Zoccolotti, P. (1995). Effectiveness of neglect rehabilitation in a randomised group-study. *Journal of Clinical and Experimental Neuropsychology, 17,* 383–389.

Bak, T. H., & Hodges, J. R. (1998). The neuropsychology of progressive supranuclear palsy. *Neurocase, 4,* 89–94.

Bench, C. J., Frith, C. D., Grasby, P. M., Friston, K. J., Paulesu, E., Frackowiak, R. S.

J., & Dolan, R. J. (1993). Investigations of the functional anatomy of attention using the Stroop Test. *Neuropsychologia, 31,* 907–922.

Benson, D. F., & Barton, M. I. (1970). Disturbances in constructional ability. *Cortex, 6,* 19–46.

Ben-Yishay, Y., Diller, L., Gerstman, L., & Haas, A. (1968). The relationship between impersistence, intellectual function and outcome of rehabilitation in patients with left hemiplegia. *Neurology, 18,* 852–861.

Berti, A., Làdavas, E., & Corte, M. D. (1996). Anosognosia for hemiplegia, neglect dyslexia, and drawing neglect: Clinical findings and theoretical considerations. *Journal of the International Neuropsychological Society, 2,* 426–440.

Blanc-Garin, J. (1994). Patterns of recovery from hemiplegia following stroke. *Neuropsychological Rehabilitation, 4,* 359–385.

Boller, F., Howes, D., & Patten, D. H. (1970). A behavioural evaluation of brain scan results with neuropathalogical findings. *Lancet, 1,* 1143–1146.

Brickenkamp, R. (1986). *Handbuch apparativer Verfahren in der psychologie.* Göttingen: Hogrefe.

Broadbent, D. B., Cooper, P. F., FitzGerald, P., & Parkes, K. R. (1982). The Cognitive Failures Questionnaire (CFQ) and its correlates. *British Journal of Clinical Psychology, 21,* 1–16.

Broks, P., Preston, G. C., Traub, M., Poppleton, P., Ward, C., & Stahl, S. M. (1988). Modelling dementia: Effects of scopolamine on memory and attention. *Neuropsychologia, 26,* 685–700.

Brooks, D. N., & McKinlay, W. (1987). Return to work within the first seven years of severe head injury. *Brain Injury, 1,* 5–15.

Brown, T. E. (1996). *Brown Attention-Deficit Disorder Scales.* San Antonio, TX: Psychological Corporation.

Burgess, P. W., Alderman, N., Evans, J., Emslie, H., & Wilson, B. A. (1998). The ecological validity of tests of executive function. *Journal of the International Neuropsychological Society, 4,* 547–558.

Burgess, P. W., Alderman, N., Wilson, B. A., Evans, J., & Emslie, H. (1996). The Dysexecutive Questionnaire (DEX). In B. A. Wilson, N. Alderman, P. W. Burgess, H. Emslie, & J. J. Evans (Eds.), *Behavioural assessment of the dysexecutive syndrome.* Bury St. Edmunds, UK: Thames Valley Test Company.

Cohen, R. A., & Kaplan, R. F. (1993). Attention as a multicomponent process—Neuropsychological validation (abstract). *Journal of Clinical and Experimental Neuropsychology, 15,* 379.

Cohen, R. M., Semple, W. E., Gross, M., Holcomb, H. J., Dowling, S., & Nordahl, T. E. (1988). Functional localization of sustained attention: Comparison to sensory stimulation in the absence of instruction. *Neuropsychiatry, Neuropsychology and Behavioral Neurology, 1,* 3–20.

Cohen, R. M., Semple, W. E., Gross, M., King, A. C., & Nordahl, T. E. (1992). Metabolic brain pattern of sustained auditory discrimination. *Experimental Brain Research, 92,* 165–172.

Corbetta, M., Miezin, F. M., Dobmeyer, S., Shulman, G. L., & Petersen, S. E. (1991). Selective and divided attention during visual discriminations of shape, color, and speed: Functional anatomy by positron emission tomography. *Journal of Neuroscience, 11,* 2383–2402.

Critchley, M. (1949). The problem of awareness or non-awareness of hemianopic field defects. *Transactions of the Ophthalmological Society of the U.K., 69,* 95–109.

Deary, I. J., Langan, S. J., Hepburn, D. A., & Frier, B. M. (1991). Which abilities does the PASAT test? *Personality and Individual Differences, 12,* 983–987.

Denes, G., Semenza, C., Stoppa, E., & Lis, A. (1982). Unilateral spatial neglect and recovery from hemiplegia: A follow-up study. *Brain, 105,* 543–552.

De Renzi, E., & Fagliono, P. (1965). The comparative efficiency of intelligence and vigilance tests in detecting hemispheric cerebral damage. *Cortex, 1,* 410–433.

Duncan, J. (1995). Attention, intelligence and the frontal lobes. In M. Gazzaniga (Ed.), *The cognitive neurosciences* (pp. 721–733). Cambridge, MA: MIT Press.

Foster, J. K., Eskes, G. A., & Stuss, D. R. (1994). The cognitive neuropsychology of attention: A frontal lobe perspective. *Cognitive Neuropsychology, 11,* 133–147.

Fullerton, J., McSherry, P., & Stout, M. (1986). Albert's Test: A neglected test of perceptual neglect. *Lancet, 8478,* 430–432.

Gainotti, G. (1972). Emotional behaviour and hemispheric side of lesion. *Cortex, 8,* 41–55.

Gialanella, B., & Mattioli, F. (1992). Anosognosia and extrapersonal neglect as predictors of functional recovery following right hemisphere stroke. *Neuropsychological Rehabilitation, 2,* 169–178.

Goodale, M. A., Milner, A. D., Jakobson, L. S., & Carey, D. P. (1990). Kinematic analysis of limb movements in neuropsychological research: Subtle deficits and recovery of function. *Canadian Journal of Psychology, 44,* 180–195.

Gottman, J. M., & Glass, G. V. (1978). Analysis of Interrupted Time Series Analysis. In T. R. Kratochwill (Ed.), *Single subject research* (pp. 197–235). New York: Academic Press.

Gray, J. M., Robertson, I. H., Pentland, B., & Anderson, S. I. (1992). Microcomputer based cognitive rehabilitation for brain damage: A randomised group controlled trial. *Neuropsychological Rehabilitation, 2,* 97–116.

Gronwall, D. M. A., & Sampson, H. (1974). *The psychological effects of concussion.* Auckland: Auckland University Press.

Halligan, P. W., Manning, L., & Marshall, J. C. (1991). Hemispheric activation vs spatio-motor cueing in visual neglect: A case study. *Neuropsychologia, 29,* 165–176.

Halligan, P. W., & Marshall, J. C. (1989). Laterality of motor response in visuo-spatial neglect: A case study. *Neuropsychologia, 27,* 1301–1307.

Heaton, R. K., & Pendleton, M. G. (1981). Use of neuropsychological tests to predict adult patients' everyday functioning. *Journal of Consulting and Clinical Psychology, 49,* 807–821.

Hecaen, H., & Albert, M. L. (1978). *Human neuropsychology.* New York: Wiley.

Heilman, K. M., Schwartz, H. D., & Watson, R. T. (1978). Hypoarousal in patients with the neglect syndrome and emotional indifference. *Neurology, 28,* 229–232.

Heilman, K. M., & Valenstein, E. (1979). Mechanisms underlying hemispatial neglect. *Annals of Neurology, 5,* 166–170.

Heilman, K. M., & Watson, R. T. (1977). The neglect syndrome—A unilateral deficit of the orienting response. In S. Harnad, R. W. Doty, L. Goldstein, J. Jaynes, & G. Krauthamer (Eds.), *Lateralization in the nervous system.* New York: Academic Press.

Heilman, K. M., Watson, R. T., Valenstein, E., & Goldberg, M. E. (1987). Attention: Behaviour and neural mechanisms. In F. Plum (Ed.), *Handbook of physiology: Section 1. The nervous system* (pp. 461–481). Bethesda, MD: American Physiological Society.

Henik, A., Rafal, R., & Rhodes, D. (1994). Visually guided saccades after lesions of the human frontal eye fields. *Journal of Cognitive Neuroscience, 6,* 400–411.

Hier, D. B., Mondlock, J., & Caplan, L. R. (1983). Recovery of behavioural abnormalities after right hemisphere stroke. *Neurology, 33,* 345–350.

Howes, D., & Boller, F. (1975). Simple reaction time: Evidence for focal impairment from lesions of the right hemisphere. *Brain, 98,* 317–322.

Janer, K. W., & Pardo, J. (1991). Deficits in selective attention following bilateral anterior cingulotomy. *Journal of Cognitive Neuroscience, 3,* 231–234.

Knight, R. T., Hillyard, S. A., Woods, D. L., & Neville, H. J. (1981). The effects of frontal cortical lesions on event-related potentials during auditory selective attention. *Electroencephalography and Clinical Neurophysiology, 52,* 571–582.

Ladavas, E., Menghini, G., & Umilta, C. (1994). A rehabilitation study of hemispatial neglect. *Cognitive Neuropsychology, 11,* 75–95.

Ladavas, E., Pesce, M. D., & Provinviali, L. (1989). Unilateral attention deficits and hemispheric asymmetries in the control of visual attention. *Neuropsychologia, 27,* 353–366.

Lawson, I. R. (1962). Visual–spatial neglect in lesions of the right cerebral hemisphere: A study in recovery. *Neurology, 12,* 23–33.

Lewin, J. S., Friedman, L., Wu, D., Miller, D. A., Thompson, L. A., Klein, S. K., Wise, A. L., Hedera, P., Buckley, P., Meltzer, H., Friedland, R. P., & Duerk, J. L. (1996). Cortical localization of human sustained attention: Detection with functional MR using a visual vigilance paradigm. *Journal of Computer Assisted Tomography, 20,* 695–701.

Loken, W. J., Thornton, A. E., Otto, R. L., & Long, C. J. (1995). Sustained attention after severe closed head injury. *Neuropsychology, 9,* 592–598.

Luria, A. R. (1966). *Higher cortical functions in man.* London: Tavistock.

Manly, T., Robertson, I. H., Anderson, V. A., & Nimmo-Smith, I. (1999). *TEA-Ch— The Test of Everyday Attention for Children.* Bury St Edmunds, UK: Thames Valley Test Company.

Mattingley, J. B., Bradshaw, J. L., Bradshaw, J. A., & Nettleton, N. C. (1994). Residual right attentional bias after apparent recovery from right hemisphere damage: Implications for a multicomponent model of neglect. *Journal of Neurology, Neurosurgery and Psychiatry, 57,* 597–604.

Mattingley, J. B., Pierson, J. M., Bradshaw, J. L., Phillips, J. G., & Bradshaw, J. A. (1993). To see or not to see: The effects of visible and invisible cues on line bisection judgements in unilateral neglect. *Neuropsychologia, 31,* 1201–1215.

McGlynn, S., & Schacter, D. L. (1989). Unawareness of deficits in neuropsychological syndromes. *Journal of Clinical and Experimental Neuropsychology, 11,* 143–205.

McLellan, D. L. (1991). Functional recovery and the principles of disability medicine. In M. Swash & J. Oxbury (Eds.), *Clinical neurology* (pp. 768–790). Edinburgh: Churchill Livingstone.

McPherson, K., Berry, A., & Pentland, B. (1997). Relationships between cognitive impairments and functional performance after brain injury, as measured by the functional assessment measure (FIM+FAM). *Neuropsychological Rehabilitation, 7,* 241–257.

Meichenbaum, D., & Cameron, R. (1973). Training schizophrenics to talk to themselves: A means of developing attentional control. *Behaviour Therapy, 4,* 515–534.

Mesulam, M. M. (1981). A cortical network for directed attention and unilateral neglect. *Annals of Neurology, 10,* 309–325.

Mirsky, A. F., Anthony, B. J., Duncan, C. C., Ahearn, M. B., & Kellam, S. G. (1991). Analysis of the elements of attention: A neuropsychological approach. *Neuropsychology Review, 2,* 109–145.

Pardo, J. V., Fox, P. T., & Raichle, M. E. (1991). Localization of a human system for sustained attention by positron emission tomography. *Nature, 349,* 61–64.

Pardo, J. V., Pardo, P., Janer, K., & Raichle, M. E. (1990). The anterior cingulate cortex mediates processing selection in the Stroop Attentional Conflict paradigm. *Proceedings of the National Academy of Science USA, 87,* 256–259.

Pizzamiglio, L., Antonucci, G., Judica, A., Montenero, P., Razzano, C., & Zoccolotti, P. (1992). Cognitive rehabilitation of the hemineglect disorder in chronic patients with unilateral right brain-damage. *Journal of Clinical and Experimental Neuropsychology, 14,* 901–923.

Ponsford, J., & Kinsella, G. (1992). The use of a rating scale of attentional behaviour. *Neuropsychological Rehabilitation, 1,* 241–257.

Posner, M. I., Inhoff, A. W., & Friedrich, F. J. (1987). Isolating attentional systems: A cognitive-anatomical analysis. *Psychobiology, 15,* 107–121.

Posner, M. I., & Petersen, S. E. (1990). The attention system of the human brain. *Annual Review of Neuroscience, 13,* 25–42.

Posner, M. I., & Snyder, C. R. R. (1975). Facilitation and inhibition in the processing of signals. In P. M. A. Rabbitt & S. Dornic (Eds.), *Attention and performance* (Vol. 5, pp. 669–682). London: Academic Press.

Posner, M. I., Walker, J. A., Fredrich, F. J., & Rafal, R. B. (1984). The effects of parietal lobe injury on covert orienting of visual attention. *Journal of Neuroscience, 4,* 1863–1874.

Riddoch, M. J., & Humphreys, G. W. (1983). The effect of cueing on unilateral neglect. *Neuropsychologia, 21,* 589–599.

Robertson, I. (1990). Does computerized cognitive rehabilitation work? A review. *Aphasiology, 4,* 381–405.

Robertson, I. H., Hogg, K., & McMillan, T. M. (1998). Rehabilitation of unilateral neglect: Improving function by contralesional limb activation. *Neuropsychological Rehabilitation, 8,* 19–29.

Robertson, I. H., Manly, T., Beschin, N., Haeske-Dewick, H., Hömberg, V., Jehkonen, M., Pizzamiglio, L., Shiel, A., Weber, E., & Zimmerman, P. (1997). Auditory sustained attention is a marker of unilateral spatial neglect. *Neuropsychologia, 35,* 1527–1532.

Robertson, I. H., & Marshall, J. C. (Eds.). (1993). *Unilateral neglect: Clinical and experimental studies.* Hillsdale, NJ: Erlbaum.

Robertson, I. H., Mattingley, J. M., Rorden, C., & Driver, J. (1998). Phasic alerting of neglect patients overcomes their spatial deficit in visual awareness. *Nature, 395,* 169–172.

Robertson, I. H., Nico, D., & Hood, B. (1995). The intention to act improves unilateral neglect: Two demonstrations. *Neuroreport, 7,* 246–248.

Robertson I. H., Nico, D., & Hood, B. M. (1997). Believing what you feel: Using proprioceptive feedback to reduce unilateral neglect. *Neuropsychology, 11,* 53–58.

Robertson, I. H., & North, N. (1992). Spatio-motor cueing in unilateral neglect: The role of hemispace, hand and motor activation. *Neuropsychologia, 30,* 553–563.

Robertson, I. H., & North, N. (1993). Active and passive activation of left limbs: Influence on visual and sensory neglect. *Neuropsychologia, 31,* 293–300.

Robertson, I. H., & North, N. (1994). One hand is better than two: Motor extinction of left hand advantage in unilateral neglect. *Neuropsychologia, 32,* 1–11.

Robertson, I. H., North, N., & Geggie, C. (1992). Spatio-motor cueing in unilateral neglect: Three single case studies of its therapeutic effectiveness. *Journal of Neurology, Neurosurgery and Psychiatry, 55,* 799–805.

Robertson, I. H., Ridgeway, V., Greenfield, E., & Parr, A. (1997). Motor recovery after stroke depends on intact sustained attention: A 2–year follow-up study. *Neuropsychology*, *11*, 290–295.

Robertson, I. H., Tegnér, R., Tham, K., Lo, A., & Nimmo-Smith, I. (1995). Sustained attention training for unilateral neglect: Theoretical and rehabilitation implications. *Journal of Clinical and Experimental Neuropsychology*, *17*, 416–430.

Robertson, I. H., Ward, A., Ridgeway, V., & Nimmo-Smith, I. (1996). The structure of normal human attention: The Test of Everyday Attention. *Journal of the International Neuropsychological Society*, *2*, 523–534.

Rorden, C., Mattingley, J. B., Karnarth, H., & Driver, J. (1997). Visual extinction and prior entry: Impaired perception of temporal order with intact motion perception after unilateral parietal damage. *Neuropsychologia*, *35*, 421–433.

Rueckert, L., & Grafman, J. (1996). Sustained attention deficits in patients with right frontal lesions. *Neuropsychologia*, *34*, 953–963.

Samuelsson, H., Hjelmquist, E., Jensen, C., Ekholm, S., & Blomstrand, C. (1988). Nonlateralized attentional deficits: An important component behind persisting visuospatial neglect? *Journal of Clinical and Experimental Psychology*, *20*, 73–88.

Samuelsson, H., Jensen, C., Ekholm, S., Naver, H., & Blomstrand, C. (1997). Anatomical and neurological correlates of acute and chronic visuospatial neglect following right hemisphere stroke. *Cortex*, *33*, 271–285.

Seron, X., Deloche, G., & Coyette, F. (1989). A retrospective analysis of a single case neglect therapy: A point of theory. In X. Seron & G. Deloche (Eds.), *Cognitive approaches to neuropsychological rehabilitation* (pp. 289–236). Hillsdale NJ: Erlbaum.

Shallice, T. (1988). *From neuropsychology to mental structure*. Cambridge, UK: Cambridge University Press.

Shallice, T., & Burgess, P. (1991). Deficit in strategy application following frontal lobe damage in man. *Brain*, *114*, 727–741.

Stone, S. P., Patel, P., Greenwood, R. J., & Halligan, P. W. (1992). Measuring visual neglect in acute stroke and predicting its recovery: The visual neglect recovery index. *Journal of Neurology, Neurosurgery and Psychiatry*, *55*, 431–436.

Stone, S. P., Wilson, B. A., Wroot, A., Halligan, P. W., Lange, L. S., Marshall, J. C., & Greenwood, R. J. (1991). The assessment of visuo-spatial neglect after acute stroke. *Journal of Neurology, Neurosurgery and Psychiatry*, *54*, 345–350.

Sturm, W., Reul, J., & Willmes, K. (1989). Is there a generalized right hemisphere dominance for mediating cerebral activation? Evidence form a choice reaction experiment with lateralized simple warning stimuli. *Neuropsychologia*, *27*, 747–751.

Sturm, W., Simone, A. D., Krause, B. J., Specht, K., Hesselmann, V., Radermacher, I., Herzog, H., Tellmann, L., Muller-Gartner, H. W., & Willmes, K. (1999). Functional anatomy of intrinsic alertness: Evidence for a fronto–parietal–thalamic–brainstem network in the right hemisphere. *Neuropsychologia*, *37*, 797–805.

Sturm, W., & Willmes, K. (1991). Efficacy of reaction training on various attentional and cognitive functions in stroke patients. *Neuropsychological Rehabilitation*, *1*, 259–280.

Sturm, W., Willmes, K., Orgass, B., & Hartje, W. (1997). Do specific attention deficits need specific training? *Neuropsychological Rehabilitation*, *7*(2), 81–103.

Stuss, D. T., & Benson, D. F. (1984). Neuropsychological studies of the frontal lobes. *Psychological Bulletin*, *95*, 3–28.

Trenerry, M. R., Crosson, B., DeBoe, J., & Leber, W. R. (1989). *Stroop Neuropsychological Screening Test.* Odessa, FL: Psychological Assessment Resources.

Vallar, G., & Perani, D. (1986). The anatomy of unilateral neglect after right-hemisphere stroke lesions: A clinical/CT scan correlation study in man. *Neuropsychologia, 24,* 609–622.

Van Zomeren, A. H., Brouwer, W. H., & Deelman, B. G. (1984). Attentional deficits: The riddles of selectivity, speed and alertness. In D. N. Brooks (Ed.), *Closed head injury: Psychological, social and family consequences* (pp. 399–415). Oxford, UK: Oxford University Press.

Van Zomeren, A. H., & Deelman, B. G. (1976). Differential aspects of simple and choice reaction time after closed head injury. *Clinical Neurology and Neurosurgery, 79,* 81–90.

Van Zomeren, A. H., & Deelman, B. G. (1978). Long-term recovery of visual reaction time after closed head injury. *Journal of Neurology, Neurosurgery and Psychiatry, 41,* 452–457.

Wagenaar, R. C., Wieringen, P. C. W. V., Netelenboss, J. B., Meijer, O. G., & Kuik, D. J. (1992). The transfer of scanning training effects in visual attention after stroke: Five single case studies. *Disability Rehabilitation, 14,* 51–60.

Whyte, J., Polansky, M., Fleming, M., Branch-Coslett, H., & Cavallucci, C. (1995). Sustained arousal and attention after traumatic brain injury. *Neuropsychologia, 33,* 797–813.

Wilkins, A. J., Shallice, T., & McCarthy, R. (1987). Frontal lesions and sustained attention. *Neuropsychologia, 25,* 359–365.

Wilson, B. A. (1996). Cognitive rehabilitation: How it is and how it might be. *Journal of the International Neuropsychological Society, 3,* 487–496.

Wilson, B. A., Alderman, N., Burgess, P. W., Emslie, H., & Evans, J. (1997). *The behavioural assessment of the dysexecutive syndrome.* Bury St. Edmunds, UK: Thames Valley Test Company.

Wilson, B. A., Cockburn, J., & Halligan, P. (1987). *The Behavioural Inattention Test.* Bury St. Edmunds, UK: Thames Valley Test Company.

Wilson, C., & Robertson, I. H. (1992). A home-based intervention for attentional slips during reading following head injury: A single case study. *Neuropsychological Rehabilitation, 2,* 193–205.

Wilson, F. C., Manly, T., Coyle, D., & Robertson, I. H. (2000). The effect of contralesional limb activation training and sustained attention training for self-care programmes in unilateral spatial neglect. *Restorative Neurology and Neuroscience, 16,* 1–4.

Woischneck, D., Firsching, R., Ruckert, N., Hussein, S., Heissler, H., Aumuller, E., & Dietz, H. (1997). Clinical predictors of the psychosocial long term outcome after brain injury. *Neurological Research, 19,* 305–310.

World Health Organization. (1980). *International classification of impairments, disabilities and handicaps: A manual of classification relating to the consequences of disease.* Geneva: Author.

World Health Organization. (1986). *Optimum care of disabled people.* Report of a WHO meeting, Turku, Finland.

Zimmermann, P., North, P., & Fimm, B. (1993). Diagnosis of attentional deficits: Theoretical considerations and presentation of a test battery. In F. Stackowiak (Ed.), *Developments in the assessment and rehabilitation of brain damaged patients.* Tubingen: G Narr Verlagg.

CHAPTER 7

Learning and Memory Impairments

ELIZABETH L. GLISKY
MARTHA L. GLISKY

Learning and memory impairments are among the most prevalent, debilitating, and intractable sequelae of neurological insult. Associated with a range of neurological conditions including traumatic brain injury, encephalitis, tumor, stroke, aneurysm, anoxic and ischemic episodes, epilepsy, Korsakoff's syndrome, and dementia, memory disorders have often been stubbornly resistant to rehabilitation efforts. At least part of the reason for the limited success of attempts at remediation relates to the lack of well-specified models of normal memory function. Whereas some cognitive domains, language, for example, have well-developed theoretical models of normal function that specify a variety of cognitive and neural components, with multiple interconnections among them, memory models have traditionally recognized only three general processes—encoding, storage, and retrieval—that are each underspecified with respect to cognitive and neural representations. Thus, it has been difficult for rehabilitation professionals to know exactly how or where to focus treatment and virtually impossible to determine the basis for improvement or failure.

In the past 20 years, however, we have learned much more about the workings of normal learning and memory, and accordingly, now have the potential to be much more sophisticated in our approaches to rehabilitation. Importantly, we have come to recognize that memory is not a unitary concept and that it can break down in a variety of ways. Thus, the notion of a single therapy for memory impairment is untenable. So, too, is the notion that memory is localized in a single brain region. Continuing technological advances, particularly in the field of neuroimaging, have implicated numerous brain regions in memory and learning, and are beginning to permit a mapping of specific memory processes onto neural structures.

Given these developments, it makes sense to adopt an *integrated approach to rehabilitation* that takes into account the kinds of memory that are spared and impaired, the particular memory processes that are compromised, and the regions of the brain that are affected. Not only will such an approach improve the likelihood of successful interventions, but it will also increase the probability of establishing cause-and-effect relations between therapies and outcomes, so that further effective treatment strategies can be developed. We also need to consider the functional consequences of memory impairment and direct our rehabilitation techniques toward eliminating or alleviating real problems in everyday life.

Neuropsychology has a key role to play in this enterprise. Assessment is clearly critical for determining which aspects of memory have been compromised and which remain intact. Knowledge of functions associated with particular brain regions is also important for deciding what cognitive and neural mechanisms might be available to help solve any particular rehabilitation problem. Armed with neuropsychological and neuroanatomical information, clinicians should be in a position to evaluate existing remedial techniques and decide which ones are most likely to be successful. Even more important, however, is the capability to develop new rehabilitation methodologies that are empirically and theoretically grounded in the new cognitive neuroscience of memory. Every neuropsychologist who is confronted with, or challenged by, memory problems can participate in this enterprise. The goal of this chapter is to provide the foundational knowledge on which to base such new approaches and techniques.

The chapter (1) outlines several models or approaches to rehabilitation, indicating their strengths and weaknesses; (2) describes selected assessment instruments, neuropsychological and behavioral, and shows how they help to give direction to rehabilitation; (3) describes a variety of existing remedial techniques and the conditions under which they are most likely to be effective; and (4) suggests some directions for interventions in the future.

APPROACHES TO REHABILITATION

Relatively little is yet known about mechanisms of recovery or how they might be affected by intervention; accordingly, the field of cognitive rehabilitation has generally lacked comprehensive models of rehabilitation (Caramazza & Hillis, 1993). Nevertheless, a number of approaches to rehabilitation have been adopted, each with different goals and assumptions, and each dictating rather different treatment methodologies. These approaches are not mutually exclusive, however, and are often combined to maximize the likelihood of success. The first two approaches to be described have focused on the repair or optimal use of damaged memory processes. These approaches are directed at the underlying impairment or cause of memory problems and aim to achieve general improvements in memory. The second two approaches, in contrast, tend to intervene directly at the behavioral level, usually targeting disability rather than impairment, and attempt to achieve specific functional outcomes (for a summary of rehabilitation approaches, see Table 7.1).

TABLE 7.1. Summary of Rehabilitation Approaches

Rehabilitation approach	Methods/goals	Limitations
Restoration of damaged function—attempts to restore damaged memory processes; targets underlying impairment	Repetitive practice drills and exercises to achieve general mnemonic benefits	No theoretical basis; not individualized; lack of generalization; regeneration of neural structures uncertain
Optimization of residual function—attempts to retrain normal memory processes; targets underlying impairment	Teaching of mnemonic strategies either to achieve general memory benefits or to learn specific information	Limited by available models of normal memory; lack of generalization; useful only for mild or moderate impairments
Compensation for lost function—compensates for or bypasses memory deficits; targets functional deficits	Use of external aids and environmental supports to solve everyday memory problems	May require extensive training
Substitution of intact function—uses intact memory processes to substitute for damaged ones; targets functional deficits	Teaching of domain-specific knowledge relevant in everyday life	Degree to which reorganization can occur at a neural level, unknown

Restoration of Damaged Function

In general, the goal of complete restoration of damaged function to premorbid levels, although clearly optimal, is probably unrealistic except in the mildest cases. Typically, this approach to rehabilitation is directed at relieving the underlying cognitive impairment, with an eye toward general mnemonic improvements. It has usually involved the stimulation or exercise of memory through extensive, repetitive practice, often with tasks or materials that have little ecological validity—digits, words, shapes, locations on computer screens and so forth—in the hope of restoring damaged cognitive and neural mechanisms.

There are several problems with this approach. First, it is a "one size fits all" approach. It is not theoretically driven, and there is no attempt to adapt training regimens to individual needs. Second, it assumes that improvements will generalize. They usually do not do so. The materials practiced within this approach often have little real-world relevance. All available evidence to date suggests that the effects of practice apply only to the materials practiced and do not generalize to other materials or contexts (Berg, Koning-Haanstra, & Deelman, 1991; Chase & Ericcson, 1981; Glisky, Schacter, & Tulving, 1986b; Godfrey & Knight, 1985). Third, the approach assumes that exercise or stimulation will induce changes at cognitive and neural levels, which should provide broad benefits to memory. Yet there is little evidence of positive outcome following drill therapies (Skilbeck & Robertson, 1992). Furthermore, even though recent evidence suggests greater plasticity in the adult human brain than was previously anticipated and the possibility of neurogenesis in brain regions that are important for memory (Eriksson et al., 1998; Kolb, 1995), the functional consequences of such plasticity and regeneration remain undetermined (Stein, 2000). Nevertheless, these findings provide some encouragement for continued research into new ways to encourage reorganization or regeneration of neural structures that might ultimately lead to restoration or improvement of function (Ogden, 2000).

Optimization of Residual Function

The goal of this approach is to find ways to optimize the use of damaged memory processes. Optimization of residual function assumes that normal memory processing mechanisms continue to exist but are reduced in efficiency and can be retrained or encouraged to function at an optimal level through intervention. The focus is on enhancing the use of specific memory processes or skills that were available premorbidly. This approach differs from the restoration model in that its goals are more specific and it is theoretically driven, but the approach is similar in that it continues to encourage people to perform memory tasks as they did prior to brain injury. It thus depends on, and is limited by, available models of normal memory. Most interventions within this framework have been concerned with training people how to use mnemonic strategies or other techniques that have proven useful for people without disabilities (Wilson, 1987).

Because this approach relies on the use of residual function, it is most appropriate for people with mild or moderate memory impairments, including those individuals who show modest declines in memory as a result of normal aging. Optimization of residual function is subject to the same criticism we mentioned earlier, however: The learning tends not to generalize across materials or contexts. Thus, although people can be trained to use encoding or retrieval strategies effectively, they tend not to use them beyond the materials or conditions of their training (Doornhein & De Haan, 1998; Wilson, 1991b). The teaching of strategies will therefore be most effective if applied to situations of importance in an individual's everyday life, such as learning people's names (Thoene & Glisky, 1995). It has been suggested that "generalization" training should itself be part of treatment programs (e.g., Sohlberg & Raskin, 1996; Wilson, 1995), but how to administer such training effectively has yet to be determined. Evidence to date still suggests that the benefits of training are confined to the training contexts.

Compensation for Lost Function

When brain damage is extensive and memory impairments are severe, rehabilitation often focuses on finding ways to help people bypass or compensate for their deficits. Typically, external supports or environmental adaptations are provided to enable people to carry out tasks important in their daily lives and thereby reduce the disabling effects of memory loss. Interventions are thus at the level of behavior; no attempt is made to affect underlying cognitive or neural processes.

The strength of this approach is its broad applicability and success in enabling people to achieve some independence in their everyday lives. Although external supports may be the only appropriate remedial tool for severely impaired individuals, they are often also recommended for people with milder memory problems and may be used in combination with some of the more cognitively demanding strategies. One caveat, however, is that many external aids—notebooks and electronic devices, for example—require extensive training before they can be used effectively.

Substitution of Intact Function

This approach (see Rothi & Horner, 1983), like the compensation for lost function approach, assumes that the cognitive and neural mechanisms required for normal memory function cannot be restored or used effectively but that other intact processes or structures not normally used for this purpose, may be recruited to serve as substitutes. Unlike the optimization of residual function model, which attempts to solve memory problems by improving the efficiency of normal memory mechanisms, this approach searches for new, alternative ways to perform memory tasks. This idea, originally suggested by Luria (1963), has been bolstered by findings that reveal plasticity in the adult human brain and by functional neuroimaging studies that have suggested the brain may compensate for losses or damage in one area by using other regions not previously or normally involved in the behavior (Buckner, Corbetta, Schatz, Raichle, & Petersen, 1996; Grady et al., 1994).

The focus of this approach has usually been on achieving specific functional outcomes, such as learning pieces of information relevant in everyday life; no generalization has been assumed or expected. Furthermore, although there is an underlying assumption with this approach that change can occur at both cognitive and neural levels, the mechanism of such change is still unknown. Because this approach attempts to tap into intact functions, it is particularly dependent on an understanding of normal memory. It also depends on careful assessment of the memory problem in order to identify which memory processes are compromised and which are spared.

ASSESSMENT

All of the approaches to memory rehabilitation can be facilitated by careful assessment of the memory deficit. At the very least, some form of assessment is needed to characterize the presence of a memory problem before treatment and to evaluate the success of the intervention after treatment. Because there are as yet no rehabilitation techniques guaranteed to be successful, it is essential that treatment outcomes be evaluated. In the acute or postacute stages of recovery, accurate assessment of treatment effects is problematic, because it is complicated by changes attributable to spontaneous recovery. For this reason, it has been extremely difficult to assess the effects of early intervention. The problem is less severe in the chronic stage, but in all cases, evaluation of the outcome of an intervention should include comparison not only to pretreatment measures but also to a control group of patients who do not receive treatment or who receive a different treatment (for a summary of assessment approaches, see Table 7.2).

The primary purpose of assessment, however, is the evaluation of the current status of the patient (neuropsychologically, behaviorally, and neuroanatomically), so that an appropriate treatment plan can be formulated. The nature of the memory problem, the cognitive strengths of the individual, the brain regions that are compromised or spared, and the person's needs in everyday life must all be considered when we try to determine reasonable treatment goals for each patient.

Neuropsychological Assessment

Neuropsychological assessment usually involves the use of standardized test instruments that allow a comparison of a patient's performance to normative data obtained from a sample of healthy individuals. Such testing is important because it provides objective measures of not only a patient's cognitive impairments but also his or her cognitive strengths, which may impact treatment planning. Objective measures are also critical for the evaluation of outcomes in order to ensure that expectations

TABLE 7.2. Summary of Assessment Approaches

Assessment approach	Strengths	Limitations
Neuropsychological—uses standardized tests to compare patient data to normative data from a sample of healthy individuals	Provides objective, quantitative measures of spared and impaired memory processes, both of which are important in treatment planning	Limited to the measures and norms available, which may lack face validity and sometimes do not predict functional capabilities or competence in everyday life
Behavioral—uses primarily interview and observational techniques to evaluate functional and everyday abilities	Can be individualized to assess patient concerns and practical problems; more predictive of real-life competencies	Self-report measures have questionable validity given the unawareness of deficit that may occur in individuals with memory impairment
Neuroanatomical—measures structural and functional abnormalities in the brain using neuroimaging techniques	Provides information about extent and location of brain damage; may be helpful in assessing recovery or reorganization of brain function	All damage is not visible on scans; lesion location is only suggestive of ensuing memory deficits; MRI cannot be used for patients with metal aneurysm clips or pacemakers

and other kinds of demand characteristics inherent in interventions do not introduce subjective biases into treatment evaluation (for a detailed discussion, see Lezak, 2000).

Both the optimization and substitution approaches are particularly dependent on neuropsychological assessment for the design of individual rehabilitation programs. The optimization model targets impaired processes for intervention and so may benefit from a careful analysis of test scores to determine as precisely as possible the underlying causes of memory impairment. The substitution approach looks additionally to intact processes to consider whether and how they might be used to substitute for damaged functions. So, for example, poor memory performance could be a function of poor executive control or attentional problems, of inadequate encoding or retrieval strategies, or of an inability to retain information in storage. Problems might affect all domains or be domain- or material-specific, and may affect some types of memory to a greater extent than others. From an optimization perspective, rehabilitation would focus on one or more of the problem areas (e.g., encoding) as a way to improve memory function. From a substitution perspective, treatment may focus on using spared functions (e.g., implicit memory) to accomplish tasks compromised by damaged functions (e.g., explicit memory).

ASSESSMENT INSTRUMENTS

The neuropsychological assessment should attempt to establish which aspects of memory are compromised and which are spared, and whether memory function is complicated by problems in other domains, such as in the areas of attention and executive function (see Lezak, 1995, for detailed description of assessment tools). The most comprehensive single battery of memory tests is the Wechsler Memory Scale—III (WMS-III; Wechsler, 1997b), which provides measures of a range of memory functions, including auditory and visual memory, recall and recognition, and working memory. Several tests are administered immediately and after a 30-minute delay, thus providing information about both encoding and storage. Special problems with retrieval can also be assessed through comparisons of recall and recognition. Various indexes of memory can be calculated, each having a mean of 100 and a standard deviation of 15, so that direct comparisons across the various measures can be made as well as to the Wechsler Adult Intelligence Scale—III (WAIS-III; Wechsler, 1997a) to determine whether memory deficits are disproportionate to any intellectual impairments.

Another test that provides multiple measures of learning and memory and is, for the most part, nonredundant with the WMS-III is the California Verbal Learning Test (CVLT; Delis, Kramer, Kaplan, & Ober, 1987). This categorized list-learning test is administered across multiple trials, thus providing a measure of learning as well as memory. In addition, the categorical structure of the list allows an assessment of strategy use in the form of semantic clustering, and the inclusion of a second list provides measures of proactive and retroactive interference.

A test that may provide additional qualitative information about memory functioning is the Buschke Selective Reminding Test (Buschke & Fuld, 1974). This test also involves word-list learning across trials, with reminders provided only for those words not recalled on the previous trial. This procedure can be administered more quickly than the CVLT and may be useful for differentiating storage from retrieval problems, although the assumptions underlying this analysis have been criticized on theoretical grounds (e.g., Feher & Martin, 1992). A variety of other abbreviated tests of list learning may be particularly appropriate for patients with very severe impairments or if time constraints are an issue. These include the Consortium to Establish a Registry for Alzheimer's Disease (CERAD) 10-word list (Morris et al., 1989), the list from the Repeatable Battery for the Assessment of Neuropsychological Status (RBANS; Randolph, 1998), and the list from the Kaplan Baycrest Neurocognitive Assessment (KBNA; Leach, Kaplan, Rewilak, Richards, & Proulx, 2000).

Fewer tests of visual memory are available other than those in the WMS-III. Nevertheless, it is important to obtain such measures in order to determine whether a memory deficit is global or confined to a particular category of materials. The Benton Visual Retention Test (Benton, 1974) and the Rey–Osterrieth Complex Figure Test (Osterrieth, 1944) examine memory for shapes and geometric designs, and the latter also provides information about planning and visual strategies. The Brief Visuospatial Memory Test—Revised (Benedict, 1997) evaluates memory for both visual designs and their spatial locations. It has six equivalent forms and includes measures of immediate and delayed recall, rate of acquisition (across three trials), and recognition. The Recognition Memory Test (Warrington, 1984) allows a comparison between recognition of words and faces, and the Three Words–Three Shapes Test (Mesulam, 1985; Weintraub et al., 2000) measures both verbal and nonverbal memory in the visual modality. This test, which is relatively short and easy to administer, includes a measure of incidental recall not available in most tests and may provide a closer simulation of a real-world memory activity. Finally, a relatively new test called Doors and People (Baddeley, Emslie, & Nimmo-Smith, 1994), which has high face validity and uses realistic materials, provides measures of immediate and delayed recall, and easy and difficult recognition in both verbal and visual domains.

As noted earlier, because of the potential impact of other cognitive functions on memory, particularly attention and executive control, and their importance in the design and success of intervention strategies, tests measuring these functions should also be included in any neuropsychological assessment (see Manly, Ward, & Robertson, Chapter 6, and Cicerone, Chapter 11, this volume).

Behavioral Assessment

Because neuropsychological assessment occurs under a variety of constraints and in somewhat artificial settings, it has been argued (Wilson, 1996a) that its results may not apply in any straightforward way to everyday life. So, for example, it is not obvious how failure to recall a list of words or to count backwards by 3's impacts the ability of an individual to function in the real world. Conversely, successful performance on neuropsychological tests may not translate into appropriate or functional behavior in everyday life. The goal of behavioral assessment, then, is to evaluate more directly how an individual may function in a natural environment. Behavioral assessment is thus concerned with the practical consequences of memory impairment rather than with the memory impairment itself. These evaluations may involve standardized tests but more commonly include less formal means such as interview and observational techniques, and self-report inventories (Knight & Godfrey, 1995).

Behavioral assessment is essential for the compensation approach, which focuses directly on achieving functional outcomes in everyday life. Although some external supports (e.g., a notebook) may be useful in a general way for everyone, no matter what their circumstances, others may need to be tailored to individual needs of daily life. The other approaches to rehabilitation can also benefit from a behavioral analysis. Because of the problems of generalization, it makes sense to ensure that rehabilitation activities are useful in and of themselves. So, for example, if one is going to practice remembering either through repetition or through the use of a mnemonic strategy, using relevant materials (e.g., the names of people in the social environment) will ensure some benefits even if training does not generalize.

ASSESSMENT INSTRUMENTS

The best-known standardized test of everyday memory is the Rivermead Behavioural Memory Test (RBMT; Wilson, Cockburn, & Baddeley, 1985). This test consists of 12 subtests, each measuring a practical aspect of memory, and includes remembering a name, the location of a hidden belonging, an appointment, a picture, a newspaper article, a face, a new route, a message, and items of orientation. A unique feature of this battery is the inclusion of tests tapping prospective memory (the ability to remember to perform actions in the future), something that is frequently required in daily life. The test is useful for identifying the kinds of everyday memory problems that might be experienced by patients with brain injury and has been found to be predictive of independent living and return to work or school (Wilson, 1991a).

In addition to the standardized tests, direct observation of patients' behavior as well as clinical interviews, questionnaires, and self-report measures can yield additional qualitative information about the kinds of problems experienced by patients in everyday life (for reviews, see Garcia, Garcia, Guerrero, Triguero, & Puente, 1998; Knight & Godfrey, 1995; Larrabee & Crook, 1996). One needs to interpret questionnaires with caution, however, because of their lack of correlation with objective tests of memory and their questionable validity, particularly in the case of self-report measures (Sunderland, Harris, & Baddeley, 1983; 1984). Because many patients with memory impairment are unaware of their deficits, their reports of everyday memory failures may be gross underestimates and often do not correlate highly with reports from caregivers. Such a lack of correlation, in fact, is often used as a measure of lack of insight into one's memory problems, a condition that may reduce motivation to participate in treatment programs (Schacter, Glisky, & McGlynn, 1990). Behavioral assessments when used judiciously, however, provide an important complement to the more objective neuropsychological assessments, supplying key information about everyday problems that should be taken into account when interventions are implemented.

Neuroanatomical Assessment

In most testing situations today, the neuropsychologist will have access to brain image analyses that can document both structural damage to the brain (computed tomography [CT] or magnetic resonance imaging [MRI]) and functional abnormalities (single-photon emission computed tomography [SPECT] or functional MRI [fMRI]). This neuroanatomical evidence can be used in conjunction with assessments to assist in the interpretation of a neuropsychological profile, to help direct or shape a remedial strategy, and to document brain-level changes that may occur as a result of an intervention. The trend recently has been toward customizing rehabilitation procedures for individual patients. Because of the variety of ways that memory may be compromised, and the variety of brain regions that might be implicated, combining neuropsychological and neuroanatomical assessment information will increase the likelihood of selecting and developing techniques that meet the needs of any individual patient.

METHODS OF REHABILITATION

A number of methods of memory rehabilitation for patients with brain damage have been tried with varying degrees of success. For the most part, these methods have not been adapted for individual use but generally have been used rather indiscriminately for patients with memory impairment. The approach to rehabilitation has been an important determinant of the kind of methods used, but within each broad category of methods, there are still numerous techniques that may be selected. Given the available assessment instruments, it should now be possible to make more informed selections of remedial methods and to tailor them more closely to the individual needs of the patients. Doing so should improve the likelihood of positive outcomes. To date, the interventions directed toward specific behavioral goals have been most successful, whereas those focused on broader achievements (i.e., improvement of memory ability in general) have had limited success. Several methods are outlined here. These are not mutually exclusive and may in fact be most effective when used in some combination (for summary of rehabilitation methods, see Table 7.3).

Practice and Rehearsal Techniques

The old adage, "Practice makes perfect," is still relevant for memory rehabilitation, but it has to be considered with appropriate caveats. There is little doubt that individuals with memory impairment require considerably more study or practice to acquire new knowledge than normal individuals, and that given such practice, almost all are able to learn at least some new information. What seems equally clear, however, is that practice does not provide general memory benefits. In other words, specific information can be acquired, but general memory ability is not restored or improved. It is therefore important that the information practiced be something relevant or useful in an individual's everyday life. There appears to be no general benefit associated with repeated practice of meaningless material (Glisky & Schacter, 1989b).

Simple repetitive practice or rote rehearsal has also long been known to be an ineffective way to ensure retention of information over the long term (Craik & Watkins, 1983). Making information meaningful through other means, for example, by relating it to information al-

TABLE 7.3. Summary of Rehabilitation Methods

Rehabilitation method	Specific techniques	Application
Practice and rehearsal	Meaningful or elaborative rehearsal, distributed practice, overlearning, spaced retrieval	Appropriate for all patients with memory impairment to assist them in learning specific pieces of information
Mnemonic strategies	Visual imagery, verbal organization, and association strategies, including story mnemonics, first-letter cueing, chaining, and PQRST	Appropriate only for those with mild or moderate deficits; helpful for learning arbitrary associations, sequences of actions, and text
Environmental supports and external aids	Labels, instructions, signage, notebooks, diaries, calendars, alarm watches, timers, electronic organizers, pagers	Appropriate for all individuals with memory impairment to assist them in independent living and in prospective memory
Domain-specific learning	Vanishing cues, errorless learning	Appropriate for patients with the most severe impairments; suited particularly to the learning of skills or tasks that can be performed implicitly

ready in the knowledge system and then practicing those meaningful relations, is more likely to be successful. Distributing several short periods of practice over time also generally leads to faster learning than long sessions of massed practice (Payne & Wenger, 1992), and overlearning (i.e., continued practice beyond the point of initial learning) appears to enhance retention even further (Butters, Glisky, & Schacter, 1993).

A distributed practice technique that has been found to be effective for even very severely impaired patients is known as *spaced retrieval* (Landauer & Bjork, 1978). This method requires people to retrieve and rehearse to-be-learned information at gradually increasing time intervals. The technique usually involves providing a piece of relevant information to a patient and then querying him or her about that information. For example, the patient might be told that she is currently in the University Rehabilitation Center. She would then immediately be asked, "Where are you?" If the patient is able to respond correctly, then a short interval of time is allowed to pass—1 minute perhaps—and then she is again asked, "Where are you?" Each time she provides a correct response, the retention interval is expanded (e.g., 1 minute, 2 minutes, 4 minutes, 8 minutes, etc.). Using this technique, researchers have successfully taught patients with memory impairment, including those with Alzheimer's disease, various kinds of information, including name–face associations, locations of objects, and items of orientation (Camp, 1989; Moffat, 1992; Schacter, Rich, & Stampp, 1985). Camp and McKitrick (1992) have speculated that spaced retrieval may rely on automatic or implicit memory processes that are often preserved in people with memory disorders.

Mnemonic Strategies

The teaching of mnemonic strategies, one of the most commonly used methods of memory rehabilitation, is based on a substantial literature documenting their efficacy in normal individuals. Nevertheless, these techniques have met with only limited success when used with neurological populations. Consistent with the idea that these strategies depend on the use of residual function, training seems to benefit only patients with mild to moderate memory disorders (Wilson, 1987). People with more extensive brain damage and severe memory loss seem unable to learn the strategies or to apply them effectively. Even those persons who can learn the techniques tend not to use them spontaneously outside of the training context, so real-world benefits have been minimal (Cermak, 1975; Wilson, 1981), although there are some exceptions (e.g., Berg et al., 1991; Wilson, 1991a). Most studies have reported that the transfer effects are quite specific, however, confined to very similar tasks and materials within the laboratory (Doornhein & De Haan, 1998). Although the use of strategies often does not seem to generalize to new materials or contexts, strategies can nevertheless be used very effectively with mildly to moderately impaired patients to help them acquire new information that might be applicable in their everyday lives.

The choice of mnemonic strategy should be based on information gained from the assessment and should be directed toward particular problems identified in everyday life by the patient. If a memory deficit is confined to the verbal domain and associated with selective damage to the left hemisphere, visual strategies are likely to be most effective. Conversely, if brain damage is on the right, affecting memory for visual information, verbal strategies are a good choice. In a general sense, most mnemonic strategies are designed to provide a meaningful way to encode information, so that it is associated either with information already in the knowledge system or with a set of cues that can be learned and regenerated at retrieval.

Strategies are particularly appropriate for patients who fail to initiate any such plans on their own, even though they are capable of making use of them when instructed. For example, a patient who does poorly in free recall on the CVLT, failing to take advantage of the categorical structure of the word list and thereby obtaining a low semantic clustering score, is likely a good candidate for strategy training. Providing such patients with a suitable strategy and training them in its application to a particular set of materials may help speed acquisition of new information. It should also benefit later access to the information to the extent that the patient is taught to regenerate encoding cues at retrieval.

There are numerous mnemonic strategies from which to choose (for reviews, see Butters, Soety, & Glisky, 1998; Glisky & Schacter, 1989b; Harris, 1992; Wilson, 1987). The few highlighted here are selected because of their application to problems in everyday life. The classic mnemonics such as the "pegword" and the "method of loci" techniques have limited application and are useful mainly for remembering unrelated lists of words—for example, shopping lists. However, constructing written lists would seem to be a more practical solution to this problem.

Visual imagery is a technique that can be used in a variety of ways to help form associations between unrelated words or objects. Its most important use in rehabilitation has been in helping patients to learn people's names—a common problem among many persons with memory disorders. Although some of these procedures require a complex series of steps and are much too difficult for most patients, simple imaging techniques, such as visualizing a face when reading a name (Glasgow, Zeiss, Barrra, & Lewinsohn, 1977), translating a name into an image (Wilson, 1982, 1987), and visualizing the face interacting with an image of the name (Thoene & Glisky, 1995), have all had some degree of success. These techniques may help to instill meaning into the arbitrary relation between a name and a face. Recently Downes and his colleagues (1997; Kalla, Downes, & van den Broek, 2001) have demonstrated increased effectiveness of imagery for the learning of face–name associations by preexposing the face and requiring patients to judge its qualities. Such a procedure may increase the familiarity and/or the meaningfulness of the face, thereby enhancing memory. Strategies that have focused on making names more meaningful (e.g., think of an object with the same name, or someone else you know with a similar name) have also proved beneficial (Milders, Deelman, & Berg, 1998). When using imagery for face–name associations, patients may need help generating the images, and some do better with actual drawings. Also, because most patients do not use the techniques spontaneously, they will require the assistance of a family member or caregiver if the strategies are to be maintained and remain useful in everyday life.

Another class of strategies focuses on principles of *organization and association*. The idea here is to organize information into natural groupings—categories, for example—that can facilitate learning and also provide cues for subsequent retrieval. Alternatively, one might devise ways to associate new, unrelated pieces of information to each other or to information already in the knowledge system. Some of these techniques (e.g., story mnemonics, first-letter cueing) have proven effective for learning unrelated lists of words, but their relevance to real-world problems once again seems limited. Two methods, however, appear to have applications in important domains of everyday life. A technique referred to as *chaining* may be particularly useful for teaching sequences of operations or actions such as those involved in many activities of daily living. In this method, complex sequences are broken down into simple steps or components and learned one at a time. As each step in the sequence is acquired, it is linked or associated in a meaningful way to the next component; those two components are practiced together until they are learned and are then linked to the next step, and so on. Long sequences of actions have been learned in this way by even quite severely impaired patients. For example, we trained a patient to learn the multiple steps of a complex data entry job using such a procedure (Glisky & Schacter, 1989a). Wilson (1996b) has used the method successfully to teach patients how to transfer from their wheelchairs to regular chairs. The method might also be appropriate for learning the various steps in traversing a route from one place to another, or for any other activity that can readily be broken down into a series of simple components.

A verbal organizational strategy that has been used effectively with mildly impaired patients for the learning of textual information (e.g., school materials, newspaper articles) is the *PQRST* method (Robinson, 1970). PQRST stands for "Preview" (i.e., get a quick overview of the reading), "Question" (i.e., formulate questions about the text), "Read" the material, "State" the answers to the questions, and "Test" for retention of the information. As with the other methods of this type, benefits are likely achieved because of the meaningful organizational structure imposed on the passages during encoding and the corresponding availability of that structure to provide cues for retrieval. The method has been used successfully with college students (Glasgow et al., 1977) and others (Wilson, 1987), although there is no evidence of maintenance of the strategy beyond training.

Although all of the mnemonic techniques are considered encoding strategies, which require people to think about and organize information in a meaningful way during input, the same organizational structures can be used to facilitate retrieval. So, for example, in the case of PQRST, regenerating the general topic of a reading and thinking back to the questions that were formulated at encoding should provide cues to facilitate retrieval of the complete text. Producing the initial word or step of a learned sequence should enable the patient to recover the entire sequence, and re-creating the original visual images associated with a face should serve to cue the name. Teaching of mnemonic strategies should therefore include instruction in the use of the same organizational techniques at retrieval that were used at encoding.

External Aids and Environmental Supports

External memory aids take a variety of forms, serve a variety of functions, and can be useful for people with a range of memory difficulties (for reviews, see Glisky, 1995b; Harris, 1992; Kapur, 1995). The choice of a compensatory device should be based on information gained from the assessments. At their simplest, they require little active participation by patients and so are useful for even the most severely impaired individuals. Environmental restructurings, including labels on cupboards, instructions on appliances, signage or other kinds of clear indicators of locations (e.g., lines on floors indicating routes), provide visible cues to help people function in their personal environments without the need for effortful memory or other control processes. Other useful aids, such as notebooks, diaries, calendars, alarm watches and timers, which may be used as reminders for future actions (i.e., prospective memory), require more active participation by the user and may require extensive training. So, for example, if a memory notebook is to be used effectively, considerable practice and role playing in both laboratory and real-world situations are usually necessary (Sohlberg & Mateer, 1989).

Recently a number of hand-held electronic memory aids or organizers, which enable people to keep track of appointments and other aspects of daily life, have become available on the market. These devices can sound an alarm as a reminder of an appointment and display a message showing the details of the activity. They also may be able to store telephone numbers and "things-to-do lists," and are potentially more effective than notebooks and alarm watches, because they provide both the signaling function of the alarm and the kinds of specific information kept in a book. These devices also tend to be highly acceptable to brain-injured patients, who are sometimes embarrassed to use aids such as notebooks. Relatively little research has been conducted in the use of these electronic aids with patient populations, however, and preliminary tests suggest that they may be useful only for mildly impaired patients; patients with severe disorders have considerable difficulty learning how to use them (Kapur, 1995; Wilson, Baddeley, & Cockburn, 1989). Some of the new learning methodologies, such as vanishing cues and errorless learning (described later in this chapter), however, may be adapted to train patients in the use of electronic aids (Wilson, Baddeley, Evans, & Shiel, 1994).

Some electronic devices, however, can be used with relatively little training provided that a caregiver or family member is available to enter the necessary information into the unit (e.g., Kim, Burke, Dowds, & George, 1999). One such device is a paging system called NeuroPage (Hersh & Treadgold, 1994), which delivers prompts and messages about daily activities through a simple pager with a small display screen. Desired information is provided to a paging company, which programs the material and delivers it via the pager at the appropriate time. Barbara Wilson and her colleagues (Wilson, Emslie, Quirk, & Evans, 1999; Wilson, Evans, Emslie, & Malinek, 1997) have tested this system and have found it effective even for patients with quite severe disorders. It requires little memory to operate and allows some patients to learn a set of routine behaviors that they can follow even after the pager is removed. Others continue to need the pager to sustain performance but are nevertheless able to carry out many daily functions that had previously been impossible. Similar findings have been obtained with an even simpler electronic device, a Voice Organizer, which has the added advantage of being inexpensive and not requiring an external agency for service (Van den Broek, Downes, Johnson, Dayus, & Hilton, 2000). The major strength of these systems is that they can be programmed to meet the precise needs of each individual patient.

Domain-Specific Learning

Recently, considerable research has been directed toward the development of learning techniques to facilitate the acquisition of new knowledge and skills by tapping into memory and learning abilities that might be preserved even in the most severely impaired patients. This approach received its initial impetus from empirical findings demonstrating that, although amnesic patients were unable to acquire new memories that could be explicitly retrieved, they were nevertheless able to retain some record of prior experience that could be expressed implicitly in their behavior (for review, see Schacter, Chiu, & Ochsner, 1993). In fact, in numerous tests of what has now been called "implicit memory," amnesic patients were found to perform within or close to normal limits. They also showed preserved procedural memory, reflected in their ability to acquire a variety of motor, perceptual, and cognitive skills in a normal fashion (for review, see Cohen & Eichenbaum, 1993).

In an effort to capitalize on these preserved memory abilities to teach patients new information, Glisky, Schacter, and Tulving (1986b) devised a faded cueing technique, *the method of vanishing cues*, designed to take advantage of patients' relatively intact implicit memory, particularly their ability to respond to partial cues. This method initially provides as much cue information as needed for correct responding and then gradually withdraws it across learning trials. Using this technique, we have been able to teach patients with memory impairment large amounts of domain-specific information relevant to their everyday lives, including computer operations (Glisky, Schacter, & Tulving, 1986a), word processing (Glisky, 1995a) and vocational tasks such as computer data entry (Glisky & Schacter, 1987; Glisky & Schacter, 1989a). Such implicit learning occurs even though patients may be unable to recollect the learning experience or to express explicitly exactly what it is that they have learned. Some examples of learning by patients with memory impairment are shown in Figure 7.1. The top half of the figure illustrates the learning of 15 computer vocabulary words by 2 patients (Glisky et al., 1986b), and the bottom half illustrates the learning of 61 word-processing responses by another severely impaired amnesic patient (Glisky, 1995a). In all cases, the number of cues needed for correct responding decreased rapidly over the first few sessions and then more gradually, until the patient was able to produce most of the information without cues.

Baddeley and Wilson (1994) suggested that part of the success of the vanishing cues method may be attributable to the fact that the cues constrain responses and thus prevent errors. In a series of studies, Wilson and colleagues have demonstrated that, compared to learning by trial and error, *errorless learning* provides benefits to a range of patients with memory impairment, including those in the early stages of Alzheimer's disease (Clare, Wilson, Breen, & Hodges, 1999). The errorless learning method has been used successfully to teach names (Kalla et al., 2001; Wilson et al., 1994), the use of an electronic memory aid, items of orientation and general knowledge (Wilson et al., 1994), the use of a memory notebook (Squires, Hunkin, & Parkin, 1996) and word-processing skills (Hunkin, Squires, Aldrich, & Parkin, 1998). Recently, it has been suggested that a combination of errorless learning and vanishing cues may provide optimal learning, although the characteristics of the individual learner also have to be considered (Komatsu, Mimura, Kato, Wakamatsu, & Kashima, 2000; Riley & Heaton, 2000). There is some evidence suggesting that the errorless learning and vanishing cues methods may be most beneficial for patients with the most severe impairments, perhaps because these patients must rely on preserved implicit memory, and may be appropriate only for tasks that can be accomplished implicitly (Evans et al., 2000; Thoene & Glisky, 1995). Further research is needed to explore in greater detail the exact limits of these learning techniques.

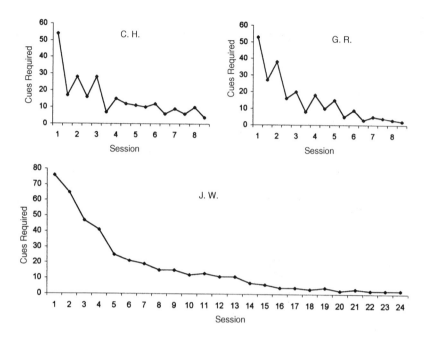

FIGURE 7.1. Number of letter cues required across sessions by 2 patients learning computer vocabulary (top) and 1 patient learning word processing (bottom). Figures adapted from Glisky, Schacter, and Tulving (1986b) and Glisky (1995a). Copyright 1986 by Swets & Zeitlinger Publishers (top portion of figure), and copyright 1995 by Lawrence Erlbaum Associates Ltd. (bottom portion of figure). Adapted by permission.

CONCLUSIONS AND FUTURE DIRECTIONS

Over the past 10 to 15 years, the focus of clinical neuropsychology has broadened considerably to encompass information that is not only important for descriptive and diagnostic purposes but also critical for treatment planning. Standard neuropsychological assessments now need to be supplemented with behavioral assessments and reinterpreted in light of the functional needs of patients and their caregivers. Although traditionally trained in assessment, neuropsychologists will increasingly be called upon to develop rehabilitation strategies, to implement them, and to evaluate their outcomes. This chapter has attempted to provide a foundation upon which such interventions may be based.

Rehabilitation in the future will be better informed. Not only is there a greater armamentarium of assessment instruments from which to characterize impairments and disabilities but there is also a growing empirical and theoretical knowledge base about normal memory that will help to focus interventions on the specific, affected memory processes. Neuroimaging techniques will provide more specific information about the neural underpinnings of memory and perhaps provide clues concerning what parts of the brain might be recruited to compensate for damaged memory structures and functions. There are also exciting new developments with respect to recovery of function and neurogenesis, as well as research into pharmacological agents and neural transplants that may one day significantly impact treatment. Neuropsychologists will need to be able to integrate information from all these sources in order to ensure the best possible therapies for their patients.

In memory rehabilitation, in the past, there has been a tendency to search for treatments that would be effective for all patients. It seems clear now, however, that the efficacy of any treatment will depend on multiple factors—the nature of the memory impairment, the severity of the problem, the extent to which other cognitive functions are implicated, the brain regions affected, and the spared cognitive and neural processes. One can easily imagine as many treatments as there are patients. Nevertheless, there must be commonalities across patients as well as differences, and it will be important to document those also. Although technological advances make customization of rehabilitation programs more attainable than in the past, the development of treatments that serve groups of patients will nevertheless be more practical and cost-effective. So, for example, one might imagine a treatment that would be appropriate for patients with frontally based retrieval problems but not suitable for patients with hippocampally based storage deficits, and vice versa. Designing two different interventions for these two broad categories of patients with memory impairment should prove more effective.

Memory rehabilitation continues to be experimental. As we have illustrated in this chapter, there is not a set of remedial techniques guaranteed to be successful with every patient. There is, however, a growing body of empirical research and theoretical principles to guide the development of further interventions. This research should take place not only in the laboratory but also in the clinic and the real world, because it is there that patients' needs are most clearly expressed and interventions have their most visible impact.

ACKNOWLEDGMENT

Preparation of this chapter was supported by Grant No. AG14792 from the National Institute on Aging.

REFERENCES

Baddeley, A., Emslie, H., & Nimmo-Smith, I. (1994). *The Doors and People Test.* Bury St. Edmonds, UK: Thames Valley Test Company.

Baddeley, A. D., & Wilson, B. A. (1994). When implicit learning fails: Amnesia and the problem of error elimination. *Neuropsychologia, 32,* 53–68.

Benedict, R. H. B. (1997). *Brief Visuospatial Memory Test—Revised.* Lutz, FL: Psychological Assessment Resources.

Benton, A. L. (1974). *The Revised Visual Retention Test.* New York: Psychological Corporation.

Berg, I. J., Koning-Haanstra, M., & Deelman, B. G. (1991). Long-term effects of memory rehabilitation. *Neuropsychological Rehabilitation, 1,* 97–111.

Buckner, R. L., Corbetta, M., Schatz, J., Raichle, M. E., & Petersen, S. E. (1996). Preserved speech abilities and compensation following prefrontal damage. *Proceedings of the National Academy of Sciences USA, 93,* 1249–1253.

Buschke, H., & Fuld, P. A. (1974). Evaluation of storage, retention, and retrieval in disordered memory and learning. *Neurology, 11,* 1019–1025.

Butters, M. A., Glisky, E. L., & Schacter, D. L. (1993). Transfer of new learning in memory-impaired patients. *Journal of Clinical and Experimental Neuropsychology, 15,* 219–230.

Butters, M. A., Soety, E. M., & Glisky, E. L. (1998). Memory rehabilitation. In P. J. Snyder & P. D. Nussbaum (Eds.), *Clinical neuropsychology* (pp. 450–466). Washington, DC: American Psychological Association.

Camp, C. J. (1989). Facilitation of new learning in Alzheimer's disease. In G. C. Gilmore, P. J. Whitehouse, & M. L. Wykle (Eds.), *Memory, aging, and dementia* (pp. 212–225). New York: Springer.

Camp, C. J., & McKitrick, L. A. (1992). Memory interventions in Alzheimer's-type dementia populations: Methodological and theoretical issues. In R. L. West & J. D. Sinnott (Eds.), *Everyday memory and aging: Current research and methodology* (pp. 155–172). New York: Springer.

Caramazza, A., & Hillis, A. (1993). For a theory of remediation of cognitive deficits. *Neuropsychological Rehabilitation, 3,* 217–234.

Cermak, L. S. (1975). Imagery as an aid to retrieval for Korsakoff patients. *Cortex, 11,* 163–169.

Chase, W. G., & Ericcson, K. A. (1981). Skilled memory. In J. R. Anderson (Ed.), *Cognitive skills and their acquisition* (pp. 141–190). Hillsdale, NJ: Erlbaum.

Clare, L., Wilson, B. A., Breen, K., & Hodges, J. R. (1999). Errorless learning of face–name associations in early Alzheimer's disease. *Neurocase, 5,* 37–46.

Cohen, N. J., & Eichenbaum, H. (1993). *Memory, amnesia, and the hippocampal system.* Cambridge, MA: MIT Press.

Craik, F. I. M., & Watkins, M. J. (1983). The role of rehearsal in short-term memory. *Journal of Verbal Learning and Verbal Behavior, 12,* 599–607.

Delis, D. C., Kramer, J., Kaplan, E., & Ober, B. A. (1987). *The California Verbal Learning Test.* San Antonio, TX: Psychological Corporation.

Doornhein, K., & De Haan, E. H. F. (1998). Cognitive training for memory deficits in stroke patients. *Neuropsychological Rehabilitation, 8,* 393–400.

Downes, J. J., Kalla, T., Davies, A. D. M., Flynn, A., Ali, H., & Mayes, A. R. (1997). The pre-exposure technique: A novel method for enhancing the effects of imagery in face–name association learning. *Neuropsychological Rehabilitation, 7,* 195–214.

Eriksson, P. S., Perfilieva, E., Bjork-Eriksson, T., Alborn, A. M., Nordbord, C., Peterson, D. A., & Gage, F. H. (1998). Neurogenesis in the adult human hippocampus. *Nature Medicine, 4,* 1313–1317.

Evans, J. J., Wilson, B. A., Schuri, U., Andrade, J., Baddeley, A., Bruna, O., Canavan, T., Della Sala, S., Green, R., Laaksonen, R., Lorenzi, L., & Taussik, I. (2000). A comparison of "errorless" and "trial-and-error" learning methods for teaching individuals with acquired memory deficits. *Neuropsychological Rehabilitation, 10,* 67–101.

Feher, E. P., & Martin, R. C. (1992). Cognitive assessment of long-term memory disorders. In D. I. Margolin (Ed.), *Cognitive neuropsychology in clinical practice* (pp. 168–203). New York: Oxford University Press.

Garcia, M. P., Garcia, J. F. G., Guerrero, N. V., Triguero, J. A. L., & Puente, A. E. (1998). Neuropsychological evaluation of everyday memory. *Neuropsychology Review, 8,* 203–218.

Glasgow, R. E., Zeiss, R. A., Barrera, M., & Lewinsohn, P. M. (1977). Case studies on remediating memory deficits in brain-damaged individuals. *Journal of Clinical Psychology, 33,* 1049–1054.

Glisky, E. L. (1995a). Acquisition and transfer of word processing skill by an amnesic patient. *Neuropsychological Rehabilitation, 5,* 299–318.

Glisky, E. L. (1995b). Computers in memory rehabilitation. In A. D. Baddeley, B. A. Wilson, & F. N. Watts (Eds.), *Handbook of memory disorders* (pp. 557–575). Chichester: Wiley.

Glisky, E. L., & Schacter, D. L. (1987). Acquisition of domain-specific knowledge in organic amnesia: Training for computer-related work. *Neuropsychologia, 25,* 893–906.

Glisky, E. L., & Schacter, D. L. (1989a). Extending the limits of complex learning in organic amnesia: Computer training in a vocational domain. *Neuropsychologia, 27,* 107–120.

Glisky, E. L., & Schacter, D. L. (1989b). Models and methods of memory rehabilitation. In F. Boller & J. Grafman (Eds.), *Handbook of neuropsychology* (Vol. 3, pp. 233–246). Amsterdam: Elsevier.

Glisky, E. L., Schacter, D. L., & Tulving, E. (1986a). Computer learning by memory-impaired patients: Acquisition and retention of complex knowledge. *Neuropsychologia, 24,* 313–328.

Glisky, E. L., Schacter, D. L., & Tulving, E. (1986b). Learning and retention of computer related vocabulary in memory-impaired patients: Method of vanishing cues. *Journal of Clinical and Experimental Neuropsychology, 8,* 292–312.

Godfrey, H. P. D., & Knight, R. G. (1985). Cognitive rehabilitation of memory functioning in amnesiac alcoholics. *Journal of Consulting and Clinical Psychology, 53,* 555–557.

Grady, C. L., Maisog, J. M., Horwitz, B., Ungerleider, L. G., Mentis, M. J., Salerno, J. A., Pietrini, P., Wagner, E., & Haxby, J. V. (1994). Age-related changes in cortical blood flow activation during visual processing of faces and location. *Journal of Neuroscience, 14,* 1450–1462.

Harris, J. E. (1992). Ways to help memory. In B. A. Wilson & N. Moffat (Eds.), *Clinical management of memory problems* (2nd ed., pp. 59–85). London: Chapman & Hall.

Hersh, N., & Treadgold, L. (1994). NeuroPage: The rehabilitation of memory dysfunction by prosthetic memory and cueing. *NeuroRehabilitation, 4,* 187–197.

Hunkin, N. M., Squires, E. J., Aldrich, F. K., & Parkin, A. J. (1998). Errorless learning and the acquisition of word processing skills. *Neuropsychological Rehabilitation, 8,* 433–449.

Kalla, T., Downes, J. J., & van den Broek, M. (2001). The pre-exposure technique: Enhancing the effects of errorless learning in the acquisition of face–name associations. *Neuropsychological Rehabilitation, 11*, 1–16.

Kapur, N. (1995). Memory aids in the rehabilitation of memory disordered patients. In A. D. Baddeley, B. A. Wilson, & F. N. Watts (Eds.), *Handbook of memory disorders* (pp. 534–556). Chichester, UK: Wiley.

Kim, H. J., Burke, D. T., Dowds, M. M., & George, J. (1999). Utility of a microcomputer as an external memory aid for a memory-impaired head injury patient during in-patient rehabilitation. *Brain Injury, 13*, 147–150.

Knight, R. G., & Godfrey, H. P. D. (1995). Behavioural and self-report methods. In A. D. Baddeley, B. A. Wilson, & F. N. Watts (Eds.), *Handbook of memory disorders* (pp. 393–410). Chichester, UK: Wiley.

Kolb, B. (1995). *Brain plasticity and behavior*. Mahwah, NJ: Erlbaum.

Komatsu, S., Mimura, M., Kato, M., Wakamatsu, N., & Kashima, H. (2000). Errorless and effortful processes involved in learning of face–name associations by patients with alcoholic Korsakoff's syndrome. *Neuropsychological Rehabilitation, 10*, 113–132.

Landauer, T. K., & Bjork, R. A. (1978). Optimum rehearsal patterns and name learning. In M. M. Gruneberg, P. E. Morris, & R. N. Sykes (Eds.), *Practical aspects of memory* (pp. 625–632). London: Academic Press.

Larrabee, G. J., & Crook, T. H. (1996). The ecological validity of memory testing procedures: Developments in the assessment of everyday memory. In R. J. Sbordone & C. J. Long (Eds.), *Ecological validity of neuropsychological testing* (pp. 225–242). Delray Beach, FL: GR Press/St. Lucie Press.

Leach, L., Kaplan, E., Rewilak, D., Richards, B., & Proulx, G. B. (2000). *The Kaplan Baycrest Neurocognitive Assessment (KBNA)*. San Antonio, TX: Psychological Corporation.

Lezak, M. D. (1995). *Neuropsychological assessment* (3rd ed.). New York: Oxford University Press.

Lezak, M. D. (2000). Nature, applications, and limitations of neuropsychological assessment following traumatic brain injury. In A.-L. Christensen & B. P. Uzzell (Eds.), *International handbook of neuropsychological rehabilitation* (pp. 67–79). New York: Kluwer Academic/Plenum.

Luria, A. R. (1963). *Restoration of function after brain injury*. New York: Macmillan.

Mesulam, M.-M. (1985). *Principles of behavioral neurology*. Philadelphia: F. A. Davis.

Milders, M., Deelman, B., & Berg, I. (1998). Rehabilitation of memory for people's names. *Memory, 6*, 21–36.

Moffat, N. (1992). Strategies of memory therapy. In B. A. Wilson & N. Moffat (Eds.), *Clinical management of memory problems* (2nd ed., pp. 86–119). London: Chapman & Hall.

Morris, J. C., Heyman, A., Mohs, R. C., Hughes, J. P., van Belle, G., Fillenbaum, G., Mellits, E. D., & Clark, C. (1989). The Consortium to Establish a Registry for Alzheimer's Disease (CERAD): Part I. Clinical and neuropsychological assessment of Alzheimer's disease. *Neurology, 39*, 1159–1165.

Ogden, J. A. (2000). Neurorehabilitation in the third millenium: New roles for our environment, behaviors, and mind in brain damage and recovery? *Brain and Cognition, 42*, 110–112.

Osterrieth, P. A. (1944). Le test de copie d'une figure complexe. *Archives de Psychologie, 30*, 206–356.

Payne, D. G., & Wenger, M. J. (1992). Improving memory through practice. In D. J. Herrmann, H. Weingartner, A. Searleman, & C. L. McEvoy (Eds.), *Memory improvement: Implications for memory theory* (pp. 187–209). New York: Springer-Verlag.

Randolph, C. (1998). *Repeatable Battery for the Assessment of Neuropsychological Status.* San Antonio, TX: Psychological Corporation.

Riley, G. A., & Heaton, S. (2000). Guidelines for the selection of a method of fading cues. *Neuropsychological Rehabilitation, 10,* 133–149.

Robinson, F. B. (1970). *Effective study.* New York: Harper & Row.

Rothi, L. J., & Horner, J. (1983). Restitution and substitution: Two theories of recovery with application to neurobehavioral treatment. *Journal of Clinical Neuropsychology, 5,* 73–81.

Schacter, D. L., Chiu, C. Y. P., & Ochsner, K. N. (1993). Implicit memory: A selective review. *Annual Review of Neuroscience, 16,* 159–182.

Schacter, D. L., Glisky, E. L., & McGlynn, S. M. (1990). Impact of memory disorder on everyday life: Awareness of deficits and return to work. In D. Tupper & K. Cicerone (Eds.), *The neuropsychology of everyday life: Assessment and basic competencies* (pp. 231–257). Boston: Kluwer.

Schacter, D. L., Rich, S. A., & Stampp, M. S. (1985). Remediation of memory disorders: Experimental evaluation of the spaced-retrieval technique. *Journal of Clinical and Experimental Neuropsychology, 7,* 79–96.

Skilbeck, C., & Robertson, I. (1992). Computer assistance in the management of memory and cognitive impairment. In B. A. Wilson & N. Moffatt (Eds.), *Clinical management of memory problems* (2nd ed., pp. 154–188). London: Chapman & Hall.

Sohlberg, M. M., & Mateer, C. A. (1989). Training use of compensatory memory books: A three stage behavioral approach. *Journal of Clinical and Experimental Neuropsychology, 11,* 871–887.

Sohlberg, M. M., & Raskin, S. A. (1996). Principles of generalization applied to attention and memory interventions. *Journal of Head Trauma Rehabilitation, 11,* 65–78.

Squires, E. J., Hunkin, N. M., & Parkin, A. J. (1996). Memory notebook training in a case of severe amnesia: Generalising from paired associate learning to real life. *Neuropsychological Rehabilitation, 6,* 55–65.

Stein, D. G. (2000). Brain injury and theories of recovery. In A.-L. Christensen & B. P. Uzzell (Eds.), *International handbook of neuropsychological rehabilitation* (pp. 3–32). New York: Kluwer Academic/Plenum.

Sunderland, A., Harris, J., & Baddeley, A. D. (1983). Do laboratory tests predict everyday memory? A neuropsychological study. *Journal of Verbal Learning and Verbal Behavior, 22,* 341–357.

Sunderland, A., Harris, J. E., & Baddeley, A. D. (1984). Assessing everyday memory after severe head injury. In J. E. Harris & P. E. Morris (Eds.), *Everyday memory, actions and absent-mindedness* (pp. 191–206). London: Academic Press.

Thoene, A. I. T., & Glisky, E. L. (1995). Learning of name–face associations in memory impaired patients: A comparison of different training procedures. *Journal of the International Neuropsychological Society, 1,* 29–38.

Van den Broek, M. D., Downes, J., Johnson, A., Dayus, B., & Hilton, N. (2000). Evaluation of an electronic memory aid in the neuropsychological rehabilitation of prospective memory deficits. *Brain Injury, 14,* 455–462.

Warrington, E. K. (1984). *Recognition Memory Test.* Windsor, UK: NFER-Nelson.

Wechsler, D. (1997a). *Wechsler Adult Intelligence Scale—III*. San Antonio, TX: Psychological Corporation.

Wechsler, D. (1997b). *Wechsler Memory Scale—III*. San Antonio, TX: Psychological Corporation.

Weintraub, S., Peavy, G. M., O'Connor, M., Johnson, N. A., Acar, D., Sweeney, J., & Janssen, I. (2000). Three Words–Three Shapes: A clinical test of memory. *Journal of Clinical and Experimental Neuropsychology, 22*, 267–278.

Wilson, B. A. (1981). Teaching a patient to remember people's names after removal of a left temporal tumor. *Behavioral Psychotherapy, 9*, 338–344.

Wilson, B. (1982). Success and failure in memory training following a cerebral vascular accident. *Cortex, 18*, 581–594.

Wilson, B. (1987). *Rehabilitation of memory*. New York: Guilford Press.

Wilson, B. A. (1991a). Long-term prognosis of patients with severe memory disorders. *Neuropsychological Rehabilitation, 1*, 117–134.

Wilson, B. A. (1991b). Theory, assessment, and treatment in neuropsychological rehabilitation. *Neuropsychology, 5*, 281–291.

Wilson, B. A. (1995). Management and remediation of memory problems in brain-injured adults. In A. D. Baddeley, B. A. Wilson, & F. N. Watts (Eds.), *Handbook of memory disorders* (pp. 451–479). Chichester, UK: Wiley.

Wilson, B. A. (1996a). The ecological validity of neuropsychological assessment after severe brain injury. In R. J. Sbordone & C. J. Long (Eds.), *Ecological validity of neuropsychological testing* (pp. 413–428). Delray Beach, FL: GR/St. Lucie Press.

Wilson, B. A. (1996b). Memory therapy in practice. In B. A. Wilson & N. Moffat (Eds.), *Clinical management of memory problems* (pp. 117–153). London: Chapman & Hall.

Wilson, B. A., Baddeley, A. D., & Cockburn, J. M. (1989). How do old dogs learn new tricks?: Teaching a technological skill to brain injured people. *Cortex, 25*, 115–119.

Wilson, B. A., Baddeley, A. D., Evans, J., & Shiel, A. (1994). Errorless learning in the rehabilitation of memory impaired people. *Neuropsychological Rehabilitation, 4*, 307–326.

Wilson, B. A., Cockburn, J., & Baddeley, A. (1985). *The Rivermead Behavioural Memory Test*. Bury St. Edmunds, UK: Thames Valley Test Company.

Wilson, B. A., Emslie, H., Quirk, K., & Evans, J. (1999). George: Learning to live independently with NeuroPage. *Rehabilitation Psychology, 44*, 284–296.

Wilson, B. A., Evans, J. J., Emslie, H., & Malinek, V. (1997). Evaluation of NeuroPage: A new memory aid. *Journal of Neurology, Neurosurgery and Psychiatry, 63*, 113–115.

CHAPTER 8

Visuoperceptual Impairments

STEVEN W. ANDERSON

VISUOPERCEPTION FOLLOWING BRAIN DAMAGE

Visuoperceptual dysfunction, common in patients referred for neuropsychological rehabilitation, can have implications for patients' participation in treatment and eventual success in vocational endeavors and other aspects of daily living. Visuoperceptual defects can result from damage to any of several brain regions, including primary visual cortex (striate cortex or Brodmann area 17), extrastriate association cortex of the occipital lobes (areas 18 and 19), visual and polymodal association cortex of the parietal and temporal lobes (e.g., areas 37 and 39), the lateral geniculate nucleus, the frontal eye fields (in the lateral aspect of area 8), and white matter pathways, including the optic radiations. Vascular disease and head trauma are the most frequent causes of visuoperceptual disorders seen in rehabilitation settings, although similar impairments may be caused by several neurological diseases (e.g., neoplasms, multiple sclerosis, hypotensive episodes, and neurodegenerative conditions).

The most common sensory and perceptual impairments that result from damage to these brain areas include the following:

- Visual field defects
- Neglect
- Impaired perceptual discrimination (e.g., form, motion)
- Visual agnosia
- Prosopagnosia
- Visuospatial disorders (e.g., location, size, orientation)
- Achromatopsia

- Visual hallucinations
- Impairment of eye movements and scanning
- Impairment of visually guided hand movements

Of these impairments, only spatial neglect has been the subject of substantial research or modeling in neuropsychological rehabilitation. The rehabilitation of neglect is discussed further in Chapter 6 of this volume. The focus of the present chapter is on models for the treatment of impairments of complex visual processing other than neglect. Somewhat surprisingly, this is a relatively undeveloped aspect of neuropsychological rehabilitation.

Although adequate visual perception is generally considered to be important for participation in rehabilitation activities and for functional independence, there has been little effort directed to the development of models to guide neuropsychological treatment of these defects. At least two factors appear to have contributed to this situation. The first is that neuropsychological rehabilitation as a field has tended to focus on neglect as the primary impairment within the realm of perception. Neglect is a relatively common, often dramatic and disabling impairment that overshadows any other co-occurring visuoperceptual defects. As a consequence, research to date on rehabilitation of perceptual disorders typically has had the goal of increasing attention to the left hemispace, and subjects have been selected on the basis of having neglect.

A second factor that seems to have contributed to the limited progress in modeling neuropsychological rehabilitation of visuoperceptual disorders is that there tends to be relatively good "spontaneous" recovery of functional abilities following acquisition of visuoperceptual disorders, along with considerable ability to compensate for residual visuoperceptual defects. It is not unusual for patients who have suffered focal visuoperceptual defects secondary to neurological injury to go on to lead quite normal lives, although certain tasks may be accomplished by means that differ from those used prior to the injury. However, despite good recovery and compensation by some patients, others suffer from chronic, non-neglect visuoperceptual disorders, with substantial secondary functional limitations. Advances in the treatment and management of these conditions will require development of more useful neuropsychological rehabilitation models.

CONTEXT FOR REHABILITATION
OF VISUOPERCEPTUAL DISORDERS

Models for the treatment and management of visuoperceptual defects need to take into account, on several levels, the context of the problem to be treated. An important level of contextual analysis when considering rehabilitation of such deficits regards the functional status of (1) the eyes (particularly in head trauma, in which visual defects often follow damage to the orbital bones, the sixth, third, and fourth cranial nerves, or the eye itself), and (2) other (nonvisual) brain areas, such as prefrontal regions involved in executive control of vision. This information is derived primarily from the neuro-ophthalmological and neuropsychological evaluations, respectively. In broad terms, these systems provide the immediate input source and output target for the activity of the visuoperceptual system, although a simple unidirectional model reflects neither the highly parallel nature of the system nor the multiple feedback mechanisms involved. Because visuoperceptual defects arising from brain damage often occur in the setting of damage to either the peripheral visual system or other brain regions, or both, specification of rehabilitation goals and procedures requires evaluation, treatment, and accommodation of comorbid visual and cognitive problems.

Perception and Vision

Processing of visual information begins with stimulation of the eyes, and knowledge of the functional integrity of a patient's eyes is necessary before beginning neuropsychological rehabilitation of visuoperceptual disorders. Neuropsychological intervention is predicated on the idea that the signal transmitted from the eyes to the patient's brain represents coding of visual input with maximum possible clarity, within the limitations of the patient's medical condition. With a neuro-ophthalmological examination as the starting point, visual impairment due to eye disease often can be treated with relative ease by means of corrective lenses or surgery, and if residual deficits still are present, they can be specified. When incorporating neuro-ophthalmological findings into rehabilitation planning, it is important not to confuse normal performance on vision screening measures with normal perception. Even when visual acuity and visual fields are normal, aging and neurological disease may cause impairments in other aspects of vision, such as contrast sensitivity, perceptual discrimination, and use of motion cues, which in turn may have implications for higher cognitive abilities (e.g., Eslinger & Benton, 1983; Rizzo, Anderson, Dawson, & Nawrot, 2000).

As Luria (1966) emphasized, there is no clear boundary between elementary and higher order visuoperceptual defects. Damage to the system at one level will have implications for processing at other levels, and, in some instances, the behavioral expression and functional implications may be indistinguishable, whether the damaged tissue is in the eye, the optic radiations, or striate cortex. For example, visual hallucinations can arise from dysfunction at virtually any level of the visual system, from the eye to primary and association cortices (e.g., Anderson & Rizzo, 1994; White, 1980). Although certain characteristics of the hallucinations, such as location within the visual field, can provide clues as to the locus of the dysfunction, these patterns are not invariant.

Perception and Cognition

Performance on real-world tasks with strong visuoperceptual demands can be influenced by not only dysfunction of the eye but also various higher order perceptual and cognitive impairments. Specification of a patient's visuoperceptual and cognitive strengths and weaknesses by means of a neuropsychological evaluation is an essential component of any model of neuropsychological rehabilitation. Assessment of visuoperceptual disorders must occur in the context of a comprehensive neuropsychological evaluation. Impairments of visuoperception can influence performances on measures of other aspects of cognition (e.g., memory, executive functions, nonverbal intellect, academic achievement, language) and, likewise, defects in these other aspects of cognition can affect performances on tests of visuoperception. A hypothesis-testing approach to evaluation of visuoperception and other cognitive abilities provides a means of systematically considering the contribution of specific impairments and strengths in these multiple domains to a patient's overall functional competence (e.g., Benton, 1994; Tranel, 1994). Neuropsychological evaluation of visuoperceptual impairments typically would consider the following general functions:

Visuoperceptual functions	*Other cognitive functions*
Static visual acuity	Visual and verbal memory
Screening of visual fields	Language
Color perception	Auditory attention
Eye movements	Constructional skills
Visually guided reaching	Verbal reasoning
Object and face recognition	Executive functions
Reading	Writing
Spatial attention	Gestural praxis
Spatial judgment	Fine motor coordination
Form discrimination	Nonverbal reasoning

Luria (1966) advocated a rehabilitative perspective for conducting neuropsychological evaluations of visuoperceptual disorders. For example, in the use of such familiar neuropsychological tasks as analysis of block patterns, he noted:

The suggestion to use aids to facilitate spatial analysis of the elements will substantially assist patients with lesions of the parieto-occipital zones but will be of no benefit to patients with frontal lesions. Conversely, the consecutive program of the patients' behavior (look at the figure; pick out the first two; count the number of elements in it; pick out the first of them, and so on), while unnecessary for patients with lesions of the parieto-occipital zones of the brain, will enable patients with frontal lesions to compensate considerably for their defect. (p. 466)

Trial "interventions" such as this, when incorporated into the neuropsychological evaluation, can help specify the nature of visuoperceptual impairments and provide guidance for the development of rehabilitation plans based on the patient's abilities and weaknesses.

For many patients, treatment of visuoperceptual disorders must be conceptualized in the context of significant coexisting cognitive impairments, one of the most important of which is neglect. The possible contribution of neglect to visuoperceptual task failure, as well as the potential benefits of treating neglect, should be considered in rehabilitation planning for visuoperceptual disorders whenever there is known or suspected right-hemisphere damage. Weinberg, Piasetsky, Diller, and Gordon (1982) have shown that patients with right-hemisphere damage but without overt neglect, may have a subtle, residual lateral attentional bias that underlies impairments on tasks requiring perceptual organization or visuoconstructional ability. These patients passed standard cancellation tasks designed to detect neglect, yet had difficulty reading and performing more complex visual tasks. Weinberg et al. further showed that interventions designed generally to increase attention to details in the left hemispace across tasks and situations can be helpful in treating such patients. Even when there is no neglect or lateral attentional bias, impairments in other aspects of visual attention (e.g., sustained attention, selective attention) may have a major influence on task performance and should be considered in the development of rehabilitation plans (see Chapter 6).

Impairments of visuoperception interact with deficits in visual memory, visuomotor skills, reading, and nonverbal reasoning. It is clear that an impairment in perceiving stimuli will negatively influence performance on tasks depending on further processing of that stimulus information (e.g., manipulating the stimulus or recalling it later). It also is true that impairments of such "higher order" visuocognitive abilities can exacerbate visuoperceptual deficits. For example, an anterograde amnesia that includes impaired memory for visual stimuli can impede learning from rehabilitation experiences structured to benefit visuoperception. Similarly, an impairment of motor control can interfere with perceptual learning in "hands-on" rehabilitation settings.

It also is common for rehabilitation of visuoperceptual defects to take place in the context of impairments of executive dysfunction. This particularly is true in cases of closed head injury with coup–contracoup injuries to prefrontal and occipitoparietal regions. Executive dysfunction can interact with and exacerbate perceptual impairments in myriad ways, for example, by dampening initiation of therapeutic and compensatory behaviors or decreasing the ability to allocate visual attention and organize scan paths. Impaired decision making due to prefrontal damage may lead patients to engage in behaviors that they are not visually competent to perform. Consideration of a patient's executive function profile is necessary if rehabilitation of visuoperceptual impairments is to succeed.

Some compensatory approaches to visuoperceptual rehabilitation place significant demands on other cognitive abilities, including language and aspects of executive function (such as awareness, self-monitoring, verbal mediation, and the ability to initiate novel behaviors). Other compensatory approaches, including the use of certain assistive devices, may be more compatible with comorbid cognitive defects. Specification of coexisting cognitive impairments and strengths by means of a comprehensive neuropsychological evaluation should provide guidance in selection of rehabilitation procedures, in addition to providing a means of monitoring patient progress. In order for the neuropsychological evaluation to be of maximum utility, it is necessary that the assessment be conducted from a rehabilitation perspective, in a manner that provides for identification of component cognitive impairments that can be targeted for intervention, as well as cognitive and behavioral strengths that can be used to the patient's advantage.

RECOVERY OF VISUOPERCEPTUAL FUNCTIONS

Certain visuoperceptual impairments can resolve without treatment, and models for visuoperceptual rehabilitation should provide guidance in distinguishing between treatment effects and spontaneous recovery. This effort currently is hampered by a paucity of longitudinal data on recovery of visuoperceptual abilities. It appears that the extent of spontaneous recovery depends in part on the nature of the visuoperceptual defects in question. For example, there is considerable capacity for spontaneous recovery of higher order visuoperceptual abilities (such as perceptual discrimination, visuospatial abilities, and visuoconstructional abilities) following brain damage (e.g., Meerwaldt, 1983; Anderson & Rizzo, 1995; Eslinger, Biddle, & Grattan, 1997), but more elementary impairments, such as visual field defects and achromatopsia, tend to show relatively little change after the acute recovery period. Visual field defects due to stroke or trauma that persist after the first few days tend to be chronic conditions. Findings from a study using serial positron emission tomography (PET) scans suggest that patients who experience good recovery from visual field defects likely have brain dysfunction outside of primary visual cortex, for example, in association cortex, subcortical nuclei, or deep white matter (Bosley et al., 1987). Although use of such methods to date has been limited, there is tremendous potential benefit in incorporating findings from structural and functional neuroimaging in models of visuoperceptual recovery and rehabilitation, and this is likely to be an area of active research in the future.

Spontaneous recovery can take various forms, and improvement in real-world visual activities can continue despite no reduction in the size of the visual field defect. Kolb (1990) applied his neuroscientific perspective to a personal encounter with recovery from a visual field defect following an occipital lobe stroke:

> My own experience suggests that field defects may show some reduction, but there was virtually no recovery after the first 50 days and virtually no improvement at all in the area of the dense scotoma after the first week. . . . In spite of the absence of a reduction in the objective size of the scotoma beyond 2 months poststroke, there is little doubt that my visual abilities continued to improve for some time. It seems likely that a major reason for this is the shift in the point of fixation. (p. 145)

As discussed later, a compensatory approach, in line with Kolb's insight, employing systematic training in eye movements into the blind visual field has proven utility.

Understanding of the functional organization of the visual system has benefited from research on nonhuman animals to a greater extent than has been the case for most other cognitive abilities. This provides an opportunity for models of neuropsychological rehabilitation of visuoperceptual disorders to draw upon relatively well-developed models, derived from animal research, of the organization of the visual system and its functional reorganization following injury. However, the applicability of these findings and models to the rehabilitation setting needs to be subjected to empirical investigation.

Some of the complexities involved in applying such work to rehabilitation can be seen in the recovery and treatment of visual field defects. Monkeys with striate cortex ablations are able visually to localize objects and make visual discriminations based on color, pattern, orientation, and luminance, likely via secondary visual pathways from the superior colliculus or lateral geniculate nucleus to extrastriate cortex. While these preserved capacities would seemingly have potential implications for recovery and rehabilitation, the findings cannot be directly generalized to naturally occurring lesions in humans, which usually involve concomitant damage to surrounding extrastriate association cortex and white matter. Similarly, because monkeys with striate cortex ablations have been reported to show reduction of visual field defects following systematic practice, patients with visual field defects have been exposed to extensive training in directing saccadic eye movements to targets in their blind visual fields. These attempts have met with mixed results (e.g., Balliet, Blood, & Bach-Y-Rita, 1985; Zihl, 1981), and there is little compelling evidence to date that patients with visual field defects substantially benefit from such procedures. However, in the context of advancing research on the plasticity of sensory and motor regions of the adult brain, it remains possible that increasingly precise identification of areas of residual vision, together with tightly targeted stimulation of scotoma border zones, will lead to greater success in this endeavor (e.g., Sabel & Kasten, 2000).

Despite potentially important differences between humans and other species in the organization of the visual system, there is little doubt that the human visual system is characterized by massively parallel processing of various stimulus features (e.g., form, motion, color, location). Felleman and van Essen (1991) described at least 30 functional representations of the visual fields in monkey cortex. Although cross-species differences are likely with regard to factors such as size, number, and location of functional areas, it is clear that processing of various visual stimulus features relies on partially distinct cortical regions. A multitude of visual cues can provide overlapping or convergent information. For example, shape can be derived from contour, shading, or motion. Brain damage often results in an uneven pattern of defects (i.e., with specific impairments in the context of relatively preserved processing of certain types of visual information). Increased reliance on preserved aspects of perceptual processing provides a putative mechanism for some spontaneous recovery.

Patients with visuoperceptual disorders also may spontaneously use language to help compensate for visuoperceptual defects, using speech or internal verbal processing as an alternative route for encoding and analyzing visual information. The tendency to compensate for acquired visuoperceptual difficulties is such a common occurrence that analysis of neurological patients' self-initiated compensatory behaviors can serve as an effective guide to understanding which stages of visuoperceptual processing are dysfunctional (Luria, 1966). It is useful in this regard not only to question the patient regarding changes in his or her approach to tasks but also to observe actual task performance, because compensatory behaviors may be employed without conscious awareness.

MODELS FOR INTERVENTION

While it is difficult to find a well-articulated model for visuoperceptual rehabilitation in the neuropsychological literature, it is possible to extract a number of guiding principles, conceptual themes, and constraints for models from extant literature and allied fields. To accommodate current practice, models for visuoperceptual rehabilitation should incorporate both *restorative* and *compensatory* methods of inducing behavioral change. Visuoperceptual defects typically are treated with some combination of restorative (or remedial) approaches that aim to improve or restore impaired function through repetitive strengthening exercises, together with compensatory approaches involving training in the use of assistive technology or alternative strategies to achieve a goal.

The general model of selective optimization with compensation (SOC) developed by Baltes and colleagues (e.g., Freund & Baltes, 1998) for conceptualization of successful coping with physical decline and other aspects of aging provides a useful framework for viewing the interaction of restorative and compensatory approaches. *Selection* processes involve decision making about where to direct one's energies, including identification of priorities and establishment of reasonable goals. *Optimization* involves developing or refining goal-related abilities, including application of restorative procedures to strengthen the impaired ability to the extent possible. *Compensation* entails development of substitutive methods of goal attainment. In line with this framework, visuoperceptual rehabilitation following brain damage can be viewed as one instantiation of adaptation to loss, in which the optimal outcome can be obtained by carefully selecting goals, optimizing residual abilities, and refining compensatory techniques.

In practice, the distinction between restorative and compensatory visuoperceptual rehabilitation procedures often is blurred, and the two approaches share important features. Independent of the subsequent course of rehabilitation, education of the patient and caregivers about the nature of the acquired impairments and the rationale for treatment is an essential component of all neuropsychological rehabilitation. Early in the course of visuoperceptual rehabilitation, it is important to address, for both patients and their families, problems with awareness of deficits, misconceptions regarding the likely course of recovery, or failure to appreciate the necessity of their taking an active role in rehabilitation. Empowering a patient with increased understanding of his or her visuoperceptual condition is sometimes the single most important step in treatment, because this can provide a basis for the patient to make practical changes in his or her behavior and in restructuring the environment (Gianutsos & Matheson, 1987).

Both restorative and compensatory approaches also require outcome measures that are based in performance of specific behavioral tasks. These tasks should reflect rehabilitation goals identified by the patient (i.e., activities the patient would like to perform but no longer can due to the perceptual consequences of his or her brain injury). Common goals include reading, locating items in the home, driving a car, shopping, and cooking, each of which involves component visual perceptual processes. Malec (1999) has described a useful means of defining and measuring progress toward individual rehabilitation goals through the method of *goal attainment scaling* (GAS), whereby the desired outcome and other possible outcomes (both good and bad) are articulated and assigned numerical values. Following operationalization of goals, it may be desirable to implement restorative procedures first to attain any possible benefit before implementing compensatory procedures. GAS can provide guidance as to when this transition should occur. A general approach for conceptualizing neuropsychological rehabilitation of visuo-perceptual disorders is provided in Figure 8.1.

Restorative Methods

Empirical support for the efficacy of restorative methods of visuo-perceptual rehabilitation remains limited, but this class of procedures has considerable potential, particularly if these methods can be interfaced with ongoing developments in technology and pharmacology. Restorative procedures have the benefit of a certain degree of face validity, in that the capacity of the normal, undamaged visual system to acquire and refine perceptual skills through repetitive practice is widely recognized. As Huxley (1942, p. 22) noted,

> Walking through a wood, a city dweller will be blind to a multitude of things which the trained naturalist will see without difficulty. At sea the sailor will detect distant objects which, for the landsman, are simply not there at all. And so on, indefinitely. In all such cases improved sensing and seeing are the result of heightened powers of perceiving, themselves due to the memory of similar situations in the past.

It is reasonable to expect that individuals with a partially damaged visual system also may be able to improve certain perceptual skills, at least somewhat, through repetitive and challenging perceptual exercises (e.g.,

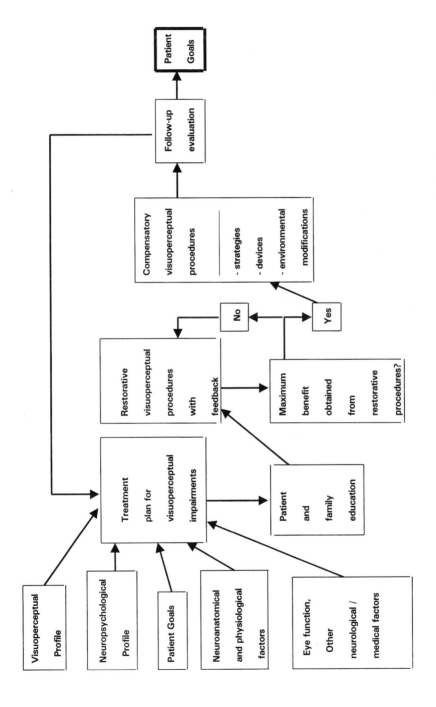

FIGURE 8.1. A general framework for neuropsychological rehabilitation of visuoperceptual disorders. *Note.* All processes are assumed to take place in a rehabilitation context and in interaction with spontaneous recovery.

Rao & Bieliauskas, 1983). Neuropsychologists can help structure activities in allied rehabilitation programs, such as physical and occupational therapies, such that tasks with visuoperceptual demands (ranging from walking to shopping and recreational activities) can be utilized for maximum learning. This may involve tailoring task demands to the patient's perceptual and cognitive profile, and incorporating targeted and repetitive visuoperceptual challenges with feedback regarding performance.

The extent to which spontaneous recovery of visuoperceptual abilities occurs following brain damage supports the notion that some degree of plasticity exists within the system, and this may provide an opportunity for restorative approaches, with repetitive, hierarchically arranged tasks to facilitate recovery. Warren (1993) has described a "bottom-up" approach to rehabilitation of visuoperceptual skills, in which elementary defects are identified and the most basic-level skills are built first, with therapy then progressing to address higher level (more complex or conflated) abilities through a developmental hierarchy. Oculomotor control, visual fields, and acuity are seen as basic-level abilities, and visual cognition (visual problem solving and planning) is at the highest level, with visual memory, scanning, and pattern recognition being intermediate-level abilities. This framework encompasses restorative and compensatory methods, but primacy is given to identifying and restoring basic component skills. This approach applies systematic repetitive training on tasks relevant to the most basic-level defect identified and also incorporates redirection of the patient's conscious, deliberate attention to the area of weakness, all within an educational context designed to facilitate generalization to real-world tasks.

Restorative methods of visuoperceptual rehabilitation typically involve provision of some form of *feedback* to the patient regarding his or her performance in order to enhance the gains from repetitive practice. Luria (1966) emphasized the importance of patients' comparing their behavioral performance to the intended output in order to assess success (e.g., evaluating proprioceptive feedback from self-produced stimulation to improve visuomotor coordination). Linking visuoperceptual experience to stimulation in another sensory modality, either auditory or tactile, provides feedback that may strengthen the representation of the experience. Recent evidence suggests that cross-modal integration may involve multiple brain areas outside of primary and association visual cortices, including prefrontal and parietal regions, and the insula (Banati, Goerres, Tjoa, Aggleton, & Grasby, 2000), providing a putative anatomical substrate for patients who have sustained damage to visual cortices, so that they may benefit from multimodal stimulation.

Provision of enhanced feedback during restorative training may have additional benefits even in the absence of any direct restoration of function. Challenging exercises in the domain of impairment, when coupled with appropriate feedback, have the potential to increase awareness of acquired visuoperceptual impairments. Unawareness of visuoperceptual defects is common following stroke and head trauma, and can be a significant impediment to rehabilitation progress. One mechanism likely contributing to unawareness of visual field defects is that cortical plasticity appears to facilitate "filling in" blind spots with information from the area surrounding the scotoma (Safran & Landis, 1996). Luria (1966) noted that right-sided visual field defects resulting from left-hemisphere lesions are typically recognized, and patients will shift their gaze to accommodate. However, left-sided visual field defects from right-hemisphere lesions are more likely to be accompanied by unawareness. We found that during the first few weeks following onset, 20% of head trauma patients denied any difficulty with their vision, despite having significant impairments on standardized measures of perception, such as Benton's tests of perceptual discrimination and spatial judgment. Among stroke patients, 85% of those with right-hemisphere lesions and 17% of those with left-hemisphere lesions denied visuoperceptual problems but were found to have significant impairments (Anderson & Tranel, 1989). Feedback during task performance is among the most direct methods of enhancing awareness of acquired visuoperceptual impairments.

Even when awareness is adequate, patients understandably may have difficulty accepting the notion of permanent vision loss. Anger and resentment can lead to rejection of compensatory devices or refusal to employ compensatory strategies. In such instances, adjustment counseling coupled with experience laboring at restorative tasks may facilitate acceptance of a visuoperceptual defect and the need to take steps to compensate for it.

Compensatory Methods

As noted earlier, compensatory efforts play an important role in the recovery of visuoperceptual abilities for many patients with acquired brain dysfunction, even if they do not receive formal rehabilitation services. For example, patients with prosopagnosia often learn on their own to recognize individuals by focusing on specific features of familiar faces (e.g., a missing tooth, facial hair, hairstyle) or paraphernalia (e.g., glasses, a hat) in a manner that bypasses the need to analyze the overall shape of the face. It is common for patients with all manner of acquired perceptual defects to take steps to reduce the complex or confusing visual demands of their environment (e.g., by eliminating night driving).

However, in addition to patient-generated compensatory efforts, systematic training in the application of compensatory strategies and the use of compensatory devices holds great promise for enhancing recovery, and these procedures must enter into models for the rehabilitation of visuoperceptual disorders.

Much can be gained in developing compensatory treatment models for neuropsychological rehabilitation of cortically based visuoperceptual defects by looking to the relatively mature field of low vision rehabilitation. Chronic, disabling, and uncorrectable visual impairment due to eye disease is relatively common in older adults, and models for the rehabilitation of these patients have elements that can be applied in the treatment of visual impairments caused by brain damage. One such example can be derived from a hierarchical systems model for rehabilitation of visual impairments (Massof, 1995). A systems model provides a generally applicable framework for organizing therapist and patient energies in coordination with available resources to progress toward attainable goals, all in the face of an underlying disease state that does not improve. This approach begins with identification of the patient's broad objectives and then specific goals that would mark progress toward those objectives. The patient's goals are linked to tasks that must be performed to attain these goals, and each is rated with regard both to its value to the patient and the degree of difficulty in attaining the goal. The effectiveness of rehabilitation is reflected in a reduced level of difficulty associated with attaining a goal, or by reduced value assigned to a goal, usually as a result of acquiring alternative strategies or otherwise adjusting to impairments.

If this type of model is to have unique value for the use of compensatory methods in neuropsychological rehabilitation of visuoperceptual disorders, it will be necessary to formulate the role of neuropsychological constructs and methods in its application. By definition, compensatory procedures rely on a patient's cognitive strengths and other available resources to counteract or minimize the consequences of a brain injury. Careful evaluation of comorbid neuropsychological deficits plays an especially important role when treatment plans include the use of compensatory methods. Impairments in other aspects of cognition (e.g., memory or executive functions) can sabotage compensatory approaches to visuoperceptual rehabilitation if not factored into selection of methods and training regimens.

Given the limited success of restorative methods for treating visual field defects, together with ability of some patients to alter spontaneously their eye movements to compensate for field defects, there is good reason to believe that systematic training in such compensatory strategies may be useful for many patients. Pommerenke and Markowitsch

(1989) provided compensatory scanning instruction to patients with chronic, stable visual field defects and found that, despite no change in the size of the field defect, improvement occurred in the efficiency, accuracy, and scope of visual search patterns. Kerkoff, Munbinger, and Meier (1994) trained patients with hemianopias, but without neglect, in methods designed to improve saccadic eye movement strategies and found significant increases in visual search field, maintenance of gains at 3-month follow-up, and good return to work among treated patients.

In addition to training patients to develop compensatory visuoperceptual skills, there can be advantages in directing rehabilitation efforts toward developing compensatory strategies based on relatively independent neurocognitive systems. For example, focal damage to posterior visual areas or right-hemisphere structures involved in visual perception can leave the language system relatively unaffected, and linguistic coding of visual information can provide an alternative route for processing information about visual elements of one's environment. There clearly are limitations to this type of approach; the rapid parallel processing of highly complex visual signals that occurs automatically during normal visual perception cannot be approximated by the relatively slow, deliberate, and largely serial processing of the language system. Furthermore, this approach assumes the presence of some sensory signal that can be verbally processed and is thus most applicable in the face of visual input that has been degraded only partially. Although systematic research on verbal compensation for non-neglect visuoperceptual disorders is lacking, such techniques have been in use for decades (e.g., Luria, 1966). We have found verbal encoding and rehearsal of visual stimulus features to be particularly useful for patients with right-hemisphere damage affecting spatial perception and visual memory. For example, we used this approach with a young woman who had substantial impairments of visuospatial perception and visual memory, resulting from a large, right-middle cerebral artery stroke, and who was unable to navigate even her immediate neighborhood without getting lost. Through extensive training in verbally encoding her routes, street names, and salient landmarks, she gradually developed the ability to travel about a medium-size city without serious complications, despite little or no improvement in her visuospatial abilities or visual memory. A similar pattern of successful compensatory verbal coding was reported for a woman with severe nonverbal memory impairments due to herpes simplex encephalitis (Eslinger, Damasio, Damasio, & Butters, 1993).

Additional potential benefits of training patients to process visual information in alternate modalities are suggested in a recent study of a visual–auditory sensory substitution system (Arno, Capelle, Wanet-Defalque, Catalan-Ahumada, & Veraart, 1999). The system employed a head-mounted camera and a mechanism whereby visual patterns were encoded in auditory signals. Following correction and feedback training in the use of this device, persons deprived of all vision were able to discriminate and identify unique visual patterns. It remains to be determined whether this type of procedure will eventually have application in the neuropsychological rehabilitation of visuoperceptual disorders. Other innovative compensatory devices that already are available include systems for electronic magnification in the form of closed-circuit television that can both enlarge text and enhance contrast, and software for personal computers that visually enlarges or converts to audio output text scanned into it (Paul, 1999). It is clear that ongoing advances in technology will provide opportunities for increasingly sophisticated compensatory devices to be integrated into visuoperceptual rehabilitation programs.

CONCLUSIONS

Patients with impairments of visuoperception are encountered frequently in neurorehabilitation settings, but models for neuropsychological rehabilitation of visuoperceptual defects are in an early stage of development. Extant models for visuoperceptual rehabilitation have emphasized remediation of neglect at the expense of other perceptual impairments, and the limited empirical work on the treatment of non-neglect perceptual defects has been guided by general or implicit models. Although more mature models from relevant fields, including low vision rehabilitation and basic visual science, have elements of value to visuoperceptual rehabilitation, these models lack a neuropsychological perspective.

A significant limitation at present is a lack of knowledge regarding the real-world significance of visuoperceptual defects. For example, it is not known if mild visuoperceptual impairments sufficiently interfere with normal daily functioning to warrant intervention. It is possible that visuoperceptual impairments cause less distress for patients and their families than do other neuropsychological problems with which they frequently co-occur (e.g., impairments of emotion, executive function, and awareness). However, defective visual perception clearly can lead to functional limitations and resultant emotional distress. Furthermore, visuoperceptual impairments often are the result of age-related disease such as stroke, with the implication that these defects will interact with other age-linked risk factors to increase susceptibility to falls and motor vehicle accidents.

Construction and application of improved models of visuoperceptual rehabilitation will require advances in knowledge of the natural course and consequences of non-neglect perceptual impairments. Increased knowledge regarding critical periods of recovery could prove to be extremely useful. It is possible that for some visuoperceptual disorders, restorative procedures may be of particular benefit in facilitating brain reorganization only during an acute recovery period, but rehabilitation neuropsychologists as yet have little empirical information to guide them in this regard.

It would seem that many of the critical elements are in place for major advances in the neuropsychological rehabilitation of visuoperceptual disorders. Although models for visuoperceptual rehabilitation presently are limited, treatment of perceptual problems may have certain advantages for model development relative to other currently more advanced aspects of neuropsychological rehabilitation. Visual perception can be relatively easily analyzed in terms of component processes, and relevant real-world goals, such as driving, can be readily measured. Useful general models already are available, and ongoing detailed study of the functional organization of the mammalian visual system should provide a basis for articulation of more neuroscientifically sophisticated models of visuoperceptual rehabilitation.

REFERENCES

Anderson, S. W., & Rizzo, M. (1994). Hallucinations following occipital lobe damage: The pathological activation of visual representations. *Journal of Clinical and Experimental Neuropsychology, 16*, 651–663.

Anderson, S. W., & Rizzo, M. (1995). Recovery and rehabilitation of visual cortical function. *NeuroRehabilitation, 5*, 129–140.

Anderson, S. W., & Tranel, D. (1989). Awareness of disease states following cerebral infarction, dementia, and head trauma: Standardized assessment. *Clinical Neuropsychologist, 3*, 327–339.

Arno, P., Capelle, C., Wanet-Defalque, M.-C., Catalan-Ahumada, M., & Veraart, C. (1999). Auditory coding of visual patterns for the blind. *Perception, 28*, 1013–1029.

Balliet, R., Blood, K. M. T., Bach-Y-Rita, P. (1985). Visual field rehabilitation in the cortically blind? *Journal of Neurology, Neurosurgery and Psychiatry, 48*, 1113–1124.

Banati, R. B., Goerres, G. W., Tjoa, C., Aggleton, J. P., & Grasby, P. (2000). The functional anatomy of visual–tactile integration in man: A study using positron emission tomography. *Neuropsychologia, 38*, 115–124.

Benton, A. L. (1994). Neuropsychological assessment. *Annual Review of Psychology, 45*, 1–23.

Bosley, T. M., Dann, R., Silber, F. L., Alavi, A., Kushner, M., Chawluk, J. B., Savino, P. J., Sergott, R. C., Schatz, N. J., & Reivich, M. (1987). Recovery of vision after ischemic lesions: Positron emission tomography. *Annals of Neurology, 21*, 444–450.

Eslinger, P. J., & Benton, A. L. (1983). Visuoperceptual performances in aging and dementia: Clinical and theoretical implications. *Journal of Clinical Neuropsychology, 3,* 213–220.

Eslinger, P. J., Biddle, K. R., & Grattan, L. M. (1997). Cognitive and social development in children with prefrontal cortex lesions. In N. A. Krasnegor, G. R. Lyon, & P. S. Goldman-Rakic (Eds.), *Development of the prefrontal cortex.* Baltimore: Brookes.

Eslinger, P. J., Damasio, H., Damasio, A. R., & Butters, N. (1993). Nonverbal amnesia and asymmetric cerebral lesions following encephalitis. *Brain and Cognition, 21,* 140–152.

Felleman, D. J., & van Essen, D. C. (1991). Distributed hierarchical processing in the primate cerebral cortex. *Cerebral Cortex, 1,* 1–47.

Freund, A. M., & Baltes, P. B. (1998). Selection, optimization, and compensation as strategies of life management: Correlations with subjective indicators of successful aging. *Psychology and Aging, 13,* 531–543.

Gianutsos, R., & Matheson, P. (1987). The rehabilitation of visual perceptual disorders attributable to brain injury. In M. Meier, A. Benton, & L. Diller (Eds.), *Neuropsychological rehabilitation.* New York: Guilford Press.

Huxley, A. (1942). *The art of seeing.* Seattle: Montana Books. (Reprinted 1975)

Kerkhoff, G., Munbinger, U., & Meier, E. K. (1994). Neurovisual rehabilitation in cerebral blindness. *Archives of Neurology, 51,* 474–481.

Kolb, B. (1990). Recovery from occipital stroke: A self-report and an inquiry into visual processes. *Canadian Journal of Psychology, 44,* 130–147.

Luria, A. R. (1966). *Higher cortical functions in man.* New York: Basic Books.

Malec, J. F. (1999). Goal attainment scaling in rehabilitation. *Neuropsychological Rehabilitation, 9,* 253–276.

Massof, R. W. (1995). A systems model for low vision rehabilitation. *Optometry and Vision Science, 72,* 725–736.

Meerwaldt, J. D. (1983). Spatial disorientation in right-hemisphere infarction: A study of the speed of recovery. *Journal of Neurology, Neurosurgery and Psychiatry, 46,* 426–429.

Paul, W. (1999). The role of computer assistive technology in rehabilitation of the visually impaired: A personal perspective. *American Journal of Ophthalmology, 127,* 75–76.

Pommerenke, K., & Markowitsch, J. H. (1989). Rehabilitation training of homonymous visual field defects in patients with post-geniculate damage of the visual system. *Restorative Neurology and Neuroscience, 1,* 47–63.

Rao, S. M., & Bieliauskas, L. A. (1983). Cognitive rehabilitation two and one-half years post right temporal lobectomy. *Journal of Clinical Neuropsychology, 5,* 313–320.

Rizzo, M., Anderson, S. W., Dawson, J., & Nawrot, M. (2000). Vision and cognition in Alzheimer's disease. *Neuropsychologia, 38,* 1157–1169.

Sabel, B. A., & Kasten, E. (2000). Restoration of vision by training of residual functions. *Current Opinion in Ophthalmology, 11,* 430–436.

Safran, A. B., & Landis, T. (1996) Plasticity in the adult visual cortex: Implications for the diagnosis of visual field defects and visual rehabilitation. *Current Opinion in Ophthalmology, 7,* 53–64.

Tranel, D. (1994). The Iowa–Benton school of neuropsychological assessment. In I. Grant & K. M. Adams (Eds.), *Neuropsychological assessment of neuropsychiatric disorders* (2nd ed.). New York: Oxford University Press.

Warren, M. (1993). A hierarchical model for evaluation and treatment of visual perceptual dysfunction in adult acquired brain injury. *American Journal of Occupational Therapy, 47,* 42–66.

Weinberg, J., Piasetsky, E., Diller, L., & Gordon, W. (1982). Treating perceptual organization deficits in nonneglecting RBD patients. *Journal of Clinical Neuropsychology, 4,* 59–75.

White, N. J. (1980). Complex visual hallucinations in partial blindness due to eye disease. *British Journal of Psychiatry, 136,* 284–286.

Zihl, J. (1981). Recovery of visual functions in patients with cerebral blindness. *Experimental Brain Research, 44,* 159–169.

CHAPTER 9

Models of Language Rehabilitation

JACQUELINE J. HINCKLEY

Rehabilitation of neurogenic language disorders has become an increasingly active area of interest for researchers, theoreticians, and practitioners. Acceptance of research methodologies, such as single-subject designs, and development of research technologies, such as neuroimaging, have created new ways to learn about language interventions. The research techniques enable observations that can contribute to the testing of theories about language and rehabilitation. The accumulation of this work begins to provide a more evidence-based context in which to apply language treatment techniques.

The purpose of this chapter is to discuss the characteristics of theoretically driven treatment, to describe theories that have served as a basis for developing interventions, and to identify the current models of language rehabilitation in the literature. The evolution of current models is described, as are the associated and characteristic assessment tools and treatment techniques. Finally, comparison and contrast of the identified models frame a discussion of future directions for theoretically based language rehabilitation.

HISTORY OF LANGUAGE REHABILITATION

Tutoring and exercises in reading, spelling, and repeating words have been used in an effort to improve the language of people with acquired disorders since at least 1673, when a patient with acquired alexia was described (LaPointe, 1983). In spite of broad interest in the neural bases of language during the last half of the 19th century, organized attempts at rehabilitation did not become widespread until World War II, relatively late in the history of our knowledge about aphasia. As many more soldiers survived gunshot wounds and other head injuries, centers were urgently created throughout the country to accommodate their rehabilitation (Wepman, 1947; Shewan, 1986). These aphasia centers were an important beginning point in the development of language rehabilitation models and techniques.

These early aphasia rehabilitation efforts were primarily derived from educational models; indeed, the speech–language pathologists and other personnel who forged the work in this area were primarily recruited from educational institutions. As a result, rehabilitation efforts were often intensive, occurring several hours each day, like a typical school day. A broad number of areas were addressed, from language skills to vocational skills. There were often large social groups that convened at least once during the day to provide a break from the study routine and to foster socialization. Some aphasia rehabilitation programs either continue or have returned to providing this kind of comprehensive and intensive training. During the 55-year interim, we have made many strides in our knowledge about the various components of rehabilitation and the success of various techniques. Although we still need to press toward the goal of identifying which treatments will be most successful with which patients, we have made some gains in establishing the general usefulness of language rehabilitation.

Recent meta-analyses and literature syntheses have all concluded that aphasia treatment, overall, is effective (Robey, 1994, 1998; Holland, Fromm, De Ruyter, & Stein, 1996). Medium-size treatment effects were obtained for treatment provided even in the chronic phase, and larger effects were obtained for treatment provided during the acute phase. Identification of which treatment, when, and for whom remain important items on the current aphasia treatment research agenda.

A THEORY OF THERAPY

Research on language rehabilitation would likely progress more readily with a meta-theory of therapy as a source of direction and testable predictions (Ferguson, 1999; Petheram & Parr, 1998; Byng & Black, 1995). Such a theory should explain the kinds of behavioral changes sought in rehabilitation, their mental and neurological underpinnings, and predict the types of change-related activities and procedures that result in particular outcomes. This type of theoretical framework would serve to unite approaches that are currently perceived as disparate and provide a common rhetoric and evaluative background from which to carry out the work of determining which treatment is best for whom.

Some have advocated use of the framework of the World Health Organization (WHO) for the International Classification of Impairment, Disability and Handicap (ICIDH-2; 1999) as a theory of therapy (Petheram & Parr, 1998). This framework presents a method of describing the levels of difficulty that are the result of a communication impairment. Specifically, the *impairment level* describes the loss or abnormality of a structure. *Activity limitations* are those activities that have been curtailed by the impairment. The extent to which one's ability to participate in society has been affected is termed *participation restrictions*. The WHO framework is able to accommodate a number of different treatment approaches and offers a helpful heuristic with which to classify desired outcomes and treatments. However, it is a purely descriptive model and as such should not properly be considered a theory of therapy.

The acknowledgment that such a theory is needed marks a change in thinking about how we should go about rehabilitation. For most of the last 60 years, research and clinical actions have evinced the belief that a necessary precursor to effective treatment is a thorough understanding of the nature of the deficit. The present search for something more suggests a dissatisfaction with simply defining further the nature of the deficit, particularly as it relates to rehabilitation. Understanding the nature of the *deficit* is a necessary (Howard, 1999) but not sufficient condition for the development of effective and efficient treatments. The overarching goal in rehabilitation is to understand the nature of *adaptive change* (i.e., plasticity) and how best to harness its benefits through interventions.

LITERATURE SYNTHESIS

Literature Synthesis: Methods

As a first step toward directly addressing the nature of change, a literature synthesis was conducted to identify contemporary approaches and obtain a sample of representative treatment studies. Specific inclusion and exclusion criteria for a systematic bibliographical search were established a priori for accepting a study into the summary list. These criteria were developed so that the outcome of the search would reflect data-based projects that contribute to our knowledge of both language rehabilitation and theoretical models.

A sample of the treatment literature was collected by conducting electronic searches of the bibliographical databases *PsycInfo*, *MedLine*, and *Linguistics and Language Behavior Abstracts* (LLBA). A majority of the journals publishing works in the area of language and rehabilitation are indexed in these three databases. Searches in all three databases were limited to 1990–2000 publication dates. Keywords used for searching included *language, language disorders, aphasia, rehabilitation*, and *treatment*, and combinations of these terms.

Literature Synthesis: Results

This initial search yielded 388 references on PsycInfo, 112 references on MedLine, and 22 references on LLBA (522 references total). Only empirical treatment studies were accepted for the purposes of this review, and search results were reviewed manually to exclude review papers, book chapters, and other nonempirical reports. Studies that focused on mental or developmental disorders, or those that emphasized non-language cognitive issues were excluded based on predetermined criteria. Of the 522 references initially selected based on search terms and publication date, 44 studies met the additional inclusion–exclusion criteria.

It is important to note that many important treatment references and studies are not included in this particular search outcome, because reviews and chapters were excluded and some important references may have appeared in journals or other publications that were not indexed in the selected databases. The resulting list of 44 studies is far from comprehensive and perforce excludes many papers that have critically affected our field's thinking in the characterization of language rehabilitation. The final 44 studies are meant only as a sample of current trends in empirically based investigations of language rehabilitation. The reference, number of subjects, brief subject description, treatment description, and major finding for each of the 44 studies appear in Table 9.1.

The final step in this synthesis was to categorize the studies into groups that reflected similar underlying models and theoretical constructs. In some cases, a theoretical or clinical model was not explicitly described but was alluded to in the background and rationale of the study. In that case, an interpretation was based on the model given in studies that were conceptually similar. The studies in Table 9.1 are grouped based on six categories that emerged from this review. The six categories included *cognitive neuropsychological approaches, cognition and learning models, compensatory approaches, linguistic models, social approaches, and neurological approaches*. Studies derived from cognitive neuropsychological, linguistic, neurological, or social approaches to language rehabilitation were the most likely to specify explicitly the underlying model for the investigated treatment. Studies characterized as using a compensatory model had in common the emphasis that the treat-

TABLE 9.1. Summary of Reviewed Studies Applying Treatment Data to Models of Language Rehabilitation

Reference	N	Subject description	Treatment description	Results
			Cognitive neuropsychological approaches	
Alimonosa, McCloskey, Goodman-Schulman, & Sokol (1993)	1	Acquired dysgraphia due to left CVA in 64-year-old	Delayed copying and spelling to dictation	Improvement for trained but not untrained words
Behrmann & McLeod (1995)	1	Aphasia due to left parietal–occipital lesion in 46-year-old	Identification of both ends of letter strings	Improved performance for letter strings; no transfer to word recognition
Conway et al. (1998)	1	Phonological alexia and mixed agraphia due to left CVA in 50-year-old	Auditory Discrimination in Depth program (phonological awareness)	Improvement in nonlexical and lexical reading at follow-up
Crerar, Ellis, & Dean (1996)	14	Aphasia due to left CVA; ages 27–74 years	Sentence training in a computerized microworld	Ss who had verb training first improved more than Ss with preposition training first.
Deloche, Hannequin, Dordain, & Metz-Lutz (1997)	18	Aphasia due to left CVA; ages 22–76 years	Written therapy	Variety of outcomes observed for oral and written picture naming.
De Partz (1995)	1	Aphasia due to left CVA in a 64-year-old; impairment of graphemic buffer	Written lexical segmentation	Trained decomposable words improved more than nondecomposable.
Eales & Pring (1998)	4	Aphasia due to left CVA, ages 49–73 years	Lexical semantic treatment; individual and group treatment	Mildly impaired Ss showed improvement and generalization in individual treatment; severely impaired Ss showed generalization in group treatment.
Greenwald, Raymer, Richardson, & Rothi (1995)	2	Aphasia due to left CVA; ages 66 and 71 years	Phonological and visual-semantic cueing for picture-naming treatment	The two treatments resulted in greater improvement and generalization than simple rehearsal.

Reference	N	Population	Treatment	Result
Haendiges, Berndt, & Mitchum (1996)	1	Aphasia due to left CVA in 53-year-old	Training to derive thematic role information	Improvement and maintenance of active but not passive voice sentences
Hillis (1993)	1	Acquired dyslexia due to left temporoparietal traumatic lesion in 48-year-old	(1) Sublexical OPO compensation; (2) holistic processing; (3) word–picture matching	All treatments were somewhat successful.
Hillis (1998)	1	Aphasia due to TBI in 22-year-old	Semantic feature training and oral reading	Improvement for trained and untrained items.
Laicono, Allamano, & Capitani (1996)	2	Aphasia due to left CVA; ages 40 and 69 years	Phonemic and graphemic cueing	Items trained improved in picture-naming task.
Le Dorze & Pitts (1995)	1	Aphasia due to left CVA in a 67-year-old	Semantic and word form training	The two treatments resulted in greater improvement than naming without cueing.
Lesser & Algar (1995)	2	Aphasia due to left CVA; ages 49 and 80 and their caregivers	Provided conversational strategies based on conversational analysis and CN assessment of impairments	There was an increased use of successful strategies in subject–caregiver conversation.
Marshall, Pring, & Chiat (1998)	1	Aphasia due to left CVA in 52-year-old	Verb facilitation and semantic cueing	Verb treatment resulted in improved sentence production.
Micell, Amitrano, Capasso, & Caramazza (1996)	2	Aphasia due to left CVA; ages 38 and 60 years	Oral reading, repetition, and picture naming	Ss improved on trained items but there was no generalization to untrained items.
Mitchum, Haendiges, & Berndt (1995)	1	Aphasia due to left CVA in 47-year-old	Thematic mapping treatment	Improved and generalization to sentence comprehension with untreated verbs and written sentences
Weinrich, Boser, & McCall (1999)	1	Aphasia due to left CVA in 65-year-old	C-VIC: training of past, present, and future tense morphology	Improvement and generalization for regular verb tense morphology but not for irregular verbs
Weinrich, Shelton, McCall, & Cox (1997)	3	Aphasia due to left CVA; ages 44, 48, and 63 years	C-VIC: computerized sentence training	Ss were unsuccessful in generalizing to multisentence narrative task.

(continued)

TABLE 9.1. (*continued*)

Reference	N	Subject description	Treatment description	Results
			Cognition and learning models	
Brush & Camp (1998)	9	Memory and language impairment due to dementia (*n* = 7) or CVA (*n* = 2)	Spaced retrieval for specific information and strategies	7 of 9 Ss successfully learned trained information and strategies
Cherney (1995)	2	Aphasia due to left CVA; ages 25 and 42 years	Oral reading	Improved accuracy and speed for oral reading of trained items; generalization unclear
Hinckley & Craig (1998)	40	Aphasia due to left CVA; ages 19–78 years	Intensive treatment; individual and group	Ss improved more during intensive treatment.
Hinckley, Patterson, & Carr (2001)	12	Aphasia due to left CVA; ages 22–78 years	Context- and skills-based treatment	Context-based treatment resulted in improvements in trained task; skills-based treatment resulted in improvements in wider range of tasks.
Katz & Wertz (1992)	43	Aphasia due to single left CVA; ages 49–74 years	Programmed computerized reading activities	Computer reading treatment resulted in more improvement and generalization than computer stimulation or no treatment.
Katz & Wertz (1997)	55	Aphasia due to left CVA; ages 48–83 years	Programmed computerized reading activities	Computer reading treatment improved more than computer stimulation or no treatment, and generalized to other language modalities.
Mackenzie (1991)	4	Aphasia due to left CVA; ages 48–67 years	Intensive individual and group treatment	Ss improved during intensive treatment more than no treatment.
Mazzoni, Vista, Geri, & Avila (1995)	26	Aphasia due to left CVA; ages 59–76 years	General; nonspecified	Treated patients made significantly more improvement in expressive language than nontreated patients.

Study	N	Population	Treatment	Outcome
Penn, Jones, & Joffe (1996)	2	Aphasia due to left CVA; ages 19 and 70 years	Hierarchical discourse therapy	Improvement in discourse outcomes as a result of discourse-based treatment
Petheram (1996)	10	Aphasia due to left CVA; 46–77 years	Home-based computerized tasks; individualized	Some improvement in computer-based tasks; no generalization to standardized language batteries
Sugishita, Seki, Kabe, & Yunoki (1993)	15	Aphasia due to left CVA; ages 27–62 years	Traditional: oral repetition and copying	3 of 15 Ss improved in response to the two treatments
Tanemura (1999)	43	Aphasia due to left CVA; ages 48–69 years	Deblocking	Most improvement in comprehension modalities
			Compensatory approaches	
Avent, Edwards, Franco, & Lucero (1995)	3	Aphasia due to left CVA; ages 31, 27, and 56 years	Verbal and nonverbal treatment	Ss responded differentially to the two treatments
Fluharty (1993)	1	Surface dysgraphia due to left temporal lobe trauma in 27-year-old	Use of electronic dictionary	Improved spelling performance on trained and untrained words
Lott, Freidman, & Linebaugh (1994)	1	Phonological alexia due to left temporoparietal CVA in 67-year-old	Kinesthetic treatment: Copying letters in palm for letter-by-letter reading	Improvement on trained and untrained items
Shelton, Weinrich, McCall, & Cox (1996)	6	Global aphasia due to left CVA; ages 46–75 years	C-VIC: computerized visual communication system with iconic lexicon	3 of 6 Ss improved on verb training
Ward-Lornegan & Nicholas (1995)	1	Global aphasia due to left CVA; 61-year-old man	Back to the Drawing Board, PACE, and functional drawing	Improvement on standardized measures of language in global aphasia (BASA)
Yoshihata, Watamori, Chujo, & Masuyama (1998)	3	Severe aphasia due to left CVA; ages 54–63 years	Gesture and drawing training, and mode interchange training	Ss communicated most effectively after being specifically trained to change modalities.

(continued)

TABLE 9.1. (*continued*)

Reference	N	Subject description	Treatment description	Results
			Linguistic models	
Drew & Thompson (1999)	4	Aphasia due to left CVA; ages 47–59 years	Semantic and orthographical–phonological treatment	2 of 4 Ss improved and generalized as a result of semantic treatment; 2 of 4 Ss improved with phonological treatment
Jacobs & Thompson (2000)	4	Agrammatic aphasia due to left CVA, ages 39–79 years	Object-cleft and passive sentence training production and comprehension	Comprehension training generalized to production; sentence production training generalized to written sentence production
Thompson, Ballard, & Shapiro (1998)	3	Agrammatic aphasia due to left CVA, ages 29–68 years	Wh- movement object clefts or who question training	Improvements on who questions; various patterns of generalization observed
Thompson, Shapiro, Tait, Jacobs, & Schneider (1996)	7	Aphasia due to left CVA; ages 39–79 years	Argument/adjunct training; wh-morpheme training	Wh- question production improved and generalized to untrained items.
			Social approaches	
Burns, Dong, & Oehring (1995)	1	Aphasia due to left CVA in 72-year-old	Traditional versus family-based treatment	The two treatments were equally effective.
Hinckley, Packard, & Bardach (1995)	15	Aphasia due to CVA and TBI; ages 19–78 years	Brief, 2-day family education seminar in conference format	Improvement in home and social integration 6 months after intervention
			Neurological approaches	
Musso, Weiller, Kiebel, Mueller, Buelau, & Rijntjes (1999)	4	Wernicke's aphasia due to left CVA; ages 55–60 years	Intense auditory comprehension training	Showed functional brain reorganization as a result of treatment in serial PET scans

Note. BASA, Boston Assessment of Severe Aphasia drawing subtest; CN, cognitive neuropsychological; CVA, cerebrovascular accident; PET, positron emission tomography; OPO, Orthographic–Phonological Output; PACE, Promoting Aphasics' Communicative Effectiveness; TBI, traumatic brain injury.

ment exploited a strength to make up for a specific language impairment, for example, successful use of an electronic dictionary to compensate for surface dysgraphia (Fluharty, 1993). Studies included under the "compensatory" model heading did not elaborate any further discussion of possible underlying mechanisms for the treatment rationale or results.

A number of studies failed to identify a specific model type or name but liberally used terminology consistent with learning theory and approaches. Phraseology such as "stimulation programmed learning" and "computer-assisted learning" (Katz & Wertz, 1992; 1997), "individualized learning tasks" (Petheram, 1996), and "modeling" (Cherney, 1995) suggested the application of a general learning approach to the development of the treatment. In other cases, specific techniques derived from learning theory, such as spaced retrieval (Brush & Camp, 1998) or massed practice (Hinckley & Craig, 1998), were cited in the studies and warranted their inclusion among those studies applying cognitive/learning models. A summary of the goals, mechanisms of change, and treatment procedures for each model is shown in Table 9.2. Further details follow in the next section.

Cognitive neuropsychologically based treatment studies made up 43% of this sample of studies, and those either explicitly or implicitly using a cognitive/learning approach comprised 27% of the sample. Fourteen percent of the sample studies was based on compensatory models of treatment, 9% was derived from linguistic theory, 5% focused on social approaches to rehabilitation, and 2% (1 study) described a neurologically based outcome of treatment.

The number of studies in each category should not be interpreted as bearing on the relative importance or acceptance of any of the models. First, as previously mentioned, the sample of studies is necessarily restricted and nonexhaustive. It is likely that newer directions in the literature will be represented with fewer studies. On the other hand, aspects of language rehabilitation that have been the subject of study for decades, such as applying aspects of learning to treatment, have become so absorbed into our understanding of treatment in general that many important findings have already been established in the literature, certainly prior to 1990. Finally, the distribution of studies according to the six models most likely does not reflect patterns of actual clinical practice, which follows the demonstration of effective therapies in the empirical literature.

Evolution of the Models: Prior Classification Systems

This sampling of treatment research extends previous work describing the status of the aphasia rehabilitation literature for articles published

TABLE 9.2. Critical Components of Current Language Rehabilitation Models

	Cognitive neuropsychological model	Cognition and learning models	Linguistic models	Compensatory models	Social approaches	Neurological models
Goals	1. Reveal the components and processes of the cognitive system through manipulation (treatment). 2. Demonstrate the usefulness of functional localization for treatment.	1. Understand the nature of cognition and learning within a disordered system. 2. Apply basic concepts about cognition and learning to language rehabilitation.	1. Understand the structure of the language system based on impaired performances. 2. Apply linguistic concepts to the matching of stimuli and patient characteristics.	Identify profiles of language strengths and weaknesses, and use strengths to develop internal or external compensatory strategies.	Target the ability to function in the world by focusing on social circles.	Identify regions of the brain associated with specific abilities, change, and various prognoses.
Mechanism of change	Remediate impaired component or develop strategies that help to compensate for the deficit.	Normal or possibly specialized learning capabilities.	Remediate or compensate for impaired language structure.	Specific, identifiable compensation for impairment.	Change occurs as a result of positive social interactions.	Neurophysiological mechanisms of brain plasticity.
Treatment procedures	Repetition of specific tasks or cueing hierarchies that are derived from an in-depth assessment.	Incorporation and adaptation of specific techniques into the intervention.	Match linguistic characteristics of stimuli to nature of the deficit.	Problem-solving approach based on the individual's strengths and weaknesses.	Family or group treatment; community-based centers; communication partners.	Choice of treatments based on nonaffected brain regions.

Note. See text for further explanation.

192

between 1972 and 1991 (Horner, Loverso, & Rothi, 1994; Horner & Loverso, 1991). A total of 152 articles published in five major journals (*Clinical Aphasiology Conference Proceedings, Aphasiology, Brain and Language, Journal of Speech and Hearing Disorders,* and *Journal of Speech and Hearing Research*) during the 20-year period were reviewed in terms of six aphasia treatment models. Their six categories included the following models: stimulation–facilitation, modality, linguistic, processing, minor-hemisphere mediation, and functional communication. A description of each of these models is provided in Table 9.3.

Interestingly, a similar classification of treatment approaches was presented by Methe, Huber, and Paradis (1993). Specific treatment procedures within stimulation approaches, behaviorist approaches, the syndrome/symptom approach, language-oriented approaches, compensatory approaches, and pharmacotherapy were catalogued and described. Note that stimulation appears in both classifications. Horner and Loverso's modality approach appears to be similar to the syndrome/symptom approach. Linguistic and language-oriented approaches refer to the same set of treatment procedures, while minor-hemisphere mediation and functional communication are included under compensatory approaches in the Methe et al. (1993) classification. Those techniques included under processing in Horner and Loverso (1991) are variously assigned to either behaviorist or language-oriented approaches. Finally, Methe et al. (1993) include pharmacotherapy as a separate approach to rehabilitation.

Evolution of the Models: Comparison of Prior and Current Classification Systems

The descriptions of some of these models are similar to those identified in the present sample. The stimulation–facilitation model had its origin in the 1960s (Schuell, Jenkins, & Jimenez-Pabon, 1964; Duffy, 1986) and reflects the stimulus–response behavioral paradigm of the same era. These specific theoretical constructs are not to be found in the current treatment literature, although remnants of the treatment procedures that follow from them are still observed and are very much in use in clinical practice. There does not appear to be any equivalent or descendant of this theoretical model in the current literature.

Although the stimulation approach to aphasia treatment is the most frequently documented procedure among all aphasia treatment studies (Robey, 1998), it is perhaps one of the least satisfying, because it does not specify the nature of the tasks or stimuli to be used. Rather, the abundance and variety of tasks (or stimulation) are the key element that follows from its underlying assumptions about language.

TABLE 9.3. Summary of the Six Aphasia Treatment Models Described by Horner and Loverso (1991)

	Stimulation–facilitation model	Modality model	Linguistic model	Processing model	Minor hemisphere mediation model	Functional communication model
Premise	Language is linked to sensory and motor modalities but is not bound by them.	Language is both linked and bound by sensory and motor modalities.	Language is a specialized, rule-governed, cognitive activity.	Language is the operation of specific modules or components and their interaction.	Some language capability is possible within the minor hemisphere.	Communication is the use of language in real contexts.
Definition of aphasia	All modalities are disturbed in aphasia in the same manner and to the same degree.	Aphasia can be described in single- or multimodality terms.	Aphasia represents disrupted linguistic processes, such as impaired syntax.	Aphasia is the disturbance of specific modules or components in the system.	Aphasia is the result of impaired dominant-hemisphere functioning and preserved minor-hemisphere functioning.	Aphasia can result in ineffective communication in naturally occurring contexts.
Treatment procedures	Intense auditory stimulation or bombardment; a variety of material to elicit responses and produce stimulation.	Remediate and reorganize modalities; pair modality strengths with impairments to "deblock" performance.	Match linguistic characteristics of stimuli to linguistic nature of the impairment.	Restore or compensate for the language component deficits.	Use minor-hemisphere capabilities to facilitate communication.	Emphasize pragmatic functions and communication through any means necessary to complete normal activities.

A modality model is based on using preserved strengths to re-mediate or compensate for impairments. A primary treatment technique, "deblocking" (Osman-Sagi, 1993), is based on the assumption that there is a preserved representation of the target that can be accessed through an appropriate channel or modality. In a recent study (Tanemura, 1999), deblocking resulted in primarily comprehension modality improvements in a group of 43 aphasic subjects. The remediation or "deblocking" component of this approach is observed in certain treatment procedures that share an underlying assumption about modality-specific language abilities. Specifically, some cognitive neuropsychological treatments use preserved modalities as means to achieve remediation of the impaired component. For example, C-VIC, a computerized visual communication system, through the support of an iconic lexicon presented and manipu-lated through the stronger visual modality, can aid globally aphasic sub-jects in performing tasks that they would otherwise be unable to do (Weinrich, Boser, & McCall, 1999; Weinrich, Shelton, McCall, & Cox, 1997).

The linguistic model has successfully persisted over the last two or three decades. A linguistic approach to language rehabilitation focuses on the language system as a specialized unit, and its structures and pro-cesses. The application of linguistic theory to treatment has become more advanced, and the manner in which the stimuli and the patient's linguistic impairment should match is increasingly being specified (e.g., Thompson, Shapiro, Tait, Jacobs, & Schneider, 1996; Thompson, Bal-lard, & Shapiro, 1998).

The operation of modules or components in the processing model are earlier relations of what we now describe as the cognitive neuropsy-chological approach (Mitchum & Berndt, 1995). A model of the cogni-tive components and operations for a specific task is identified, and an in-depth assessment of a patient's abilities vis-à-vis the model is con-ducted. As a result, treatment can be specified to this functional localiza-tion. These approaches have become very specific, and quite a body of literature derived from this approach is developing.

The minor-hemisphere mediation model purports that rehabilita-tion can make use of abilities ascribed to the minor hemisphere to facili-tate communication (Horner & Fedor, 1983). Since that time, a number of studies documenting various patterns of brain plasticity have been completed, many of which demonstrate change in both major and minor hemispheres. A neurological model properly accommodates change throughout the brain but owes much to earlier work that evidenced the role of the right hemisphere in language abilities.

Finally, the functional communication model has become more de-veloped in the last 10 years as a result of advances in treatment research.

The functional approach originated in philosophical ideas about the nature of language and the reality and importance of everyday events (Holland & Hinckley, in press). It has developed from its original emphasis on pragmatic abilities and skills to the communication abilities required to perform everyday activities (Elman & Bernstein-Ellis, 1995). The functional approach has become an industry standard in that third-party payers emphasize "functional" outcomes and gains in their reimbursement patterns. Therefore, compensatory techniques that assist the patient in carrying out normal activities have often been clinically incorporated into functional treatment.

A further advance in the functional approach is the social approach, which capitalizes on the wealth of social interaction for improvement in communication and psychosocial status. These social approaches have also grown out of the use of language in context and emphasize the social contexts that are important to the patient as both a means and an end of rehabilitation efforts (e.g., Penn, Jones, & Joffe, 1996).

The six models identified by Horner and Loverso (1991) have naturally evolved over the last 10 years. Current models reflect this history and growth. Each of the six current categories of language treatment models are reviewed, with their representative studies from the literature synthesis, and augmented by additional literature pertinent to each model. The theoretical background and concepts of the mechanisms for change are described for each of the six models. These elements are particularly important for considering the nature of change and a theory of therapy. Representative assessment tools and treatment procedures are provided as examples.

COGNITIVE NEUROPSYCHOLOGICAL APPROACHES

Background

Cognitive neuropsychological (CN) approaches infer impairment of particular theorized components of the cognitive system based on profiles of task performances. These task performances can be integrated with neurological data to demonstrate behavioral patterns consistent with particular brain lesions (e.g., Roeltgen & Heilman, 1985). The logic of this approach is based on assumptions about double dissociations and the modularity of components, including information encapsulation and domain specificity (Mitchum & Berndt, 1995).

A CN approach to patient performance and specifically to rehabilitation has as a primary goal to inform our theoretical models about the structure of cognition and its disorders (e.g., Nickels, 1995; Martin,

Gagnon, Schwartz, Dell, & Saffran, 1996; Raymer et al., 1997). A secondary goal is to develop intervention techniques.

Many proponents of the CN approach have been skeptical about whether any contribution can effectively be made to rehabilitation theories and models (Baddeley, 1993; Hillis, 1993; Mitchum & Berndt, 1995). A CN approach does not specify the nature or mechanism of change. Mitchum and Berndt (1995, p. 6) wrote that the CN approach "has been criticized for the fact that even the most detailed analysis of the functional impairment fails to point to the most appropriate intervention strategy."

Mechanisms of Change

Two possible mechanisms for change have been suggested within the CN literature. It is possible that either the targeted component is strengthened as a result of training or some internal compensatory strategy is developed (e.g., Greenwald, Raymer, Richardson, & Rothi, 1995). These two ideas about how improvement comes about as a result of intervention are consistent with traditional ideas about the workings of change over the course of rehabilitation (Rothi & Horner, 1983). Indeed, some authors have suggested that the CN approach as currently carried out cannot make a contribution to theories of therapy (Hillis, 1998).

Assessment Tools and Techniques

The CN approach relies on comprehensive assessment of each individual subject; therefore, single-subject experimental design methodologies have been a primary mode of investigation. The development and use of complete and well-controlled assessment are a hallmark of the CN approach. Stimuli items are controlled for parameters such as word frequency, imageability, age of acquisition, and length, among others. These items are then presented within tasks that tap the theorized language components. The combination of tasks follows the logic of the approach and enables the experimenter to "zero in" on the impaired components and processes (e.g., Kerr, 1995).

Examples of the kinds of tasks used in a typical naming investigation include spoken word–picture matching, written word–picture matching, oral naming, written naming, oral reading, and repetition, with stimuli in each task carefully controlled. Input, output, and semantic components are assessed in detail. A typical standardized aphasia battery, for example, assesses certain gross aspects of language capabilities, without an in-depth analysis of the component processes that contribute to task completion. At the end of such an assessment, a clinician has little evidence for the origin of a picture-naming problem; it could be due to deficits in object recognition, phonological output lexicon, or semantic system impairments.

A commercially available assessment kit that offers such a set of controlled tasks is the Psycholinguistic Assessment of Language Processing in Aphasia (PALPA; Kay, Lesser, & Coltheart, 1992). This battery provides a set of 60 already created tasks that a clinician can use to delve into the more in-depth aspects of a patient's impairment. Although some of these tasks do have normative data, others do not, and the clinician must use these tasks descriptively.

Treatment Procedures

Treatment is individualized based on the in-depth assessment results. An overview of the common procedures used in CN treatment studies shows that the actual treatment methods are rarely, if ever, novel; the advantage of the CN approach is that the treatment methods are matched more specifically to the patient's impairment; therefore, a positive and perhaps more efficient outcome should result.

For example, naming treatments have commonly employed cueing hierarchies based on semantic cueing or phonological cueing of targets, depending on the nature of the subject's impairment (e.g., Le Dorze & Pitts, 1995). Both of these types of cueing approaches have long been applied in aphasia rehabilitation but perhaps much less discriminately.

Mapping treatment, a verb-based approach to therapy for sentence production, applies an essentially didactic method; that is, the patient is taught techniques for constructing sentence forms through the manipulation of written words on cards and similar materials. In this case, as in previous examples, the nature of the patient's impairment is much better described and matched to the therapy goal, but the actual treatment procedures incorporated are long-standing (Byng, Nickels, & Black, 1994; Schwartz, Saffran, Fink, Myers, & Martin, 1994).

COGNITION AND LEARNING MODELS

Background

Models of learning have actually been the basis for aphasia treatment since its onset (Backus, 1945), when special educators and speech-language pathologists were recruited to staff aphasia centers serving World War II veterans. Treatment for aphasia has always incorporated techniques from current theories of learning. For example, during the 1960s, various reinforcement patterns and even punishment was investigated as means to elicit verbal behavior change among adults with aphasia

(Brookshire, 1967; Holland, 1972). As theories of learning have changed over the decades, so have our treatment procedures.

Lately, the press for a theory of therapy has led some researchers to consider theories of learning as appropriate candidates for such a role (Ferguson, 1999). At present, this has amounted to a call for identification of the theory of learning that is being applied in any given treatment study. Others have gone further and explicitly aligned themselves with theories of skill acquisition (Hinckley, Patterson & Carr, 2001), suggesting parallels between normal language learning and the rehabilitation model (Basso, Burgio, & Prandoni, 1999; Ptak, Gutbrod, & Schnider, 1998).

It follows from such an approach that various cognitive abilities, such as attention, memory, and executive function, would be considered critical to the rehabilitation process. Indeed, a growing body of literature defines "aphasia" as an impairment of the relationship between language and attention, for example, and the various attentional deficits of aphasic patients have been documented (for a review, see Murray, 1999). Others have taken this a step further and suggested that intervention targeting cognitive abilities can result in language improvements (Helm-Estabrooks, 1998).

Mechanisms of Change

When we borrow techniques from theories of learning and skills acquisition, we are implicitly or explicitly assuming that the treatment process is a learning process. Because people with aphasia have been observed to improve their communication skills, we can probably deduce that adults with aphasia can learn language-related skills and strategies. Investigations of the word- and category-learning abilities of adults with aphasia suggest patterns characteristic of the type of aphasia and locus of lesion but confirm that such learning is possible. For example, Grossman and Carey (1987) showed that anterior aphasics learned the semantic characteristics of a new word better than they learned the syntactic use of the word and posterior aphasic patients had some difficulty acquiring the semantic borders of the word, but no difficulty with its syntactic characteristics.

Assessment Tools and Techniques

Unfortunately, many treatment studies that have relied on ideas borrowed directly from theories of learning have often not considered the cognitive abilities of the aphasic subjects in question. Most studies have assessed and described thoroughly only the language capabilities of the subjects. A notable exception is the work of Martin and Saffran (1999), in which the interrelatedness of language and working memory is investigated among aphasic adults.

Attentional assessments that may be useful with language-impaired subjects include the Test of Everyday Attention (Robertson, Ward, Rigeway, & Nimmo-Smith, 1994), the Paced Auditory Serial Addition Test (Gronwall, 1977), and the Stroop Test (Trenerry, DeBoe, & Leber, 1989). Memory tests often rely on verbal capabilities, such as the Rey Auditory Verbal Learning Test or even digit span tasks. Digit span recognition and pointing span tasks are available as subtests of the PALPA (Kay, Lesser, & Coltheart, 1992). A shortened version of the Rivermead Behavioral Memory Test (Wilson, Cockburn, & Baddeley, 1985) has been shown to be sensitive to memory deficits and insensitive to language deficits (Cockburn, Wilson, Baddeley, & Hiorns, 1990). Executive function tasks such as the Wisconsin Card Sorting Test (Grant & Berg, 1993) can also be useful for assessing the capabilities of language-impaired patients.

Raven's Colored Progressive Matrices (Raven, Court, & Raven, 1979) has been a widely used tool to assess the nonverbal reasoning abilities of adults with aphasia, all the more so because it is a component of the Western Aphasia Battery (Kertesz, 1982). This assessment, and others like it, tend to demonstrate the preserved nonverbal reasoning skills of adults with aphasia.

Treatment Procedures

Many treatment procedures are derived from a cognitive and learning approach; however, they are not often done so explicitly. For example, in the computerized treatment study of Katz and Wertz (1997), reference is made to programmed stimulation. This approach has been a part of our clinical procedures for some time and has its origin in learning theory (LaPointe, 1983).

More recently, direct intervention of attention has been identified as a possible treatment approach. Attentional treatment among aphasic adults has resulted in both improvement on auditory and visual attention tasks, with no generalization to other cognitive measures (Sturm & Willmes, 1991), and observable language improvement (Helm-Estabrooks, Connor, & Albert, 2000).

COMPENSATORY APPROACHES

Background

Compensatory approaches probably have as their origin a no-nonsense, problem-solving attitude toward coping with a communication disorder.

They also achieve the primary goal of a functional approach, in which effective message communication is prioritized over specific language component or modality performance.

Compensatory approaches assume that patients have preserved cognitive or other abilities with which they can learn strategies that enable them to accomplish communication tasks using alternative strategies. Message communication can be accomplished through drawing, gesture, or other alternative modalities. Electronic solutions can also help to achieve basic communication or to accomplish desirable tasks, such as e-mail, writing checks or letters, or ordering items over the Internet.

Mechanisms of Change

The use of a compensatory strategy can achieve a functional outcome and allows the individual to accomplish tasks that he or she would not otherwise be able to do. This occurs because it is assumed that the patient has the cognitive capability to retain the trained strategy and retrieve it at appropriate times. In some cases, the use of an alternative modality has been shown to facilitate production in the natural or primary mode. For example, Hanlon, Brown, and Gerstman (1990) showed that gesture can facilitate oral naming. Similarly, other strategies, such as drawing (Ward-Lornegan & Nicholas, 1995; Morgan & Helm-Estabrooks, 1987; Lyon & Helm-Estabrooks, 1987) and the use of augmentative or assistive electronic devices (Fluharty, 1993; Shelton, Weinrich, McCall, & Cox, 1996), often result in improvements in the area that was targeted for compensation. Thus, compensatory approaches may provide not only an avenue for effective communication but also a bridge that facilitates improvement in other language modalities.

Assessment Tools and Techniques

As with the cognition and learning approaches, the compensatory approach appears to rely quite heavily on the cognitive ability of the patient to actually learn and use these strategies, some of which can be quite complex and require a high degree of executive functioning. Given that assumption, it is surprising that studies investigating this approach have typically not assessed subjects' cognitive abilities other than to provide a language profile. Typically, language strengths and weaknesses are assessed so that appropriate strategies can be developed.

For example, in the Back to the Drawing Board technique, appropriate candidates should achieve a particular scoring criterion on the Boston Assessment of Severe Aphasia drawing subtest (BASA; Helm-Estabrooks, Ramsberger, Morgan, & Nicholas, 1989; Helm-Estabrooks

& Albert, 1991). Other compensatory approaches have not routinely specified exact criteria for candidacy.

Treatment Procedures

In the compensatory approach, preserved strengths are exploited to achieve communication. Using alternative visual representations for lexical items and combinations is a successful approach for some aphasia types (Goodenough-Trepagnier, 1995; Shelton et al., 1996). Nonverbal treatment, such as gesture, drawing, and their combinations, are also routine procedures (Avent, Edwards, Franco, & Lucero, 1995; Lott, Freidman, & Linebaugh, 1994; Yoshihata, Watamori, Chujo, & Masuyama, 1998). For patients with severe aphasia, direct training to address the ability to change from one alternative modality to another can be needed and successful (Yoshihata et al., 1998).

LINGUISTIC APPROACHES

Background

The field of linguistics has been a useful field of inquiry and application for aphasiology for decades (Jakobson, 1956; Goodglass & Blumstein, 1973). In that time, there has been a steady linguistic pursuit of aphasic deficits relative to linguistic constructs. Data from aphasic patients have been used as a basis to modify theoretical models (e.g., Grodzinsky, 1986; Cornell, Fromkin, & Mauner, 1993; Shapiro, 1997).

While many linguistically oriented studies delve into the nature of aphasic deficit, others have applied linguistic theory to the development of treatments. In particular, current linguistic approaches emphasize treatment for agrammatism, or the use of agrammatism as a model in which to test theoretical predictions (e.g., Caramazza & Miceli, 1991).

Assessment Tools and Techniques

A detailed analysis of performances on linguistics-based tasks is essential to the approach. Often, sentence–picture matching or production tasks serve as part of an initial assessment and/or baseline measures.

Use of grammatical structures in discourse is assessed using specific elicitation, coding, and analysis procedures. Picture description has been used as both an elicitation context (Whitworth, 1995) and a narrative discourse (Saffran, Berndt, & Schwartz, 1989). A key part of the logic in analyzing these treatments is whether generalization has occurred to other linguistic structures that are theoretically linked to the trained structure.

Treatment Procedures

In what has been dubbed "movement therapy," Thompson and colleagues (Jacobs & Thompson, 2000; Thompson, Ballard, & Shapiro, 1998; Thompson, Shapiro, Tait, Jacobs, & Schneider, 1996) have developed a technique for training movement of the noun phrase in a declarative sentence to produce *wh-* questions. This approach is based on the trace deletion hypothesis and Chomsky's government and binding theory. The linguistic theory predicts that movement for production of *who* questions, for example, should generalize to *what* questions, but not to *when* or *where* questions. These unique patterns of generalization have been documented in the Thompson et al. research. The treatment is conducted with the use of cue cards that have targeted pictures and sentence words. The client is guided through the movement of the appropriate words in the sentence to produce the target item. Thus far, these techniques have been very productive for the development of treatment procedures for agrammatism as well as confirmation of theoretical relationships.

SOCIAL APPROACHES

Background

The long-lasting psychosocial difficulties of living with chronic aphasia are well known and include depression, vocational loss or change, social isolation, family stress and adjustment, and reduction of leisure activities (Sarno, 1993). These psychosocial difficulties come about as a result of neurological and psychological changes within the individual and social changes within the family due to role reversals and adaptations (Gainotti, 1997). Social approaches constitute an aggressive effort on the part of interventionists to address these persistent and catastrophic changes.

A natural outgrowth of the functional approach's emphasis on communication effectiveness is inclusion of the social network in which communication occurs. Social approaches emphasize the social context of communication and therefore include caregivers and significant others, as well as social peers, with and without aphasia, as fundamental components of their procedures. The emphasis here, beyond the effective communication of the message, is the effective participation of the individual in social activities that are typical and appropriate.

An important relationship exists between social approaches to language rehabilitation and the disability movement (Worrall, 1992; Jordan & Kaiser, 1996). Proponents of the disability movement take exception to the typical rehabilitation goal of moving toward independence and would prefer to focus on autonomy—being in control of activities and the support necessary to accomplish them. The typical independence goals of rehabilitation are perceived as a move toward "cure" rather than acceptance of people as they are (French, 1993).

In such a framework, then, there is a focus on the consumer, and clinician and client work cooperatively to achieve goals set by and important to the client (Parr, 1996; Horton, Mudd, & Lane, 1998). An emphasis on consumer satisfaction is a real-world result of health care financial structure changes and competition among providers (Rao, Blosser, & Huffman, 1998). The change in viewpoint from "patient" as recipient of treatment chosen by the clinician, to "consumer and active partner" in rehabilitation efforts is evidenced by the developing interest in participant observation and ethnographic research approaches in aphasiology (Damico, Simmons-Mackie, Oelschlager, Elman, & Armstrong, 1999), and the development of consumer-oriented outcome tools (e.g., John, 1998). Indeed, discourse between the clinician and the client can be viewed as an institutionalized routine that may establish the role of the patient as a responder and recipient of treatment (Simmons-Mackie, 1999).

Mechanisms of Change

The social approach has as its goal changing the behavior and attitudes of those who interact with people with aphasia, as well as targeting behavioral change in the individual with aphasia. The attitudes and behaviors of friends and community members can be effectively changed with appropriate training in conversational techniques (Kagan, 1998; Lyon et al., 1997). Similarly, information and strategy training can impact both family relationships and communication effectiveness within the family unit (Williams, 1993; Lesser & Algar, 1995; Hinckley & Packard, 2001). These attitudinal and behavioral changes seem to be a result of direct training that is focused on the current knowledge and needs of significant others and community members. There also appears to be an effect of experience with people with aphasia; that is, the combination of information and training, as well as the experience of seeing people with aphasia communicate competently, creates a new view of the person, and this perceptual change is manifested in more supportive and natural conversational exchanges.

The individual with aphasia also changes as a result of socially based interventions. Important improvements in functional abilities, perceived wellness, and quality of life have been reported for various social treatments. Some socially based treatments, such as group therapy, are associated with specific language improvements and social benefits

(Elman & Bernstein-Ellis, 1999; Brumfitt & Sheeran, 1997). These kinds of outcomes are attributable to the sharing, social support, and peer interactions inherent in these interventions.

Although a theoretical base for learning in these approaches has not typically been explicitly explored, social cognitive theory (Bandura, 1977, 1978) may serve as a useful theoretical foundation for such work. In this model, social effects, such as modeling, persuasion, and stress reduction due to social support, figure prominently. According to the theory, specific sources of task choice and persistence that result in mastery can be manipulated in tested training procedures (Berry & West, 1993). Such a model might prove to be an important way to organize and test predictions within a social approach.

Assessment Tools and Techniques

Interactional analysis and, specifically, conversational analysis are important assessment tools for measuring the effects of social interventions. Such analyses can be conducted on both (or all) conversational partners and therefore capture the essence of this treatment approach. Conversational analysis has been successfully applied to document the unique communication situations of individuals and changes associated with communication training (Damico, Oelschlager, & Simmons-Mackie, 1999; Boles & Bombard, 1998; Galski, Tompkins, & Johnston, 1998).

Organized discourse assessments are also available and often take the form of checklists. Both the Discourse Abilities Profile (Terrell & Ripich, 1989) and the Assessment Profile of Pragmatic Linguistic Skills (Gerber & Gurland, 1989) offer structured analyses of narrative and conversational discourse. Successful interactions, breakdowns, and repairs can be monitored, and strategies for improving the ability to recognize and repair communication breakdowns can be a source of treatment goals and tasks.

Various rating scales and questionnaires are well suited to measurement of the perceived wellness and quality of life that are often outcomes of this approach. The Communicative Effectiveness Index (CETI; Lomas et al., 1989) is completed by the primary caregiver and captures his or her perceptions about the patient's ability to perform various communication tasks. Actual social activities and participation can be assessed through questionnaires such as the Community Integration Questionnaire (Willer, Rosenthal, Kreutzer, Gordon, & Rempel, 1993), which measures home and social integration as well as productivity. Assessment tools such as the McMaster Family Assessment Device (Epstein, Baldwin, & Bishop, 1983) and the Functional Life Scales (Sarno, Sarno, & Levita, 1973) assess participation in social activities and social functioning.

Treatment Procedures

The elements of this approach require the inclusion of family members, community members, or at least peers, in the treatment procedures. No social approaches can occur in individual therapy without the inclusion of family or important others. Family-based intervention often occurs in the home (Lesser & Algar, 1995; Burns, Dong, & Oehring, 1995), in groups (Kagan, 1998), or in educational seminars (Borenstein, Linell, & Wahrborg, 1987; Hinckley, Packard, & Bardach, 1995). Aphasia groups can offer peer training and support. Finally, aphasia centers can provide training to individuals with aphasia, their families, and community members within the center's programs (Kagan, 1998).

Family-based intervention procedures typically identify and target individualized communication strategies through clinician modeling, direct training, and supervised practice. The Communication Partners approach (Lyon et al., 1997) matches the individual with aphasia to a volunteer from the community, and the pair participate in shared interests, such as bowling or cooking. This approach foregrounds social participation and interaction above other traditional goals of aphasia intervention. Kagan (1998) has developed materials and specific conversational techniques to enable trained partners to support the communication effectiveness of individuals with severe aphasia.

NEUROLOGICAL APPROACHES

Background

These approaches emphasize the lesioned and spared areas of the brain and associated functions as a starting point for the rehabilitation process. This rehabilitation approach is probably most consistent with typical medical models that identify organic disease and impairment, and change to the underlying biological process is the goal and standard.

Mechanisms of Change

Brain plasticity and the neurobiological and behavioral processes that facilitate changes in brain activity patterns are the primary focus. In the last decade, the development of sophisticated brain imaging techniques has produced radical changes in our view of adult brain plasticity after injury. It has not been long since rehabilitation professionals believed that little or no change occurs in adult brain functioning. As Stein, Brailowsky, and Will (1995) wrote:

. . . most people, including physicians, neuroscientists (like ourselves), and health-care professionals, were taught to believe that brain injury is permanent, that the brain cannot be repaired. This explains why, until very recently, people with brain damage could receive virtually no treatment. The widely held belief that nothing can be done about brain damage leads to a vicious circle as far as patient care is concerned. If you presume that it is useless to waste time and precious medical resources trying to repair the brain, then nothing will be done. Since it is often the case that doing nothing effectively results in nothing changing, the belief in the inevitability of permanent brain damage goes unchallenged. (p. 3)

We now have a growing body of literature that documents various brain changes associated with treatment and recovery (Musso et al., 1999; Small, Flores, & Noll, 1998; Thulborn, Carpenter, & Just, 1999). It may also be that adults with aphasia who have good recovery experience a period of brain activation in the contralateral hemisphere, with a return of language functioning to the ipsilateral hemisphere, particularly to regions surrounding the original infarct (Cao, Vikingstad, George, Johnson, & Welch, 1999). These preliminary data may suggest ongoing brain changes years after an injury, with possible relationships to efficiency and automaticity of behavioral functioning.

Some evidence obtained in animal models of rehabilitation has suggested that plasticity mechanisms that occur as a result of practice and use may be sensitive to particular recovery times postonset (Schallert et al., 2000). The grand majority of literature (e.g., Robey, 1998) in aphasia treatment supports the general idea of more and faster improvements during the acute phase (typically defined as the first 3 months after onset). We do not know, however, if there are particularly good or bad outcomes associated with specific periods within the acute phase, or whether specific types or amounts of treatments might alter ultimate recovery and brain function patterns. For example, Murray and Holland (1995) found that patients with aphasia who received 45 minutes of didactic and conversational therapy during the first 4–6 weeks of inpatient rehabilitation performed less well at hospital discharge than a matched group of patients who received 15 minutes of conversational therapy. However, both groups performed equally well at 3-month follow-up. Additional research of this type might help us to determine beneficial amounts and types of treatments during particular recovery windows.

Assessment Tools and Techniques

Neuroimaging and electrophysiological techniques provide a window to brain functioning. Evoked potentials provide excellent temporal resolution, and brain mapping via electrophysiology can add the power of localization (Lauter, 1991). Wave form morphology can suggest typical or atypical processing patterns. These techniques have been investigated for both their potential prognostic power and their ability to assess change over time.

Functional neuroimaging such as positron emission tomography (PET) and functional magnetic resonance imaging (fMRI) are more broadly applied because of their strengths in localization and visualization of signs of brain activation patterns. In both cases, the underlying assumption is that brain regions that are active for task completion will have increased blood flow, and the correlates of this blood flow are used as the basis for measurement and imaging (George, Vikingstad, & Cao, 1998). The fMRI is particularly appealing because of its high spatial resolution and relative safety of use with neurologically impaired patients.

Treatment Procedures

The work of Naeser and colleagues (Frumkin, Palumbo, & Naeser, 1994) based treatment-type decisions on computed tomography (CT) scan and lesion analysis. They assessed the lesion extent and characteristics, and developed a rating scale. Those patients with scores in the lower range, signifying brain injury in areas necessary for speech recovery, were assigned to nonverbal treatment approaches, whereas high-scoring patients, who did not have damage in those critical areas, were recommended for verbal treatment. Lesion information is prioritized above other signs or prognosticators for treatment-type decisions. They confirmed their neurological observations by correlating good and poor response to the verbal and nonverbal treatment approaches to brain injuries as visualized on CT. They were able to identify several important brain regions that appeared related to response to treatment. In spite of the promise of this approach, it appears to be difficult to implement in actual clinical practice, because CT scans at the beginning of outpatient language intervention (2–3 months postonset) are typically not medically necessary, not covered by insurance, and therefore are unavailable to the practicing clinician for treatment decision making.

Some behavioral aphasia treatments have been based on the assumption that practice in forms typically handled by the minor hemisphere would facilitate or exploit preserved functions and result in improved language. Melodic Intonation Therapy (MIT) originally offered this rationale (Sparks, Helm-Estabrooks, & Albert, 1974; Albert, Sparks, & Helm-Estabrooks, 1973). In this treatment, patients intone common words and phrases, leading to functional speech production. Indeed, patients with right-hemisphere lesions were found to be poor candidates for this treatment. Recently, researchers (Carlomagno et al., 1997) found that activation in undamaged areas of the left hemisphere, including Broca's area, prefrontal cortex, angular and Heschl's gyri, and the temporal pole, were associated with word repetition with intonation, after a course of MIT training, and no increase in right hemisphere activation. This neurological finding may support the notion that use of preserved abilities such as intonation may facilitate recovery.

DISCUSSION

The six general treatment approaches described in this chapter can be compared and contrasted with regard to their theoretical foundation, the assumed mechanism for change, and the aspects of the cognitive system that are the focus of the treatment. When it comes to the development of a theory of therapy, these are perhaps the most important parameters to consider.

Theoretical foundations differ across these treatment models, and as mentioned throughout the chapter, many language rehabilitation studies and models do not necessarily specify the underlying theory. Linguistic and cognitive neuropsychological approaches are generally linked most explicitly to theoretical foundations, and recent work in these categories has used intervention results to shed light on theoretical models. In these cases, the theory provides testable predictions regarding both the stimuli used in treatment and the outcomes that should result according to the model.

Cognitive/learning and social approaches derive from sound models, but intervention researchers in these categories infrequently link their work to the theoretical foundations. The connections between the treatment procedures and the theoretical models are typically implicit, although often well-grounded. It would be helpful if work in these areas used the available theoretical bases to make predictions about the nature of intervention and expected outcomes. Such an approach would produce strong clinical results and have potential implications for the development of theoretical models related to intervention.

Compensatory and neurological approaches are based on even less obvious theoretical ground. Compensatory approaches tend to be practical, "no-nonsense" techniques for adapting to a communication problem. Neurological models are based on a strong body of clinical evidence that describes important relationships among brain functions, behavior, and recovery, but is not typically associated with any particular theoretical model. Treatment research in these areas tends to be the most descriptive.

Linguistic, CN, and neurological approaches are based on models of underlying language, cognition, or brain structures. Explorations of the results of interventions help us to determine which components are interrelated, or which behaviors should change relative to the internal structures.

Compensatory and social approaches do not require a structural proposal before treatment procedures are generated. Rather, the starting point is identification of a functional or social problem with a direct, ecologically valid link to a process addressing the problem. Applying the WHO ICIDH-2 (1999) framework, linguistic, CN, and neurological approaches emphasize the impairment, and compensatory and social approaches address the activity limitations and participation restrictions associated with aphasia.

Should practitioners simply identify whether an impairment, activity, or participation-based problem is a clinical priority and choose an intervention that addresses that level of functioning? (Of course, such a therapeutic process would require its own series of investigations on effectiveness). Instead of only a symptom-oriented classification of treatment procedures, such a view offers an outcome-oriented, decision-making process for clinicians—quite a benefit in today's results-oriented health care market.

However, we lose a view of the organization and operation of the mental representations that comprise the system we hope to improve, and continue on in the absence of detailed hypotheses about the nature of change. Linguistic and CN approaches focus on the language and/or cognitive system components specifically relevant to language production and processing, typically without considering other cognitive or social factors (Parisi, 1985). Similarly, compensatory and social approaches can be equally myopic in regard to language and cognitive components. All of these aspects of the affected individual—language, cognition, and the social system—contribute to change and improvement. A "levels" approach such as the ICIDH-2 framework risks continued segmentation of parts of the individual.

Finally, we are no further along in the identification of theories that can explain and predict the mechanisms of change. A review of Table 9.2 reveals that the two approaches specifying change mechanisms in greatest detail are cognitive/learning and neurological theories. CN and linguistic approaches, although they differ in treatment tasks and stimuli, are not different in regard to the processes that subserve learning and change. Compensatory models and social approaches identify the externally observable behavior or support that facilitates improvement, without hypothesizing about requisite internal workings.

Cognitive/learning approaches are based on theories of learning and skill acquisition that detail the cognitive mechanisms of change. Similarly, neurological approaches are built on neurochemical and biological observations related to behavioral change.

The theories underlying these two approaches, then, may offer the best hope for explicating rehabilitation. Indeed, learning mechanisms specified in these learning models apply wherever change is observed and are therefore equally relevant to change that comes as a result of linguistic, CN, compensatory, or social approaches. A careful consideration of these approaches may demonstrate their potential usefulness for a theory of therapy.

FUTURE RESEARCH NEEDS

As the focus of rehabilitation research moves toward the mechanisms of change, underlying similarities between the six approaches described in this chapter may become more apparent. Establishing the commonalities among intervention types will enable us to specify in new ways the characteristics and procedures that make certain treatments unique in their mechanisms and outcomes. Two treatments may share the rationale that practice on a specific skill will increase the strength of associations and result in an overall improvement in the targeted skill. However, the means of achieving this goal may differ in the two treatments. One treatment may target linguistically relevant stimuli within sentences, for example, while another may target didactic strategies for sentence construction, without deriving stimulus choices from linguistic theory. Conceptualizing differences in treatment strategies in this way will alert us to the need to assess outcomes of various types and help us create research projects that can detect more sensitive differences in treatment outcomes as predictable differences in treatment procedures. This philosophical shift in emphasis of treatment research is necessary to achieve the goal of determining the treatment of choice for any particular individual with a language disorder.

A shared perspective on treatment procedures should be extended to different etiologies, language disorders, and severities. Different treatment approaches and rationales have been used in treatments for aphasia versus cognitive–linguistic disorder due to traumatic brain injury. Whereas linguistic impairments have been emphasized in one approach, cognitive impairments have been emphasized in the other. Yet in both disorders we observe cognitive and linguistic impairments. A theoretical perspective on the mechanisms underlying change would provide both a unification of certain treatment approaches and better specification as to which activities result in which types of outcomes for various populations. Finally, a disproportionate amount of clinical research has focused on procedures to use with persons who have severe and moderate aphasia. Individuals with mild aphasia, although able to do basic "survival" communication skills, may be the ones with the best chance of returning to work or otherwise reducing the burden of disability on society overall. With regard to persons with traumatic brain injury (TBI), vocational rehabilitation has been an important topic. While part of this difference lies in the typical age distribution of the individuals affected by stroke and TBI, therapy from a theory of change and skills acquisition perspectives should be applicable to a variety of disorder groups and might offer the opportunity to direct research to multiple populations and severity levels in theoretically cohesive ways.

This can be accomplished when treatment research includes various levels and types of outcome measurements within the research designs. Much of the existing rehabilitation literature is based on the use of specific assessment tools that reflect the single underlying theory or predicted result, without testing a broad range of possible outcomes. The WHO ICIDH-2 framework has encouraged the examination of change on each of the three levels, impairment, activity, and participation, rather than just measuring potential changes in impairment by a standardized aphasia battery. Generalization of targeted behaviors should continue to be a major focus in treatment research, particularly because various theories about change might offer different predictions about generalization patterns. Finally, treatment research should include more measurement of the efficiency of response. In a time-pressured world, accurate performance that requires abnormally long periods of response time may not be functional, and treatment should take into account the viability as well as the accuracy of the speed of response.

With all of these treatment research questions to pursue, we are faced with a harsh reality about the resources available for treatment. We must not only work toward determining which treatment for whom but also ask questions. How fast can we do it? When is the best time for the treatment in relation to onset? In what format can it be accomplished most efficiently—individual therapy, group therapy, and/or home practice? Can certain aspects of efficient treatment programs be provided by support personnel? To accomplish these goals, researchers should apply theoretical models about learning and tap into the resources of learning and change developed in other fields. Models of second-language acquisition and other skills theories will provide us with a foundation of testable predictions and give future research in language rehabilitation a fresh perspective.

SUMMARY

Important developments in the empirical and theoretical bases for rehabilitation have been achieved over the last 55 years. A sample of the current language treatment literature yielded six descriptive categories of treatment approaches, differentiated by their emphases on various aspects of the communication process and the degree to which they are founded on theoretical predictions. They can be coherently linked by emphasizing the nature of change rather than the nature of the deficit. It is argued that cognitive/learning theories, in conjunction with neurological evidence, offer the best current step toward a theory of therapy.

ACKNOWLEDGMENTS

This work was supported in part by a grant from the James S. McDonnell Foundation (JSMF 97-44, Pilot Studies in Cognitive Rehabilitation Research) and by a Research and Creative Scholarship Grant from the University of South Florida.

REFERENCES

Albert, M., Sparks, R., & Helm-Estabrooks, N. (1973). Melodic intonation therapy for aphasia. *Archives of Neurology, 29,* 130–131.

Aliminosa, D., McCloskey, M., Goodman-Schulman, R., & Sokol, S. M. (1993). Remediation of an acquired dysgraphia as a technique for testing interpretations of deficits. *Aphasiology, 7,* 55–69.

Avent, J, R., Edwards, D. J., Franco, C. R., & Lucero, C. J. (1995). A verbal and nonverbal treatment comparison study in aphasia. *Aphasiology, 9,* 295–303.

Backus, O. (1945). The rehabilitation of aphasic veterans. *Journal of Speech Disorders, 10,* 149–155.

Baddeley, A. (1993). A theory of rehabilitation without a model of learning is a vehicle without an engine: A comment on Caramazza and Hillis. *Neuropsychological Rehabilitation, 3,* 235–244.

Bandura, A. (1977). Self-efficacy: Toward a unifying theory of behavioral change. *Psychological Review, 84,* 191–215.

Bandura, A. (1978). The self system in reciprocal determinism. *American Psychologist, 77,* 344–358.

Basso, A., Burgio, F., & Prandoni, P. (1999). Acquisition of output irregular orthographic representations in normal adults: An experimental study. *Journal of the International Neuropsychological Society, 5,* 405–412.

Behrmann, M., & McLeod, J. (1995). Rehabilitation for pure alexia: Efficacy of therapy and implications for models of normal word recognition. *Neuropsychological Rehabilitation, 5,* 149–180.

Berry, J. M., & West, R. L. (1993). Cognitive self efficacy in relation to personal mastery and goal setting across the lifespan. *International Journal of Behavioral Development, 16,* 351–379.

Boles, L., & Bombard, T. (1998). Conversational discourse analysis: Appropriate and useful sample sizes. *Aphasiology, 12,* 547–560.

Borenstein, P., Linell, S., & Wahrborg, P. (1987). An innovative therapeutic program for aphasia patients and their relatives. *Scandinavian Journal of Rehabilitation Medicine, 19,* 51–56.

Brookshire, R. H. (1967). Speech pathology and the experimental analysis of behavior. *Journal of Speech and Hearing Disorders, 32,* 215–221.

Brumfitt, S. M., & Sheeran, P. (1997). An evaluation of short-term group therapy for people with aphasia. *Disability and Rehabilitation, 19,* 221–230.

Brush, J. A., & Camp, C. J. (1998). Using spaced retrieval as an intervention during speech–language therapy. *Clinical Gerontologist, 19,* 51–64.

Burns, M. S., Dong, K. Y., & Oehring, A. K. (1995). Family involvement in the treatment of aphasia. *Topics in Stroke Rehabilitation, 2,* 68–77.

Byng, S., & Black, M. (1995). What makes a therapy?: Some parameters of therapeutic intervention in aphasia. *European Journal of Disorders of Communication, 30,* 303–316.

Byng, S., Nickels, L., & Black, M. (1994). Replicating therapy for mapping deficits in agrammatism: Remapping the deficit? *Aphasiology, 8,* 315–341.

Cao, Y., Vikingstad, E. M., George, K. P., Johnson, A. F., & Welch, K. M. A. (1999). Cortical language activation in stroke patients recovering from aphasia using functional MRI. *Stroke, 30,* 2331–2340.

Caramazza, A., & Miceli, G. (1991). Selective impairment of thematic role assignment in sentence processing. *Brain and Language, 41,* 402–436.

Carlomagno, S., Van Eeckhout, P., Blasi, V., Belin, P., Samson, Y., & Deloche, G. (1997). The impact of functional neuroimaging methods on the development of a theory for cognitive remediation. *Neuropsychological Rehabilitation, 7,* 311–326.

Cherney, L. R. (1995). Efficacy of oral reading in the treatment of two patients with chronic Broca's aphasia. *Topics in Stroke Rehabilitation, 2,* 57–67.

Cockburn, J., Wilson, B., Baddeley, A., & Hiorns, R. (1990). Assessing everyday memory in patients with dysphasia. *British Journal of Clinical Psychology, 29,* 353–360.

Conway, T. W., Heilman, P., Rothi, L. J. G., Alexander, A. W., Adair, J., Crosson, B. A., & Heilman, K. M. (1998). Treatment of a case of phonological alexia with agraphia using the Auditory Discrimination in Depth (ADD) program. *Journal of the International Neurological Society, 4,* 608–620.

Cornell, T. L., Fromkin, V. A., & Mauner, G. (1993). A linguistic approach to language processing in Broca's aphasia: A paradox resolved. *Current Directions in Psychological Science, 2,* 47–52.

Crerar, M. A., Ellis, A. W., & Dean, E. C. (1996). Remediation of sentence processing deficits in aphasia using a computer-based microworld. *Brain and Language, 52,* 229–275.

Damico, J. S., Oelschlaeger, M., & Simmons-Mackie, N. (1999). Qualitative methods in aphasia research: Conversation analysis. *Aphasiology, 13,* 667–679.

Damico, J. S., Simmons-Mackie, N., Oelschlaeger, M., Elman, R., & Armstrong, E. (1999). Qualitative methods in aphasia research: Basic issues. *Aphasiology, 13,* 651–665.

Deloche, G., Hannequin, D., Dordain, M., & Metz-Lutz, M. (1997). Diversity of patterns of improvement in confrontation naming rehabilitation: Some tentative hypotheses. *Journal of Communication Disorders, 30,* 11–22.

De Partz, M. (1995). Deficit of the graphemic buffer: Effects of a written lexical segmentation strategy. *Neuropsychological Rehabilitation, 5,* 129–147.

Drew, R. L., & Thompson, C. K. (1999). Model-based semantic treatment for naming deficits in aphasia. *Journal of Speech, Language, and Hearing Research, 42,* 972–989.

Duffy, J. R. (1986). Schuell's stimulation approach to rehabilitation. In R. Chapey (Ed.), *Language intervention strategies in adult aphasia.* Baltimore: Williams & Wilkins.

Eales, C., & Pring, T. (1998). Using individual and group therapy to remediate word finding difficulties. *Aphasiology, 12,* 913–918.

Elman, R., & Bernstein-Ellis, E. (1995). What is functional? *American Journal of Speech–Language Pathology, 4,* 115–117.

Elman, R., & Bernstein-Ellis, E. (1999). The efficacy of group communication treatment in adults with chronic aphasia. *Journal of Speech, Language, and Hearing Research, 42,* 411–419.

Epstein, N. B., Baldwin, L. M., & Bishop, D. S. (1983). The McMaster Family Assessment Device. *Journal of Marital and Family Therapy, 9,* 171–180.

Ferguson, A. (1999). Learning in aphasia therapy: It's not so much what you do, but how you do it! *Aphasiology, 13,* 125–132.

Fluharty, G. (1993). Use of an electronic dictionary to compensate for surface dysgraphia. *Journal of Cognitive Rehabilitation, 11,* 28–30.

French, S. (1993). What's so great about independence? In J. Swain, V. Finkelstein, S. French, & M. Olver (Eds.), *Disabling barriers—Enabling environments.* London: Open University Press.

Frumkin, N. L., Palumbo, C. L., & Naeser, M. A. (1994). Brain imaging and its application to aphasia rehabilitation: CT and MRI. In R. Chapey (Ed.), *Language intervention strategies in adult aphasia.* Baltimore: Williams & Wilkins.

Gainotti, G. (1997). Emotional, psychological and psychosocial problems of aphasic patients: An introduction. *Aphasiology, 11,* 635–650.

Galski, T., Tompkins, C., & Johnston, M. V. (1998). Competence in discourse as a measure of social integration and quality of life in persons with traumatic brain injury. *Brain Injury, 12,* 769–782.

George, K. P., Vikingstad, E. M., & Cao, Y. (1998). Brain imaging in neurocommunicative disorders. In A. F. Johnson & B. H. Jacobson (Eds.), *Medical speech–language pathology: A practitioner's guide.* New York: Thieme.

Gerber, S. K., & Gurland, G. B. (1989). Applied pragmatics in the assessment of aphasia. *Seminars in Speech and Language, 10,* 14–25.

Goodenough-Trepagnier, C. (1995). Visual analogue communication: An avenue of investigation and rehabilitation of severe aphasia. *Aphasiology, 9,* 321–341.

Goodglass, H., & Blumstein, S. (1973). *Psycholinguistics and aphasia.* Baltimore: Johns Hopkins Press.

Grant, D. A., & Berg, E. A. (1993). *Wisconsin Card Sorting Test.* Los Angeles: Western Psychological Services.

Greenwald, M. L., Raymer, A. M., Richardson, M. E., & Rothi, L. J. G. (1995). Contrasting treatments for severe impairments of picture naming. *Neuropsychological Rehabilitation, 5,* 17–49.

Grodzinsky, Y. (1996). Language deficits and the theory of syntax. *Brain and Language, 27,* 135–159.

Gronwall, D. M. A. (1977). Paced Auditory Serial Addition Task: A measure of recovery from concussion. *Perceptual and Motor Skills, 44,* 367–373.

Grossman, M., & Carey, S. (1987). Selective word learning deficits in aphasia. *Brain and Language, 32*, 306–324.

Haendiges, A. N., Berndt, R. S., & Mitchum, C. C. (1996). Assessing the elements contributing to a "mapping" deficit: A targeted treatment study. *Brain and Language, 52*, 276–302.

Hanlon, R. E., Brown, J. W., & Gerstman, L. J. (1990). Enhancement of naming in nonfluent aphasia through gesture. *Brain and Language, 38*, 298–314.

Helm-Estabrooks, N. (1998). A "cognitive" approach to treatment of an aphasic patient. In N. Helm-Estabrooks & A. L. Holland (Eds.), *Approaches to the treatment of aphasia.* San Diego: Singular.

Helm-Estabrooks, N., & Albert, M. L. (1991). *Manual of aphasia therapy.* Austin, TX: Pro-Ed.

Helm-Estabrooks, N., Connor, L. T., & Albert, M. L. (2000, October). *Training attention to improve auditory comprehension in aphasia.* Paper presented at the meeting of the Academy of Aphasia, Montreal, Quebec, Canada.

Helm-Estabrooks, N., Ramsberger, G., Morgan, A., & Nicholas, M. (1989). *Boston Assessment of Severe Aphasia.* San Antonio, TX: Special Press.

Hillis, A. E. (1993). The role of models of language processing in rehabilitation of language impairments. *Aphasiology, 7*, 5–26.

Hillis, A. E. (1998). Treatment of naming disorders: New issues regarding old therapies. *Journal of the International Neuropsychological Society, 4*, 648–660.

Hinckley, J. J., & Craig, H. K. (1998). Influence of rate of treatment on the naming abilities of adults with chronic aphasia. *Aphasiology, 12*, 989–1006.

Hinckley, J. J., & Packard, M. E. W. (2001). Family education seminars and social functioning of adults with chronic aphasia. *Journal of Communication Disorders, 34*, 241–254..

Hinckley, J. J., Packard, M. E. W., & Bardach, L. G. (1995). Alternative family education programming for adults with chronic aphasia. *Topics in Stroke Rehabilitation, 2*, 53–63.

Hinckley, J. J., Patterson, J. P., & Carr, T. H. (2001). Differential effects of context- and skill-based treatment: Preliminary findings. *Aphasiology, 15*, 463–476.

Holland, A. (1972). Case studies in aphasia rehabilitation. *Journal of Speech and Hearing Disorders, 37*, 3–10.

Holland, A. L., Fromm, D. S., De Ruyter, F., & Stein, M. (1996). Treatment efficacy: Aphasia. *Journal of Speech and Hearing Research, 39*, S27–S36.

Holland, A. L., & Hinckley, J. J. (in press). Assessment and treatment of pragmatic aspects of communication in aphasia. In A. E. Hillis (Ed.), *Handbook on adult language disorders: Integrating cognitive neuropsychology, neurology, and rehabilitation.* Philadelphia: Psychology Press.

Horner, J., & Fedor, K. H. (1983). Measuring aphasia treatment effects: Large-group, small-group, and single-subject studies. In F. Plum (Ed.), *Language, communication, and the brain.* New York: Raven Press.

Horner, J., & Loverso, F. L. (1991). Models of aphasia treatment in *Clinical Aphasiology* 1972–1988. In T. E. Prescott (Ed.), *Clinical aphasiology,* (pp. 61–75). Austin, TX: Pro-Ed.

Horner, J., Loverso, F. L., & Rothi, L. G. (1994). Models of aphasia treatment. In R. Chapey (Ed.), *Language intervention strategies in adult aphasia.* Baltimore: Williams & Wilkins.

Horton, S., Mudd, D., & Lane, J. (1998). Is anyone speaking my language? *International Journal of Language and Communication Disorders, 33*(Suppl.), 126–133.

Howard, D. (1999). Learning theory is not enough. *Aphasiology, 13,* 140–143.

Jacobs, B. J., & Thompson, C. K. (2000). Cross-modal generalization effects of training noncanonical sentence comprehension and production in agrammatic aphasia. *Journal of Speech, Language, and Hearing Research, 43,* 5–20.

Jakobson, R. (1956). Two aspects of language and two types of aphasic disturbances. In R. Jakobson & M. Halle (Eds.), *Fundamentals of language.* The Hague: Mouton.

John, A. (1998). Measuring client and career perspectives. *International Journal of Language and Communication Disorders, 33*(Suppl.), 132–137.

Jordan, L., & Kaiser, W. (1996). *Aphasia—A social approach.* London: Chapman & Hall.

Kagan, A. (1995). Family perspectives from three aphasia centers in Ontario, Canada. *Topics in Stroke Rehabilitation, 2,* 33–52.

Kagan, A. (1998). Supported conversation for adults with aphasia: Methods and resources for training conversation partners. *Aphasiology, 12,* 816–831.

Katz, R. C., & Wertz, R. T. (1992). Computerized hierarchical reading treatment in aphasia. *Aphasiology, 6,* 165–177.

Katz, R. C., & Wertz, R. T. (1997). The efficacy of computer-provided reading treatment for chronic aphasic adults. *Journal of Speech and Hearing Research, 40,* 493–507.

Kay, J., Lesser, R., & Coltheart, M. (1992). *Psycholinguistic assessments of language processing in aphasia.* Philadelphia: Psychology Press.

Kerr, C. (1995). Dysnomia following traumatic brain injury: An information-processing approach to assessment. *Brain Injury, 9,* 777–796.

Kertesz, A. (1982). *Western Aphasia Battery.* New York: Grune & Stratton.

Laiacona, M., Allamano, N., & Capitani, E. (1996). Performance consistency in picture naming: A study of the rehabilitation effect on two aphasic patients. *Journal of Clinical and Experimental Neuropsychology, 18,* 923–933.

LaPointe, L. L. (1983). Aphasia intervention with adults: Historical, present, and future approaches. *ASHA Reports, 12,* 127–136.

Lauter, J. L. (1991). Visions of speech and language: Noninvasive imaging techniques and their applications to the study of human communication. In H. Winitz (Ed.), *Human communication and its disorders: A review.* Timonium, MD: York Press.

Le Dorze, G., & Pitts, C. (1995). A case study evaluation of the effects of different techniques for the treatment of anomia. *Neuropsychological Rehabilitation, 5,* 51–65.

Lesser, R., & Algar, L. (1995). Towards combining the cognitive neuropsychological and the pragmatic in aphasia therapy. *Neuropsychological Rehabilitation, 5,* 67–92.

Lomas, J., Pickard, L., Bester, S., Elbard, H., Finalyson, A., & Zoghabib, C. (1989). The communicative effectiveness index: Development and psychometric evaluation of a functional communication measure for adult aphasia. *Journal of Speech and Hearing Disorders, 54,* 113–124.

Lott, S. N., Freidman, R. B., & Linebaugh, C. W. (1994). Rationale and efficacy of a tactile–kinaesthetic treatment for alexia. *Aphasiology, 8,* 181–195.

Lyon, J., & Helm-Estabrooks, N. (1987). Drawing: Its communicative significance for expressively restricted aphasic adults. *Topics in Language Disorders, 8,* 61–71.

Lyon, J. G., Cariski, D., Keisler, L., Rosenbek, J., Levine, R., Kumpula, J., Ryff, C., Coyne, S., & Blanc, M. (1997). Communication partners: Enhancing participation in life and communication for adults with aphasia in natural settings. *Aphasiology, 11,* 693–708.

Mackenzie, C. (1991). Four weeks of intensive aphasia treatment and four weeks of no treatment. *Aphasiology, 5,* 435–437.

Marshall, J., Pring, T., & Chiat, S. (1998). Verb retrieval and sentence production in aphasia. *Brain and Language, 63,* 159–183.

Martin, N., Gagnon, D. A., Schwartz, M. F., Dell, G. S., & Saffran, E. M. (1996). Phonological facilitation of semantic errors in normal and aphasic speakers. *Language and Cognitive Processes, 11,* 257–282.

Martin, N., & Saffran, E. M. (1999). Effects of word processing and short-term memory deficits on verbal learning: Evidence from aphasia. *International Journal of Psychology, 34,* 339–346.

Mazzoni, M., Vista, M., Geri, E., & Avila, L. (1995). Comparison of language recovery in rehabilitated and matched, non-rehabilitated aphasic patients. *Aphasiology, 9,* 553–563.

Methe, S., Huber, W., & Paradis, M. (1993). Inventory and classification of rehabilitation methods. In M. Paradis (Ed.), *Foundations of aphasia rehabilitation.* New York: Pergamon Press.

Micell, G., Amitrano, A., Capasso, R., & Caramazza, A. (1996). The treatment of anomia resulting from output lexical damage: Analysis of two cases. *Brain and Language, 52,* 150–174.

Mitchum, C. C., & Berndt, R. S. (1995). The cognitive neuropsychological approach to treatment of language disorders. *Neuropsychological Rehabilitation, 5,* 1–16.

Mitchum, C. C., Haendiges, A. N., & Berndt, R. S. (1995). Treatment of thematic mapping in sentence comprehension: Implications for normal processing. *Cognitive Neuropsychology, 12,* 503–547.

Morgan, A. L. R., & Helm-Estabrooks, N. (1987). Back to the Drawing Board: A treatment program for nonverbal aphasic patients. In R. H. Brookshire (Ed.), *Clinical aphasiology* (Vol. 17). Minneapolis: BRK Publishers.

Murray, L. L. (1999). Attention and aphasia: Theory, research and clinical implications. *Aphasiology, 13,* 91–111.

Murray, L. L., & Holland, A. L. (1995). The language recovery of acutely aphasic patients receiving different therapy regimens. *Aphasiology, 9,* 387–405.

Musso, M., Weiller, C., Kiebel, S., Mueller, S. P., Buelau, P., & Rijntjes, M. (1999). Training-induced brain plasticity in aphasia. *Brain, 122,* 1781–1790.

Nickels, L. (1995). Getting it right?: Using aphasic naming errors to evaluate theoretical models of spoken word recognition. *Language and Cognitive Processes, 10,* 13–45.

Osman-Sagi, J. (1993). Psychological mechanisms of speech rehabilitation in aphasic patients. *Acta Neurologica, 56,* 85–90.

Parisi, D. (1985). A procedural approach to the study of aphasia. *Brain and Language, 26,* 1–13.

Parr, S. (1996). Everyday literacy in aphasia: Radical approaches to functional assessment and therapy. *Aphasiology, 10,* 469–503.

Penn, C., Jones, D., & Joffe, V. (1996). Hierarchical discourse therapy: A method for the mild patient. *Aphasiology, 11,* 601–613.

Petheram, B. (1996). Exploring the home-based use of microcomputers in aphasia therapy. *Aphasiology, 10,* 267–282.

Petheram, B., & Parr, S. (1998). Diversity in aphasiology: Crisis or increasing competence? *Aphasiology, 12,* 435–447.

Ptak, R., Gutbrod, K., & Schnider, A. (1998). Association learning in the acute confusional state. *Journal of Neurology, Neurosurgery and Psychiatry, 65,* 390–392.

Rao, P., Blosser, J., & Huffman, N. P. (1998). Measuring consumer satisfaction. In C. Frattali (Ed.), *Measuring outcomes in speech–language pathology.* New York: Thieme.

Raven, J. C., Court, J. H., & Raven, J. (1979). *Manual for Raven's Progressive Matrices and Vocabulary Scales.* London: Lewis.

Raymer, A. M., Foundas, A. L., Maher, L. M., Greenwald, M. L., Morris, M., Rothi, L. J. G., & Heilman, K. M. (1997). Cognitive neuropsychological analysis and neuroanatomic correlates in a case of acute anomia. *Brain and Language, 58,* 137–156.

Robertson, I. H., Ward, T., Ridgeway, V., & Nimmo-Smith, I. (1994). *Test of Everyday Attention.* Gaylord, MI: Northern Speech Services.

Robey, R. R. (1994). The efficacy of treatment for aphasic persons: A meta-analysis. *Brain and Language, 47,* 585–608.

Robey, R. R. (1998). A meta-analysis of clinical outcomes in the treatment of aphasia. *Journal of Speech, Language, and Hearing Research, 41,* 172–187.

Roeltgen, D. P., & Heilman, K. M. (1985). Review of agraphia and a proposal for an anatomically-based neuropsychological model of writing. *Applied Psycholinguistics, 6,* 205–230.

Rothi, L. J., & Horner, J. (1983). Restitution and substitution: Two theories of recovery with application to neurobehavioral treatment. *Journal of Clinical Neuropsychology, 5,* 73–81.

Saffran, E. M., Berndt, R. S., & Schwartz, M. F. (1989). The quantitative analysis of agrammatic production: Procedure and data. *Brain and Language, 10,* 282–297.

Sarno, J. E., Sarno, M. T., & Levita, E. (1973). The Functional Life Scale. *Archives of Physical Medicine and Rehabilitation, 54,* 214–220.

Sarno, M. T. (1993). Aphasia rehabilitation: Psychosocial and ethical considerations. *Aphasiology, 7,* 321–334.

Schallert, T., Bland, S. T., Leasure, J. L., Tillerson, J., Gonzales, R., Williams, L., Aronowski, J., & Grotta, J. (2000). Motor rehabilitation, use-related neural events, and reorganization of the brain after injury. In H. S. Levin & J. Grafman (Eds.), *Cerebral reorganization of function of the brain after injury.* New York: Oxford University Press.

Schuell, H., Jenkins, J. J., & Jimenez-Pabon, E. (1964). *Aphasia in adults: Diagnosis, prognosis, and treatment.* New York: Harper & Row.

Schwartz, M. F., Saffran, E. M., Fink, R., Myers, J., & Martin, N. (1994). Mapping therapy: A treatment programme for agrammatism. *Aphasiology, 8,* 19–54.

Shapiro, L. P. (1997). Tutorial: An introduction to syntax. *Journal of Speech and Hearing Research, 40,* 254–272.

Shelton, J. R., Weinrich, M., McCall, D., & Cox, D. M. (1996). Differentiating globally aphasic patients: Data from in-depth language assessment sand production training using C-VIC. *Aphasiology, 10,* 319–342.

Shewan, C. (1986). The history and efficacy of aphasia treatment. In R. Chapey (Ed.), *Language intervention strategies in adult aphasia* (2nd ed.). Baltimore: Williams & Wilkins.

Simmons-Mackie, N. (1999). Social role negotiation in aphasia therapy: Competence, incompetence and conflict. In D. Kovarsky & J. Duchan (Eds.), *Constructing (in)competence: Disabling evaluations in clinical and social interaction.* Mahwah, NJ: Erlbaum.

Small, S. L., Flores, D. K., & Noll, D. C. (1998). Different neural circuits subserve reading before and after therapy for acquired dyslexia. *Brain and Language, 62,* 298–308.

Sparks, R., Helm-Estabrooks, N., & Albert, M. (1974). Aphasia rehabilitation resulting from melodic intonation therapy. *Cortex, 10,* 303–316.

Stein, D. G., Brailowsky, S., & Will, B. (1995). *Brain repair.* New York: Oxford University Press.

Sturm, W., & Willmes, K. (1991). Efficacy of a reaction training on various attentional and cognitive functions in stroke patients. *Neuropsychological Rehabilitation, 1,* 259–280.

Sugishita, M., Seki, K., Kabe, S., & Yunoki, K. (1993). A material-control single-case study of the efficacy of treatment for written and oral naming difficulties. *Neuropsychologia, 31,* 559–569.

Tanemura, J. (1999). Aphasia therapy using the deblocking method and Kanji/Kana issues. *Topics in Stroke Rehabilitation, 6,* 23–32.

Terrell, B. Y., & Ripich, D. N. (1989). Discourse competence as a variable in intervention. *Seminars in Speech and Language, 10,* 282–297.

Thompson, C. K., Ballard, K. J., & Shapiro, L. P. (1998). The role of syntactic complexity in training wh-movement structures in agrammatic aphasia: Optimal order for promoting generalization. *Journal of the International Neuropsychological Society, 4,* 661–674.

Thompson, C. K., Shapiro, L. P., Tait, M. E., Jacobs, V. J., & Schneider, S. L. (1996). Training wh-question production in agrammatic aphasia: Analysis of argument and adjunct movement. *Brain and Language, 52,* 175–228.

Thulborn, K. R., Carpenter, P. A., & Just, M. A. (1999). Plasticity of language-related brain function during recovery from stroke. *Stroke, 30,* 749–754.

Trenerry, M. R., Crosson, B., DeBoe, J., & Leber, W. R. (1989). *Stroop Neuropsychological Screening Test.* Odessa, FL: Psychological Assessment Resources.

Ward-Lornegan, J. M., & Nicholas, M. (1995). Drawing to communicate: A case report of an adult with global aphasia. *European Journal of Communication Disorders, 30,* 475–491.

Weinrich, M., Boser, K. I., & McCall, D. (1999). Representation of linguistic rules in the brain: Evidence from training an aphasic patient to produce past tense verb morphology. *Brain and Language, 70,* 144–158.

Weinrich, M., Shelton, J. R., McCall, D., & Cox, D. M. (1997). Generalization from single sentence to multisentence production in severely aphasic patients. *Brain and Language, 58,* 327–352.

Wepman, J. (1947). The organization of therapy for aphasia: I. The inpatient treatment center. *Journal of Speech Disorders, 12,* 407.

Whitworth, A. (1995). Characterising thematic role assignment in aphasic sentence production: Procedures for elicited and spontaneous output. *European Journal of Disorders of Communication, 30,* 384–399.

Willer, B., Rosenthal, M., Kreutzer, J. S., Gordon, W. A., & Rempel, R. (1993). Assessment of community integration following rehabilitation for traumatic brain injury. *Journal of Head Trauma Rehabilitation, 8,* 75–87.

Williams, S. E. (1993). The impact of aphasia on marital satisfaction. *Archives of Physical Medicine and Rehabilitation, 74,* 361–367.

Wilson, B. A., Cockburn, J., & Baddeley, A. D. (1985). *The Rivermead Behavioral Memory Test.* Titchfield, UK: Thames Valley Test Company.

World Health Organization. (1999). *ICIDH-2: International Classification of Functioning and Disability* (Beta-2 Draft, Full Version). Geneva: Author.

Worrall, L. (1992). Functional communication assessment: An Australian perspective. *Aphasiology*, 6, 105–110.

Yoshihata, H., Watamori, T., Chujo, T., Masuyama, K. (1998). Acquisition and generalization of mode interchange skills in people with severe aphasia. *Aphasiology*, 12, 1035–1045.

Yosihata, H., Watamori, T., Chujo, T., & Masayuma, K. (1998). Acquisition and generalization of mode interchange skills in people with severe aphasia. *Aphasiology*, 12, 1035–1045.

CHAPTER 10

Apraxia

CAROLINE VAN HEUGTEN

Apraxia is one of the four classical neuropsychological deficits—such as agnosia, amnesia, and aphasia—that cause restrictions in the ability to carry out purposeful and learned activities. Steinthal (1871) first used the term "apraxia," and Hughlings-Jackson first described the symptoms 5 years later (Kolb & Whishaw, 1990). Geschwind (1975) offered a modern definition of the apraxias: "disorders of the execution of learned movements which cannot be accounted for by either weakness, incoordination, or sensory loss, nor by incomprehension of or inattention to commands" (p. 188).

Since Steinthal, much has been written about apraxia and many empirical data have accumulated. Unfortunately, apraxia remains a difficult concept for both clinicians and researchers because of the following limitations: (1) There is not one accepted taxonomy or classification of the forms of apraxia; (2) concepts and terminology are poorly defined; (3) testing procedures and scoring methods are inconsistent and confusing; and (4) recovery and treatment of apraxia have hardly been the subject of many research studies (Tate & McDonald, 1995). Indeed, Tate and McDonald referred to apraxia as "the clinician's dilemma" and with regard to the assessment of apraxia, this is still true to a large extent. Both improved clinical batteries and reliable diagnostic criteria are needed. For treatment of apraxia, this is less true, because recent intervention studies have shed some light on the issues, and positive treatment effects have been found to reduce the disrupting influence of apraxia on everyday life (Goldenberg & Hagman, 1998a; van Heugten et al., 1998; Donkervoort, Dekker, Stehmann-Saris, & Deelman, in press). These in-

222

tervention attempts are directed toward more applied, functional, and pragmatic treatment approaches in natural environments. This line of research on the efficacy of apraxia treatment clearly follows suggestions already made by others that apraxia treatment requires further study (Maher & Ochipa, 1997).

OCCURRENCE AND PREVALENCE OF APRAXIA

Apraxia is most often found in stroke patients, but the deficit is also seen in patients with Alzheimer's disease (Ochipa, Gonzalez-Rothi, & Heilman, 1992; Taylor, 1994). In addition, apraxia is one of the symptoms of corticobasal degeneration (Leiguarda, Lees, Merello, Starkstein, & Marsden, 1994; Jacobs, Adair, Macauley, Gold, Gonzalez-Rothi, & Heilman, 1999) and is also reported in individuals with Huntington's disease (Shelton & Knopman, 1991). In patients with corticobasal degeneration, apraxia is a key finding for the differential diagnosis, but the features found are most probably not the same as those exhibited by patients with a left-hemisphere stroke with apraxia (Merians et al., 1999). Apraxia and aphasia frequently coexist, and the association between the two deficits is likely due to the fact that contiguous structures are involved (De Renzi, 1989; Tate & McDonald, 1995). Only a few single-case studies support the independence of apraxia from aphasia (Selnes, Pestronk, Hart, & Gordon,1991). In a sample of 699 right-handed patients with left-hemisphere lesions, Papagno, Della Sala, and Basso (1993) studied a double aphasia–apraxia dissociation and found 10 patients to be apractic but not aphasic, and 149 patients to be aphasic but not apractic. These results were based on the use of the Token test for language comprehension and a 24-item test for ideomotor apraxia.

Although apraxia is one of the more common consequences of left-hemispheric lesions, little is known about the exact prevalence of apraxia. De Renzi (1989) concluded that approximately one third of patients with left-brain damage were found to be apractic. This left-hemispheric dominance was noticed first by Liepmann (1908), who found apraxia in 50% of his patients with left-hemispheric damage, while none of the patients with right-brain damage were found to be apractic. Liepmann concluded that the left hemisphere is dominant for motor control. Later studies have supported this claim (e.g., Pieczuro & Vignolo, 1967; De Renzi, Pieczuro, & Vignolo, 1968; Basso, Luzatti, & Spinnler, 1980; Kertesz & Ferro, 1984; Heilman & Gonzalez-Rothi, 1985). Goldenberg conducted two studies in which the prevalence of apraxia was investigated for the imitation of gestures (Goldenberg,

1996) and tool use (Goldenberg & Hagman, 1998b). In both studies, patients with left-brain damage were found to be more apractic than patients with right-brain damage. In a recent study on the prevalence of apraxia (Donkervoort, Dekker, van den Ende, Stehmann-Saris, & Deelman, 2000) after an intensive literature search, researchers concluded that 8 of only 10 studies found on the prevalence of apraxia were published by two collaborating Italian research groups; this could imply that the studies concern overlapping or even the same patient groups. Donkervoort, Dekker, van den Ende, et al. (2000) therefore investigated the prevalence of apraxia among patients with a first left-hemisphere stroke hospitalized in rehabilitation centers and nursing homes in the Netherlands. They found that, among a total of 492 patients, the prevalence of apraxia was 28% in rehabilitation centers and 37%. in nursing homes. No relationship was found between the prevalence of apraxia and age, gender, or type of stroke (i.e., hemorrhage or infarction). This percentage confirms earlier estimations by De Renzi (1989).

Table 10.1 presents an overview of the studies on the prevalence of apraxia

TABLE 10.1. Overview of Studies on the Prevalence of Apraxia

Author	% apraxia	
	LBD	RBD
Liepmann (1908)	50	0
Pieczuro & Vignolo (1967)	46	9
De Renzi, Pieczuro, & Vignolo (1968)	28	0
Basso, Luzatti, & Spinler (1980)	39	—[a]
De Renzi, Motti, & Nichelli (1980)	50	20
De Renzi, Faglioni, & Sorgato (1982)	32/34[b]	2/6[b]
Kertesz & Ferro (1984)	55/45	—
Basso, Faglioni, & Luzatti (1985)	45	—
Basso, Capitani, Della Sala, & Laiacona (1987)	43	—
Barbieri & De Renzi (1988)	57	34
	50	13
Goldenberg (1996)	43	13
Goldenberg & Hagman (1998b)	55	—[c]
Donkervoort, Dekker, van den Ende, et al. (2000)	28/37[d]	—

Note. LBD, left brain damaged; RBD, right brain damaged.
[a]No patients with right-brain damage were included in the study.
[b]Imitation and object use pantomime were tested respectively.
[c]RBD patients were tested, but the percentages cannot be derived from the publication.
[d]Patients were tested in rehabilitation centers and nursing homes, respectively.

FORMS OF APRAXIA

Many different classifications, taxonomies, and forms of apraxia are described in the literature. However, an accepted taxonomy for the apraxias is not available (Tate & McDonald, 1995). Liepmann (1920) formulated the first, now-classic theory, in which he proposed three different types of apraxia: ideational, motor, and limb-kinetic. These forms were characterized by impairments in the proper sequence of intact movements, especially the composition of single movements into action. The forms differ in the presumed mechanisms underlying them: Ideational apraxia was thought to be an inability to conjure up a concept or mental image of the intended action; motor apraxia was an inability to translate this concept or mental image into actions; limb-kinetic apraxia was due to a loss of visuokinetic engrams that exist for a limited range of highly practiced routine actions and are stored for the opposite hand in each of the hemispheres. Luria (1966) also discussed three forms of apraxia: frontal, premotor, and kinesthetic apraxia. In the first two types, again, the sequencing of movements is improper. In kinesthetic apraxia, the sequencing stays intact, but the kinesthetic sensitivity disappears (i.e., the sense of limb position and limb movement).

Liepmann's and Luria's classifications have in common impairments of the limbs per se. Apraxia can also be classified in terms of the body part that is affected; for example, buccofacial or oral apraxia. In these cases, the voluntary movements of the face, mouth, lips, tongue, or larynx are impaired (Heilman & Gonzalez-Rothi, 1985). In addition, many forms of apraxia are described in relation to the activity that is disturbed, for example, walking apraxia (Gerstman & Schilder, 1926), constructional apraxia (Kleist, 1934), and dressing apraxia (Brain, 1941). Most types of apraxia have been the object of research studies; some forms have been dismissed or at least disputed as separate forms of apraxia, such as dressing apraxia.

Ideational and ideomotor apraxia have been the object of most apraxia studies in recent years and are sometimes labeled as the two classic forms (Tate & McDonald, 1995). A patient with ideational apraxia (IA) does not know what to do; the very concept or idea of the motor act is lacking or not accessible from memory (De Renzi & Lucchelli, 1988; De Renzi, 1989). In another definition of these two forms, originally proposed by Morlaas (1928), that has been endorsed by others, IA concerns the actual use of tools and objects, whereas ideomotor apraxia concerns gestures without a real object present (including pantomime of object use; Goldenberg & Hagman, 1998b). IA patients who have problems organizing performance will, for instance, first put on their shoes and then try putting on the socks, or keep putting food in their mouths without swallowing (Arnadottir, 1990). Because the plan or idea of the act is missing, patients do not know what to do with objects: They might brush their teeth with a spoon and comb their hair with a toothbrush (Singu, Cohen, Duhamel, Pillon, Dubois, & Agid, 1995). Because the plan is missing it might not be possible for the IA patient to combine an activity's component parts into a total sequence of movements; in these cases, the components are performed normally (Poeck, 1983; De Renzi & Lucchelli, 1988). The type of errors observed are omissions, mislocation or misuse of objects, and sequence mistakes (De Renzi & Lucchelli, 1998).

In ideomotor apraxia (IMA), the idea or plan of action is not impaired (i.e., the patient does know what to do), but the implementation of the movement sequence into a proper mode of action is disrupted (i.e., the patient does not know how to do it; De Renzi, 1989). IMA patients would use the comb to comb their hair but might place the comb upside down on their heads. The most frequent errors made by IMA patients include the use of body parts as objects, spatial orientation problems, inappropriate hand postures, perseverative errors, and content errors (Heilman & Gonzalez-Rothi, 1985; Miller, 1986; Shelton & Knopman, 1991). The movements are generally regarded as clumsy and inflexible (Arnadottir, 1990). A most striking observation in IMA is the fact that a patient may not be able to perform on command but might execute perfectly the same activity in a natural setting (De Renzi, Motti, & Nichelli, 1980).

There are many discussions in the literature about the autonomy, definitions, and manifestations of both IA and IMA. Distinctions between the two forms have been defended on the basis of many theoretical claims and neuroanatomical models. Some authors, however, conclude that to differentiate between the forms of apraxia on the basis of abstract theoretical claims is not recommended; instead, one should use descriptive terminology and focus on the specific, observable problems in daily functioning (Arnadottir, 1990; Lezak, 1995).

ASSESSMENT

Concerning testing procedures, a large number of studies have reported many different levels of task demands. Task demands vary depending on the part of the movement system involved (limb vs. axial movements), the type of movement (dynamic vs. posture), the type of limb gesture (transitive vs. intransitive, symbolic vs. nonsymbolic, meaningful vs. meaningless), the input modality (verbal vs. visual vs. tactile, command vs. imitation), and the complexity of the movement (single vs. complex, single vs. multiple object use; Roy, Square-Storer, Hogg, & Adams,

1991; Tate & McDonald, 1995). IMA is most commonly tested by asking the patient to imitate gestures (De Renzi et al., 1980). Typically, IA is examined in tests requiring the use of objects (De Renzi, Faglioni, & Sorgato, 1982; De Renzi & Lucchelli, 1988).

Besides numerous different task demands, many different quantitative and qualitative scoring methods have been applied to measure the extent to which apraxia is present (Tate & McDonald, 1995). Quantitative methods are used mostly in research studies. Qualitative scoring methods offer more information concerning the nature of the problems in performance but are less reliable. Error analyses have provided some insight into apractic performance (McDonald, Tate, & Rigby, 1994).

Most of the methods mentioned, however, are found mainly in empirical studies, and application in clinical practice is troublesome or not sufficiently informative. Clinicians attempting to diagnose apraxia are thus confronted with additional problems. The existing testing procedures are often merely part of a neuropsychological battery not specifically aimed at apraxia; many clinicians rely on intuition, clinical impression, and personal experience (Poeck, 1985). In addition, apraxia is frequently accompanied by other cognitive deficits such as aphasia; further on, patients often fail when performance is requested, but they may act correctly in spontaneous situations. Finally, apraxia is often defined by what it is not, which implies that it can only be diagnosed if a full battery of neuropsychological tests is used.

Rehabilitation of patients is concerned with the consequences of the disease and the implications for the patient's daily life. In 1980, the World Health Organization (WHO) published the International Classification of Impairments, Disabilities and Handicaps (ICIDH), classifying the consequences of diseases at three levels of health experience: (1) loss or abnormality of psychological, physiological, or anatomical structures or functions (impairments); (2) restriction or lack of ability to perform activities in the manner or within the range considered normal for a human being (disabilities); and (3) disadvantages for individuals that limit or prevent fulfillment of a role that is normal (handicaps). Although the ICIDH model does not completely fit the area of psychology, it is a useful framework in clinical practice for the purpose of rehabilitation. Assessing apraxia and its consequences can be done by studying behavioral performance in a neuropsychological apraxia test conducted in a highly standardized context, in order to try to capture the praxis functions as closely as possible (i.e., impairment level): The consequences of apraxia for everyday life—the disabilities—can be assessed by observation of activities of daily living (ADL) conducted in a more ecologically valid context resembling real-life situations as much as possible. Neuropsychological tests can help to differentiate between apraxia and other impairments, but the results do not readily generalize to performance in daily life. Recently, in two studies on assessment and treatment of apraxia, researchers used a diagnostic procedure consisting of these two complementary levels: (1) clinical assessment of apraxia, including imitation of gestures, pantomime, and use of objects; and (2) standardized ADL tests in which activities from the domains of grooming, dressing, and eating were observed (Goldenberg & Hagman, 1998a; van Heugten et al., 1998). Both research groups executed reliability and validity studies on these instruments, which turned out to be good (Goldenberg & Hagman, 1998a; van Heugten, Dekker, Deelman, Stehmann-Saris, & Kinebanian, 1999a, 1999b; Van Heugten, Dekker, Deelman, van Dijk, et al., 2000). Goldenberg and Hagman (1998a) investigated the interrater reliability of the ADL test, which turned out to be good (correlation coefficients ranging from .83 to .96). The relationship of their ADL test to clinical apraxia tests showed significant correlations, indicating that the failure on ADL was primarily related to the severity of the apraxia and not to the severity of the aphasia, which was established with the Token test. Van Heugten et al. (1999a, 1999b; van Heugten, Dekker, Deelman, van Dijk, et al., 2000) examined (1) the internal consistency (alpha = .96) and diagnostic value of the apraxia test (sensitivity and specificity > 80%); (2) the internal consistency (alpha = .94) and interrater reliability of the ADL observations (kappa ranges from .44 to .95); and (3) the relationship between the apraxia test, motor functioning, the ADL observations, and the Barthel index (good construct and clinical validity for the ADL observations).

This interplay of standardized tests and observation techniques is important in practice and clinical research. The underlying deficits can be made explicit to a certain degree, but the subjective elements in behavior are also taken into account. Especially when subjects perform daily activities, it is necessary to consider their background, family, and cultural influences. In certain religious cultures, for instance, the use of a kitchen knife is restricted to the adult men in the family. A woman handling a kitchen knife in a strange way is therefore not a case of apractic behavior. Performance is not by definition inadequate if it is not within the range of possibilities determined by the clinician. Self-report devices and interviews with patients and their families should be equally appreciated in diagnostic settings. Combining the diagnostic findings of the neuropsychologist with those of the occupational, speech, and physical therapists, nurses and social workers, is advisable in light of these issues.

TREATMENT

Current Status of Interventions on Apraxia

Although the incidence of apraxia after acquired brain damage is considerable, the literature on recovery and treatment is very minimal. Maher and Ochipa (1997) identified several reasons why so little has been written about the management and treatment of apraxia. First, patients with apraxia often seem to be unaware of their deficit and rarely complain (Rothi, Mack, & Heilman, 1990). This can be the result of two associated disorders: (1) Hemiplegia of the dominant hand can force patients to use their nondominant hand, which leads to deficits that are not labeled apractic; and (2) the presence of nonfluent aphasia could limit patients' ability to express concern over their poor performance. Second, many researchers believe that recovery from apraxia is spontaneous (Basso, Capitani, Della Sala, Laiacona, & Spinnler, 1987). Recent studies suggest that although some aspects of apraxia are persistent, others show improvement over time (Foundas, Rayner, Maher, Rothi, & Heilman, 1993; Maher, Rayner, Foundas, Rothi, & Heilman, 1994). Third, some authors believe that apraxia only occurs when performance is requested of patients in testing conditions, and that patients display the correct, spontaneous behavior in natural settings (De Renzi et al., 1980; Geschwind & Damasio, 1985; Poeck, 1985), which indicates that apraxia has no negative impact on everyday life and that therapy is unnecessary. This claim has been challenged in recent years. Bjorneby and Reinvang (1985) assessed at different stages of recovery the degree of self-care in patients who had suffered a stroke. All apraxia variables appeared to be significant predictors of subsequent dependence: The relationship between initial apraxia measures and long-term dependence after rehabilitation (4–6 months poststroke) is especially strong. Sundet, Finset, and Reinvang (1988) reported similarly that variables related to apraxia at the start of rehabilitation correlate significantly with the level of ADL dependence after discharge. Foundas et al. (1995) observed a significant, positive correlation between the degree of apraxia severity and the number of action errors in mealtime behavior. In addition, Goldenberg and Hagman (1998a) concluded that apraxia has an adverse influence on ADL independence in patients with right-sided hemiplegia with apraxia. Finally, Saeki, Ogata, Okubo, Takahashi, and Hoshuyama (1993) reported that apraxia is one of the factors influencing return to work after stroke in Japan. These studies all confirm the adverse ecological impact of apraxia on patients' lives and the potential importance of intervention research for the treatment of apraxia. By now, there is agreement that apraxia hinders ADL independence, and treatment of apraxia should definitely be part of the overall neurorehabilitation program after brain damage.

Recovery of Apraxia

Not much is known about the natural recovery course of apraxia. This is probably because the negative influence of apraxia on everyday life had been denied for such a long time. Basso et al. (1987) did investigate the recovery from IMA in acute stroke patients and assessed variables capable of predicting the evolution of ideomotor apraxia. They found that improvement often required a long period of time and was not related to age, sex, education, type of aphasia, or initial severity or the size of the lesion. Recovery did seem to be related to the site of the lesion: Patients with anterior lesions had a better chance of recovery. Thirteen of the 26 acute patients were still apractic at the second examination, at least 5 months later. The evolution of IMA was correlated more with the evolution of oral apraxia than with other neuropsychological variables. Finally, the presence of a second lesion in the right hemisphere did not have the negative influence on recovery that might have been expected.

Maher et al. (1994) looked at the pattern of recovery of limb apraxia over a period of 6 months. They found differential patterns of recovery for intransitive (e.g., waving goodbye) and transitive gestures (e.g., tool use). For intransitive gestures, there was a spontaneous decrease in the number of content errors, while for transitive gestures, the number of unidentifiable production errors decreased (perseverations, unrecognizable or no responses). Spatial and temporal errors were found to be persistent. The authors suggested that the natural recovery course of apraxia is seen in the areas of meaningfulness and recognizability of the gestures, because that is were performance improves.

Sunderland, Tinson, and Bradley (1994) reported preliminary findings on differences in recovery of constructional apraxia 5 months poststroke between patients with left- and right-hemispheric damage. Constructional apraxia refers to a visuomotor disorder in which patients are unable to perform activities such as assembling, building and drawing (Kolb & Whishaw, 1990). It appeared that the group with left-hemipsheric damage showed more improvement and also greater variability in amount of recovery within the group. Constructional apraxia, however, is not discussed further in this chapter.

Treatment Models

Although no specific literature states that apraxia is irreversible, the fact that it is not plausible to restore higher cognitive functions completely is widely acknowledged (Miller, 1984; Moffat, 1984). It is unlikely that the adult nervous system possesses sufficient plasticity for complete restoration. Recovery of all practical behaviors is therefore not a realistic goal for therapy, neither by aiming for spontaneous recovery, nor by repeatedly stimulating brain structures through cognitive retraining. Cognitive retraining (or drill and practice) was actually found to be ineffective in various studies (e.g., Ericsson & Chase, 1982; Prigatano et al., 1984; Berg, 1993; van Zomeren & Brouwer, 1994). The main treatment aim therefore, is best focused on therapies in which patients deal with the existing impairment more efficiently in order to obtain improved functioning. Research on the effectiveness of rehabilitation in apraxia is sparse, but it suggests that compensatory strategies may be the most effective approach (Wilson, 1988; Pilgrim & Humphreys, 1994; Butler, 1997; van Heugten et al., 1998; Donkervoort, Dekker, Stehmann-Saris, & Deelman, in press). It has also been proposed that verbal and visual mediation are needed to facilitate movement in apraxia: verbalizing what one wants to do and looking at what one is doing (Croce, 1993; Butler, 1996a, 1996b).

Measurement of Treatment-Related Effects

SINGLE-CASE STUDIES

Occasionally, a single-case study on the rehabilitation of a patient with apraxia is reported. Wilson (1988) described a case of remediation of apraxia following an anesthetic accident leading to both physical and cognitive deficits for which neuropsychological testing was not even possible. To improve the self-help skills of the patient, a treatment program was developed in which tasks such as drinking from a cup were broken down into small steps. Treatment started 4 months after the accident and took place during daily occupational therapy sessions. The patient was able to learn tasks once she had been through the sequence a few times, possibly supported by covert verbalization. Natural recovery could not account for the rapid success of the program, concludes Wilson, because the patient had never learned to complete self-help tasks without a similar structured program.

Maher, Rothi, and Greenwald (1991) studied the effects of treatment on a 55-year-old man with IMA and preserved gesture recognition subsequent to a stroke. Daily, 1-hour therapy sessions over a 2-week period consisted of presenting the patient with multiple cues; the patient was to demonstrate the use of the target tool. Immediate accuracy feedback and correction of errors were given, and the cues were systematically withdrawn. A substantial improvement in the quality of gesture production was found for both treated and untreated gestures. Because no conclusions could be drawn as to which features of the treatment were most effective, Ochipa, Maher, and Rothi (1995) developed a treatment program aimed at specific error types. Praxis performance was studied in two chronic stroke patients with left-hemispheric damage both having Broca's aphasia and IMA. The treatment, the training of gestures for common tool/household items, was specifically designed to address the error types of each patient. It appeared that both patients achieved considerable improvements in performance, but the observed effects were treatment specific: Treatment of a specific error type did not improve across untreated gestures.

Pilgrim and Humphreys (1994) presented the case of a left-handed, head-injured patient with IMA of his left upper limb. The rehabilitation strategy was a modified form of conductive education (CE), which is an educational approach for the rehabilitation of children and adults with brain damage, aimed at functional motor goals (Cotton & Sutton, 1986). The principle of this treatment was to restore performance through restructuring the functional system by involving the role of speech in motor actions. This means that a "conductor" (i.e., the therapist) provides rhythmically verbalized, goal-directed instructions simultaneously with the patient's serial performance of the component parts of an action. The therapy showed a positive effect in terms of an improvement in the use of objects but little carryover to daily life. Bergego, Bradat-Diehl, Taillefer, and Migeot (1994) also published a paper on the treatment of a single apractic patient; again, reeducation of the use of objects during ADL functioning appeared to be successful.

Butler (1997) conducted a case study exploring the effectiveness of tactile and kinesthetic stimulation as an intervention strategy, in addition to verbal and visual mediation input, in the rehabilitation of a man with IMA and IA following a head injury. In practice, the intervention strategy involves cueing people with apraxia to look at what they are doing and where they are going, and demonstrating activities and movements, thereby providing a visual model. In addition, the patient is encouraged to verbalize performance and its results. Evaluation of the motor performance in an ABA design showed mixed results related to an intervention effect. The hypothesis that additional sensory stimulation could increase motor performance was supported partially. The study, however, had some limitations, because the results could in part be explained by motor recovery and some ceiling effects were present.

QUASI AND PREEXPERIMENTAL EFFECT STUDIES

Goldenberg and Hagman (1998a) published a study in which an ADL therapy was evaluated in 15 apractic patients who made errors in performance. The researchers distinguished between fatal errors, which prevented successful completion of the activity, and reparable errors, which could be deleted during training sessions. It appeared that the number of errors correlated with clinical measures of apraxia (such as imitation, pantomime, and object use). The aim of therapy was restoration of ADL independence through training of ADL activities. The training was given by an occupational therapist five times a week. Fifteen patients who made fatal errors in at least two out of three activities were admitted to the therapy study. Each week, patients were trained in one of the three activities and given maximum support in the other two activities during daily routines. Two approaches were combined during training : (1) giving support in order that patients achieve errorless completion of the whole activity and (2) training of details of the activity. Every week, patients were trained in another activity and administered ADL tests. After therapy, with a mean duration of about 4 weeks, 10 patients could perform all three activities without fatal errors, and 3 patients made only one fatal error (see overall results in Table 10.2). Elimination of fatal errors was restricted to the week the activity was trained, which means that no generalization of training effects from trained to nontrained activities was shown. It appeared that there was no spontaneous recovery of ADL capacities, but specific training could restore ADL independence for trained activities. The training effect was preserved after 6 months only in those patients who kept practicing in their home situation.

In order to evaluate a therapy program for stroke patients with apraxia, Van Heugten et al. (1998) conducted a noncontrolled pre–posttest study based on teaching patients strategies to compensate for the presence of apraxia during the rehabilitation phase. They expected

TABLE 10.2. Influence of a Therapy of ADL Activities on Fatal Errors during Performance (Goldenberg & Hagman, 1998)

	55 weeks of activities with therapy	110 weeks of activities without therapy
Elimination of fatal error	26	10
No change	28	94
Occurrence of fatal error	1	6

Note. Fifteen patients were treated for a total of 55 weeks. Each week, therapy was given for one activity, while the other two activities were without therapy. Thus, each week yielded 3 weeks of measurement, one for each activity. The values give the number of weeks in which the respective change-of-error scores were observed. From Goldenberg and Hagman (1998a). Copyright 1998 by Psychology Press. Reprinted by permission of Psychology Press Ltd., Hove, UK.

changes in the patients' performance of ADL activities after treatment. More specifically, they expected improvements in ADL functioning but no changes, or only small changes, in the severity of apraxia, because restoration of the praxis function was not plausible. Recovery of apraxia was not a goal for therapy; rather, the therapy program was designed for assessment and treatment by occupational therapists. Thirty-three stroke patients were treated at occupational therapy (OT) departments in three hospitals, eight rehabilitation centers, and five nursing homes for a period of 12 weeks; the number of treatments was determined by the therapist and varied from three to five training sessions per week. During the treatment period, patients were trained in activities that were relevant to (re)learn, the program focused on disabilities resulting from apraxia, thereby hindering daily-life functioning. Every 2 weeks an activity was chosen. The specific interventions administered during treatment corresponded with the specific problems assessed during standardized ADL observations. ADL activities were conceptualized as being composed of three successive events: selection of the proper plan of action as well as the correct objects (initiation), followed by adequate performance of the plan (execution), evaluated in terms of the result (control and, if necessary, correction of the activity). The specific interventions in the form of instructions, assistance, and feedback were presented to the occupational therapists in a protocol. The following measurements were conducted before and after the 12-week training program: an apraxia test, a test of motor functioning, standardized observation of four activities of daily living, the Barthel index, and an ADL-questionnaire for the patients and the therapists. The neuropsychological apraxia test consisted of two subtests: demonstration of the use of objects and imitation of gestures. The standardized ADL observations consisted of four activities scored on four aspects: independence, initiation, execution, and control. Subsequently, the four measures were added to arrive at a total ADL score. The results showed large improvements in ADL functioning on all measures and small improvements on the apraxia test and motor functioning test (Table 10.3). The effect sizes for the disabilities, ranging from 0.92 to 1.06, were large compared to the effect sizes for the apraxia test (0.34) and motor functioning (0.19). The significant effect of treatment was also seen when researchers considered patients' individual and subjective improvement. These results suggest that the therapy program seems to be successful in teaching patients compensatory strategies that enable them to function more independently, despite the lasting presence of apraxia. The conclusions of this study, however, remain tentative, because no control group was present. However, spontaneous recovery was not possible, because the patients entered this study more than 2 months poststroke and a differential effect was found between the measurements. In addition, multivariate analyses further sup-

TABLE 10.3. Treatment Outcome in a Sample of Stroke Patients Receiving 12 Weeks of Strategy Training (van Heugten et al., 1998)

Tests	N	Baseline		Posttreatment		p	Effect sizes
		Mean	(SD)	Mean	(SD)		
Motor functioning	33	7.6	(6.2)	8.8	(6.3)	.03	0.19
Apraxia	31	58.1	(28.0)	67.6	(26.9)	<.001	0.34
ADL observations	25	1.0	(0.7)	0.4	(0.5)	<.001	0.92
Barthel Index	28	10.1	(5.5)	14.9	(5.0)	<.001	0.86
ADL Questionnaire (OT)	28	5.4	(1.6)	7.0	(1.8)	<.001	1.06

From van Heugten, Dekker, Deelman, van Dijk, et al. (1998). Copyright 1998 by *Clinical Rehabilitation*. Reprinted by permission.

port the findings. But the results of this study should indeed be tested in a controlled study.

EXPERIMENTAL EFFECT STUDIES

Poole (1998) published a study examining the ability of participants with left-hemisphere stroke to learn one-handed shoe tying. Participants included 5 stroke patients with apraxia, 5 stroke patients without apraxia, and 5 control patients. Apraxia was determined using De Renzi's apraxia test (De Renzi et al., 1968), with a cutoff point of 17. The researcher demonstrated and verbalized the instructions of the task. Retention was assessed after a 5-minute interval, during which participants performed other tasks. All groups differed significantly in regard to the number of trials needed to learn the task of shoe tying with one hand. However, on the retention task, the stroke patients with apraxia required significantly more trials than the other two groups. All groups required fewer trials on the retention tasks than on the learning task. Poole concluded that stroke patients with apraxia have difficulty learning and retaining a functional sequencing task. These findings confirm clinical observations showing that apractic patients have difficulties learning new ADL techniques.

Recently two randomized control trials (RCTs) on the rehabilitation of apraxia were conducted. Treatment effects in RCTs could be accounted for by generic occupational factors because of the equal number of hours of therapy in all groups. Demographic or clinical factors were well balanced. Spontaneous recovery was not liable because of the time since injury, which was at least 2 months poststroke. One study on limb apraxia was conducted by Smania, Girardi, Domenicali, Lora, and Aglioti (2000). Thirteen patients with acquired brain injury in the left hemisphere and limb apraxia lasting more than 2 months were randomly assigned to a study group receiving experimental training for limb apraxia, or to a control group receiving conventional treatment for aphasia. The experimental training involved a behavioral training with gesture-production exercises. The program was made up of three sections dedicated to the treatment of gestures, with and without symbolic value, and related or nonrelated to the use of objects. Thirty-five 50-minute sessions were conducted. IA was tested by requiring the use of real objects (see De Renzi et al., 1968). IMA was tested by using De Renzi's test involving symbolic and nonsymbolic intransitive gestures (De Renzi et al., 1980). Recognition of gestures was tested by showing the patients pictures. The patients receiving the experimental training showed a significant improvement in performance on IA and IMA tests. They also showed a reduction of errors on both tests. Control patients did not show any significant change in performance. The authors concluded that their specific training program was possibly effective for the treatment of limb apraxia. In addition, the improvement was not restricted to trained items, but extended to gestures requested during assessment, suggesting some generalizalibity. This study, however, also leaves at least one important question to be answered: Is this specific rehabilitation program also useful in improving gestural performance under daily-life conditions?

The goal of the study by Donkervoort, Dekker, Stehmann-Saris, et al. (in press) was to determine in a controlled study the efficacy of strategy training in left-hemispheric stroke patients with apraxia. The main hypotheses to be tested were as follows: (1) that strategy training incorporated into the usual treatment by occupational therapists would lead to more independence than the usual treatment alone; (2) that there would be no differential effect with regard to the apractic impairment itself; and in addition, (3) that the usual treatment by occupational therapists would lead to more improvement in motor functioning, because more time was available for training motor functions. A randomized, single-blind, controlled trial design was used to compare OT treatment for apraxia, with or without strategy training incorporated. The group of patients receiving strategy training were given the same training as that in the study by van Heugten et al. (1998). The main focus of the therapy for the control group of patients was on (sensori)motor impairments, and disabilities due to these impairments. This treatment was mainly based on trial and error, and experience of the therapist. Patients were assessed on cognitive (apraxia test, verbal comprehension, star cancellation, Cognitive Screening Test), motor (Motricity index, Functional Motor Test) and daily-life functioning (ADL observations, Barthel index, Rivermead ADL scale for OT and patient) at baseline, posttreatment (8 weeks) and follow-up (20 weeks). During the study, 315 patients with apraxia were referred for OT treatment; of the 113 patients eligible for the study, 56 were allocated to strategy training and 57 to the usual treatment. During the study, several patients dropped out for diverse reasons. The amount of therapy did not differ significantly between the treatment groups, nor did the content of treatment in terms of training for motor impairments, cognitive training, advice, splinting, aid, and housing adjustments. The use of other therapies was equally divided over both groups, but the strategy training group received more ADL training, which was expected. Table 10.4 shows the changes from baseline, and the differences between the groups and effect sizes. Patients in the strategy training group improved more on the primary outcome measure ($p = .03$). The matching effect size (0.37) indicates that strategy training is associated with a small to medium effect on ADL functioning. The Barthel index showed a significant medium effect (0.48) in favor of strategy training. These results confirm the previous findings of van Heugten et al. (1998) that the strategy training was successful in teaching patients ways to function more independently. The larger improvement in motor functioning in the control group was not found. At the 20-week follow-up, no significant differences between the two groups were found (Table 10.5), showing that the control group improved further, but the experimental group remained at the same level of functioning. The absence of this long-term, specific effect could be due to the fact that more patients in the control group received OT.

Indications for Treatment

Identification of patients who will benefit more than others from a specific treatment is important for caregivers, in order to set realistic treatment goals and to allocate health care services efficiently. Perhaps even

TABLE 10.4. Posttreatment Outcome in the Donkervoort, Dekker, Stehmann-Saris, et al. study (2000) during 8-Week Follow-Up Measures

| | Change from baseline | | | | |
| | Strategy training | | Usual treatment | | |
Tests	N	Mean	N	Mean	Effect sizes
Motricity Index	44	5.2	49	6.0	−0.03
Functional Motor Test	45	0.6	49	0.3	0.18
Apraxia Test	44	4.2	48	2.2	0.20
ADL observations	43	0.2	39	0.1	0.37
Barthel Index	45	2.4	47	1.1	0.48
ADL Questionnaire (OT)	47	0.9	48	1.1	−0.14

From Donkervoort, Dekker, Stehman-Saris, and Deelman (in press). Copyright by Psychology Press. Reprinted by permission of Psychology Press Ltd., Hove, UK.

TABLE 10.5. Follow-Up Outcome in the Donkervoort, Dekker, Stehmann-Saris, et al. study (2000) during 20-Week Follow-Up Measures

| | Change from baseline | | | | |
| | Strategy training | | Usual treatment | | |
Tests	N	Mean	N	Mean	Effect sizes
Motricity Index	41	6.3	40	7.9	−0.06
Functional Motor Test	41	0.5	40	0.5	0.03
Apraxia Test	40	6.3	39	3.7	0.20
ADL observations	37	0.2	34	0.2	−0.02
Barthel Index	41	2.8	38	2.8	−0.03
ADL Questionnaire (OT)	35	1.2	35	1.5	−0.22

From Donkevoort, Dekker, Stehman-Saris, and Deelman (in press). Copyright by Psychology Press. Reprinted by permission of Psychology Press Ltd., Hove, UK.

more importantly, patients and their families should be informed adequately about the expected outcome. Most prognostic studies, however, do not differentiate between spontaneous recovery and the effects of treatment. Basso et al. (1987) studied which variables were capable of predicting the evolution of IMA. They found that recovery was related only to the site of the lesion: patients with anterior lesions appeared to have a better chance of recovery. Sundet et al. (1988) found that variables associated with apraxia at the start of rehabilitation correlated significantly with the level of help patients needed for managing at home alone after discharge: Apraxia on admission predicted significantly higher patient dependence on aids and other persons. The effect of rehabilitation or spontaneous recovery cannot, however, be differentiated from these studies. To help address this dilemma, in part, Van Heugten, Dekker, Deelman, Stehmann-Saris, et al (2000) investigated which additional cognitive and motor impairments are present in stroke patients with apraxia, and which of these factors influence the effects of treatment. For the group of 33 stroke patients with apraxia who received strategy training (see van Heugten et al., 1998), the following variables were analyzed: (1) additional neuropsychological deficits (comprehension of language, dementia-like cognitive impairments, neglect, and short-term memory), (2) level of motor functioning, (3) severity of apraxia, (4) ADL performance, and (5) relevant patient characteristics (gender, age, type of stroke, time since stroke, and location of treatment). The results showed that the presence of apraxia was associated with additional cognitive and motor impairments: Concerning comprehension of language, dementia-like cognitive impairments, and short-term memory functioning, the patients with apraxia scored significantly lower than the norms of control groups without apraxia. However, the successful outcome of strategy training was not prevented by cognitive comorbidity. The outcome seemed to be more prominent in more severely impaired patients at the start of rehabilitation, in terms of the degree of motor impairments, the severity of apraxia, and the initial ADL dependence. Demographic variables, specifically, age, did not predict the outcome of treatment. This study suggests that neither the presence of additional cognitive impairments nor the severity of motor problems or old age should be an indication to refrain from treating apraxia. There was no indication that the effect of treatment was weaker in more severely disabled patients.

Donkervoort, Dekker, Stehmann-Saris, et al. (in press) conducted subgroup analyses with respect to the primary outcome measures to determine specific treatment effects. The results suggested that strategy training is more beneficial in patients with more severe forms of apraxia. However, the interaction between treatment and the severity of apraxia was not found to be significant.

The expectation that most patients with apraxia have additional, other impairments apparently holds, but these negative influences on daily functioning do not disturb the outcome of treatment.

FUTURE RESEARCH AND DEVELOPMENT

Maher and Ochipa (1997) conclude their chapter on management and treatment of apraxia with the notion that the efficacy of treating limb apraxia requires further study. Apparently, this is still true, although more evaluation studies have clearly been conducted in the last few years. One of the issues that still remains to be solved after most of the studies cited is that of generalization: Does the positive effect of treatment generalize to other tasks and situations other than those trained? Maher and Ochipa noticed some common elements in apraxia treatment studies that might relate to the lack of generalization. First, to control for spontaneous recovery, most studies involve chronic patients. Perhaps treating more acute patients might lead to more generalization. Second, in the treatment studies, most patients with apraxia are also aphasic, which could have a negative influence on daily functioning in general. Finally, Maher and Ochipa speculated that a more substitutive approach involving compensatory strategies—instead of a restitutive approach— might have generalized more. A substitutive approach was chosen in the studies by van Heugten et al. (1998) and Donkervoort, Dekker, Stehmann-Saris, et al. (in press). In these studies strategy training was chosen over different methods for cognitive rehabilitation for two reasons. First, strategy training is aimed at improving daily activities instead of basic cognitive functions, which are more difficult to reverse. And second, strategy training is aimed at teaching methods that can be used during performance, instead of teaching a specific task. This implies that the results of the training should generalize to other activities and situations. In terms of therapeutic gains, task and context specificity are not of benefit for the ecological impact of the treatment outcome. In many studies, it was not possible to show generalization effects (e.g., Pilgrim & Humphreys, 1994; Ochipa et al., 1995; Goldenberg & Hagman, 1998a). The experimental design by Goldenberg and Hagman (1998a) involved training of another activity every week; a reduction of errors in the trained activity was considered to reflect the effect of therapy, whereas improvement on the other activities reflected either spontaneous recovery or the effect of generalization. The results showed that the majority of weeks without therapy was not associated with any change in fatal errors. This means that the effect of therapy remained specific to the activity being trained. Goldenberg and Hagman hypothesized that the absence of generalization of therapeutic gains comes from the cognitive basis of object use and mechanical skills. It is possible, however, that methodological constraints caused the lack of generalization. In many neuropsychological effect studies, the effect is executed only once: One task, one test, or one activity is scored to determine the effect of treatment. In other research fields, it is known that skills acquisition follows the power law of learning: The higher the number of practice trials, the shorter the time needed to complete the task. This principle of the transfer of learning could be applied in future studies on the effect of generalization.

SUMMARY AND CONCLUSIONS

In this chapter, I have provided an overview of literature on treatment and management of apraxia. After a short introduction, some notes on the occurrence, prevalence, and forms of apraxia were presented. The focus of this chapter was mainly on ideational and ideomotor apraxia, sometimes labeled the classical forms of apraxia. Assessment was then described, concluding with the preference for a diagnostic procedure consisting of different levels of measurement, including (1) a neuropsychological apraxia test that can help to differentiate between persons with and without apraxia, and (2) standardized tests for observing ADL activities through which the consequences of the apraxia for daily life are determined. Clinicians and researchers are encouraged to take into account the subjective elements in behavior as well: in performing daily activities, subjects' backgrounds and their family and cultural norms and values can strongly influence behavior. Heteroanamnesis (i.e., assessing and interviewing the patients' family members) that involves the family in therapy and multidisciplinary teamwork is essential in diagnosing and treating patients with apraxia.

Many recent studies have confirmed the ecological impact of apraxia on patients' lives. By now, there is agreement that apraxia hinders ADL independence, and treatment of apraxia should definitely be part of the overall rehabilitation program. Unfortunately, not much is known about the natural course of apraxia, but recent studies on the effectiveness of rehabilitation have shown that compensatory strategies may be the most effective approach. Treatment should be focused on functional activities that are structured and practiced using errorless learning approaches. Recovery of apraxia should probably not be the main goal of therapy: Instead, therapy should be geared to help patients function more independently despite the probably lasting presence of apraxia. The most important variables to measure in outcome studies are those related to functional activities. Some recent studies have shown that the functional approach can be successful, but further studies on pragmatic treatment approaches in natural environments are certainly needed. Patients who show severe apraxia at the start of rehabilitation, or present themselves with other cognitive and motor impairments, should be treated as well, because there is no indication that the effect of strategy training is weaker in more severely disabled persons. Patients should be considered for treatment of apraxia at all phases after stroke, because the studies do not show differentiation in effect of treatment as a result of time since stroke. Advising about frequency and length of treatment is difficult, because the intervention studies described in this chapter are not unequivocal on this point. The lack of generalization of treatment effects to nontrained activities and situations should definitely be a challenge for future research.

ACKNOWLEDGMENTS

I would like to thank Georg Goldenberg and Peter van de Sande for commenting on draft versions of this chapter.

REFERENCES

Arnadottir, G. (1990). *The brain and behavior.* St. Louis: Mosby.
Barbieri, C., & De Renzi, E. (1988). The executive and ideational components of apraxia. *Cortex, 24,* 535–543.
Basso, A., Capitani, E., Della Sala, S., Laiacona, M., & Spinnler, H. (1987). Recovery

from ideomotor apraxia: A study on acute stroke patients. *Brain, 110,* 747–760.

Basso, A., Faglioni, P., & Luzzatti, C. (1985). Methods in neuroanatomical research and an experimental study on limb apraxia. In E. A. Roy (Ed.), *Neuropsychological studies of apraxia and related disorders.* Amsterdam: North-Holland.

Basso, A., Luzzatti, C., & Spinnler, H. (1980). Is ideomotor apraxia the outcome of damage to well-defined regions of the left-hemipshere?: Neuropsychological study of CAT correlations. *Journal of Neurology, Neurosurgery and Psychiatry, 43,* 118–126.

Berg, I. J. (1993). *Memory rehabilitation for closed head injured patients.* Doctoral dissertation, University of Groningen, The Netherlands.

Bergego, C., Bradat-Diehi, P., Taillefer, C., & Migeot, H. (1994). Evaluation et reeducation de l'apraxie d'utilisation des objets. In D. El Gall & G. Aubin (Eds.), *L'apraxie.* Marseille: Solal.

Bjorneby, E. R., & Reinvang, I. R. (1985). Acquiring and maintaining self-care skills after stroke: The predictive value of apraxia. *Scandinavian Journal of Rehabilitation Medicine, 17,* 75–80.

Brain, W. R. (1941). Visual disorientation with special reference to lesions in the right cerebral hemisphere. *Brain, 64,* 244–272.

Butler, J. (1996a). Does sensory input influence recovery in ideomotor apraxia? *Brain Research Association Abstracts, 13,* 66.

Butler, J. (1996b). Intervention in a case of ideomotor apraxia. *Proceedings of the British Psychological Society, 4*(1), 55.

Butler, J. (1997). Intervention effectiveness: Evidence from a case study of ideomotor and ideational apraxia. *British Journal of Occupational Therapy, 60*(11), 491–497.

Cotton, E., & Sutton, A. (1986). *Conductive education: A system of overcoming motor disorder.* Beckenham, UK: Croom Helm.

Croce, R. (1993). A review of the neural basis of apractic disorders with implications for rehabilitation. *Adapted Physical Activity Quarterly, 10,* 173–215.

De Renzi, E. (1989). Apraxia. In F. Boller & J. Grafman (Eds.), *Handbook of neuropsychology* (Vol. 2). Amsterdam: Elsevier.

De Renzi, E., Faglioni, P., & Sorgato, P. (1982). Modality-specific and supramodal mechaisms of apraxia. *Brain, 105,* 301–312.

De Renzi, E., & Lucchelli, F. (1988). Ideational apraxia. *Brain, 111,* 1173–1185.

De Renzi, E., Motti, F., & Nichelli, P. (1980). Imitating gestures: A quantitative approach to ideomotor apraxia. *Archives of Neurology, 37,* 6–18.

De Renzi, E., Pieczuro, A., & Vignolo, L. A. (1968). Ideational apraxia: A quantitative study. *Neuropsychologia, 6,* 41–52.

Donkervoort, M., Dekker, J., van den Ende, E., Stehmann-Saris, J. C., & Deelman, B. G. (2000). Prevalence of apraxia among patients with a first left-hemisphere stroke in rehabilitation centers and nursing homes. *Clinical Rehabilitation, 14,* 130–136.

Donkervoort, M., Dekker, J., Stehmann-Saris, J. C., & Deelman, B. G. (in press). Efficacy of strategy training in left hemisphere stroke patients with apraxia: A randomized clinical trial. *Neuropsychological Rehabilitation.*

Ericsson, K. A., & Chase, W. G. (1982). Exceptional memory. *American Scientist, 70,* 607–615.

Foundas, A. L., Macauley, B. C., Rayner, A. M., Maher, L. M., Heilman, K. M., & Rothi, L. J. G. (1995). Ecological implications of limb apraxia: Evidence from mealtime behaviour. *Journal of the International Neuropsychological Society, 1,* 62–66.

Foundas, A. L., Rayner, A. M., Maher, L. M., Rothi, L. J. G., & Heilman, K. M. (1993). Recovery in ideomotor apraxia. *Journal of Clinical and Experimental Neuropsychology, 15*, 44.

Gerstman, J., & Schilder, P. (1926). Uber eine besondere gangstorung bei Stinhirnerkrankung. *Wine. Med. Wschr., 76*, 97–102.

Geschwind, N. (1975). The apraxias: Neural mechanisms of disorders of learned movements. *American Scientist, 63*, 188–195.

Geschwind, N., & Damasio, A. R. (1985). Apraxia. In J. A. M. Frederiks (Ed.), *Handbook of clinical neurology.* New York: Elsevier.

Goldenberg, G. (1996). Defective imitation of gestures in patients with damage in the left or right hemispheres. *Journal of Neurology, Neurosurgery and Psychiatry, 61*, 176–180.

Goldenberg, G., & Hagman, S. (1998a). Therapy of activities of daily living in patients with apraxia. *Neuropsychological Rehabilitation, 8*(2), 123–141.

Goldenberg, G., & Hagman, S. (1998b). Tool use and mechanical problem solving in apraxia. *Neuropsychologia, 36*(7), 581–589.

Heilman, K. M., & Gonzalez-Rothi, L. J. (1985). Apraxia. In K. M. Heilman & E. Valenstein (Eds.), *Clinical neuropsychology* (2nd ed.). Oxford, UK: Oxford University Press.

Jacobs, D. H., Adair, J. C., Macauley, B., Gold, M., Gonzalez-Rothi, L. J., & Heilman, K. M. (1999). Apraxia in corticobasal degeneration. *Brain and Cognition, 40*(2), 336–354.

Kertesz, A., & Ferro, J. M. (1984). Lesion size and location in ideomotor apraxia. *Brain, 107*, 921–333.

Kleist, K. (1934). *Gehirnpathologie vornehmlich auf grund der Kriegerfahrungen.* Leipzig: Barth.

Kolb, B., & Whishaw, I. Q. (1990). *Fundamentals of human neuropsychology* (3rd ed.). New York: Freeman.

Leiguarda, R., Lees, A. J., Merello, M., Starkstein, S., & Marsden, C. D. (1994). The nature of apraxia in corticobasal degeneration. *Journal of Neurology, Neurosurgery and Psychiatry, 57*, 455–459.

Lezak, M. D. (1995). *Neuropsychological assessment.* New York: Oxford University Press.

Liepmann, H. (1908). *Drei aufsatze aus dem apraxiegebiet.* Berlin: Krager.

Liepmann, H. (1920). Apraxie. *Erg. gesamt. Med., 1*, 516–543.

Liepmann, H. (1980). The left hemisphere and action. In D. Kimura (Ed. & Trans.) *Translations from Liepmann's essays on apraxia.* London, Canada: University of Western Ontario. (Original work published 1905)

Luria, A. R. (1966). *Higher cortical functions in men.* New York: Basic Books.

Maher, L. M., & Ochipa, C. (1997). Management and treatment of limb apraxia. In L. J. G. Rothi & K. M. Heilman (Eds.), *Apraxia: The neuropsychology of action.* Hove, UK: Psychology Press.

Maher, L. M., Rayner, A. M., Foundas, A., Rothi, L. J. G., & Heilman, K. M. (1994). *Patterns of recovery in ideomotor apraxia.* Paper presented at the annual meeting of the International Neuropsychological Society, Cincinatti, OH.

Maher, L. M., Rothi, L. J. G., & Greenwald, M. L. (1991). Treatment of gesture impairment: A single case. *ASHA, 33*, 195.

McDonald, S., Tate, R. C., & Rigby, J. (1994). Error types in ideomotor apraxia: A qualitative analysis. *Brain and Cognition, 25*, 250–270.

Merians, A. S., Clark, M., Poizner, H., Jacobs, D. H., Adair, J. C., Macauley, B., Gonzalez-Rothi, L. J., & Heilman, K. M. (1999). Apraxia differs in corticobasal degeneration and left parietal stroke: A case study. *Brain and Cognition, 40*(2), 314–335.

Miller, E. (1984). *Recovery and managements of neuropsychological impairments.* New York: Wiley.

Miller, N. (1986). *Dyspraxia and its management.* London: Croom Helm.

Moffat, N. (1984). Strategies of memory therapy. In B. A. Wilson & N. Moffat (Eds.), *Clinical management of memory problems.* London: Croom Helm.

Morlaas, J. (1928). *Contribution a l'etude de l'apraxie.* Paris: Amedee Legrand.

Ochipa, C., Maher, L. M., & Rothi, L. J. G. (1995). Treatment of ideomotor apraxia. *Journal of the International Neuropsychological Society, 2,* 149.

Ochipa, C., Gonzalez-Rothi, L. J., & Heilman, K. M. (1992). Conceptual apraxia in Alzheimer's disease. *Brain, 115,* 1061–1071.

Papagno, C., Della Sala, S., & Basso, A. (1993). Ideomotor apraxia without aphasia, aphasia without apraxia: The anatomical support for a double dissociation. *Journal of Neurology, Neurosurgery and Psychiatry, 56,* 286–289.

Pieczuro, A., & Vignolo, L. A. (1967). Studio sperimentale sul'aprasiaideomtoria. *Sist. nerv., 19,* 131–143.

Pilgrim, E., & Humphreys, G. W. (1994). Rehabilitation of a case of ideomotor apraxia. In M. J. Riddoch & G. W. Humphreys (Eds.), *Cognitive neuropsychology and cognitive rehabilitation.* Hove, UK: Erlbaum.

Prigatano, G. P., Fordyce, D., Zeiner, H., Roueche, J., Pepping, M., & Wood, B. (1984). Neuropsychological rehabilitation after closed head injury in young adults. *Journal of Neurology, Neurosurgery and Psychiatry, 47,* 505–513.

Poeck, K. (1983). Ideational apraxia. *Journal of Neurology, 230,* 1–5.

Poeck, K. (1985). Clues to the nature of disruptions in limb apraxia. In E. A. Roy (Ed.), *Neuropsychological studies of apraxia and related disorders.* New York: North-Holland.

Poole, J. (1998). Effect of apraxia on the ability to learn one-handed shoe tying. *Occupational Therapy Journal of Research, 18*(3), 99–104.

Rothi, L. J. G., Mack, L., & Heilman, K. M. (1990). Unawareness of apraxic errors. *Neurology, 40*(1), 202.

Roy, E. A., Square-Storer, P., Hogg, S., & Adams, S. (1991). Analysis of task demands in apraxia. *International Journal of the Neurosciences, 56,* 177–186.

Saeki, S., Ogata, H., Okubo, T., Takahashi, K., & Hoshuyama, T. (1993). Factors influencing return to work after stroke in Japan. *Stroke, 24,* 1182–1185.

Selnes, O. A., Pestronk, A., Hart, A., & Gordon, B. (1991). Limb apraxia without aphasia in a left sided lesion in a right handed patient. *Journal of Neurology, Neurosurgery and Psychiatry, 54,* 734–733.

Shelton, P. A., & Knopman, D. S. (1991). Ideomotor apraxia in Huntington's disease. *Archives of Neurology, 48,* 35–41.

Singu, A., Cohen, L., Duhamel, J. R., Pillon, B., Dubois, B., & Agid, Y. (1995). A selective impairment of hand posture for object utilization in apraxia. *Cortex, 31,* 41–55.

Smania, N., Girardi, F., Domenicali, C., Lora, E., & Aglioti, S. (2000). The rehabilitation of limb apraxia: A study in left-brain damaged patients. *Archives of Physical Medicine and Rehabilitation, 81,* 379–388.

Steinthal, P. (1871). *Abris der Sprachwissenschaft.* Berlin: Krager.

Sunderland, A., Tinson, D., & Bradley, I. (1994). Differences in recovery from constructional apraxia after right and left hemisphere stroke? *Journal of Clinical and Experimental Neuropsychology, 16*(6), 916–920.

Sundet, K., Finset, A., & Reinvang, I. R. (1988). Neuropsychological predictors in stroke rehabilitation. *Journal of Clinical and Experimental Neuropsychology,* *10*(4), 363–379.

Tate, R. L., & McDonald, S. (1995). What is apraxia?: The clinician's dilemma. *Neuropsychological Rehabilitation, 5*(4), 273–297.

Taylor, R. (1994). Motor apraxia in dementia. *Perceptual and Motor Skills, 79,* 523–528.

van Heugten, C. M., Dekker, J., Deelman, B. G., van Dijk, A. J., Stehmann-Saris, J. C., & Kinebanian, A. (1998). Outcome of strategy training in stroke patients with apraxia: A phase II study. *Clinical Rehabilitation, 12,* 294–303.

van Heugten, C. M., Dekker, J., Deelman, B. G., Stehmann-Sairs, J. C., & Kinebanian, A. (1999a). A diagnostic test for apraxia in stroke patients: Internal consistency and diagnostic value. *Clinical Neuropsychologist, 13*(2), 182–192.

van Heugten, C. M., Dekker, J., Deelman, B. G., Stehmann-Saris, J. C., & Kinebanian, A. (1999b). Assessment of disabilties of stroke patients with apraxia: Internal consistency and inter-observer reliability. *Occupational Therapy Journal of Research, 19*(1), 55–74.

van Heugten, C. M., Dekker, J., Deelman, B. G., van Dijk, A. J., Stehmann-Saris, J. C., & Kinebanian, A. (2000). Measuring disabilities in stroke patients with apraxia: A validation study of an observational method. *Neuropsychological Rehabilitation, 10*(4), 401–414.

van Heugten, C. M., Dekker, J., Deelman, B. G., Stehmann-Saris, J. C., & Kinebanian, A. (2000). Rehabilitation of stroke patients with apraxia: The role of additional cognitive and motor impairments. *Disability and Rehabilitation, 22*(2), 547–555.

van Zomeren, A. H., & Brouwer, W. H. (1994). *Clinical neuropsychology of attention.* Oxford, UK: Oxford University Press.

Wilson, B. (1988). Sarah: Remediation of apraxia following an anaesthetic accident. In J. West & P. Spinks (Eds.), *Case studies in clinical psychology.* Bristol: John Wright.

World Health Organization. (1980). *International classification of impairments, disabilities and handicaps.* Geneva: Author.

CHAPTER 11

The Enigma of Executive Functioning
Theoretical Contributions to Therapeutic Interventions

KEITH D. CICERONE

The rehabilitation of executive functions can be enigmatic. Remedial interventions for acquired cognitive impairments often emphasize the acquisition of specific compensations in controlled situations, and responsibility for the selection and application of compensatory strategies may rest with the therapist. In contrast, disturbances of executive functioning are most likely to be evident when the patient is required to assume responsibility for the application of compensatory strategies (Shallice & Burgess, 1991) or to cope with novel situations (Godefrey & Rousseaux, 1997). The development of effective therapeutic interventions for dysexecutive symptoms must therefore rely on an adequate conceptualization of the nature of executive abilities and their dissolution. The primary goal of this chapter is to describe briefly several theoretical perspectives on executive functioning, particularly those that may have a direct application to remedial intervention approaches. It should be noted that the concepts of frontal lobe function and executive functioning have been intimately related, and the theoretical positions that I discuss have generally relied on the analysis of frontal lobe function and dysfunction. While this perspective is relevant and valuable for heuristic purposes, it should be noted that these anatomical and behavioral concepts are dissociable, and disturbances of executive functioning can be observed without observable frontal lobe damage, and with various forms of focal or diffuse damage throughout the cerebral axis.

TEUBER'S COROLLARY DISCHARGE

Perhaps the first modern formulation of executive functioning was provided by Teuber (1964), who noted that most previous clinical descriptions of symptoms after frontal lobe damage had relied on "sensationalistic" psychological concepts, such as a disturbance of "will." In contrast to the "classical tendency to start all considerations of brain function from the sensory side" (p. 418). Teuber proposed that the critical function of the frontal lobes is in maintaining a "corollary discharge—i.e., a discharge from motor to sensory structures—which prepares the sensory structures for an anticipated change" (p. 418). In establishing a motor, or *executive*, role in higher cortical functioning, Teuber provided a neurophysiological mechanism that could serve as the basis for volitional behavior, and for the disturbances of volitional behavior that appeared to characterize lesions of the frontal lobes. In this view, all voluntary behavior involves two neural correlates, the activation of impulses to the effector organs and a simultaneous corollary discharge to central neural receptors, which preset these receptors for the detection of changes occurring as a consequence of the particular behavior. The corollary discharge therefore establishes an internal representation of behavior independent of the external response (a concept that is not dissimilar to current notions of working memory as the temporary activation of a mental representation to guide cognition and behavior when the relevant environmental markers are not present; Goldman-Rakic, 1988). According to Teuber, then, "it is not in the reaction to incoming stimuli, *but in the prediction of them* . . . that the significance of frontal structures lies" (p. 440, emphasis added). A disturbance in these anticipatory processes may be particularly apparent in nonroutine situations (Karnath, Wallesch, & Zimmerman, 1991) and thus reflect one of the fundamental characteristics of executive dysfunction.

This conceptualization of executive functioning, derived from the mechanism of corollary discharge, has several important implications for rehabilitation. First, it suggests that improving the patient's ability to predict his or her own behavior and its consequences should, in principle, help to reestablish the intentional character of thinking and acting. Second, this same process should establish a feedback mechanism and allow for the monitoring of discrepancies among intentions, actions, and behavioral outcomes (Fink et al., 1999). Once it becomes possible to predict the consequences of one's actual behaviors, it is also possible to predict the consequences of potential behaviors and the consideration of alternative courses of action, allowing for the establishment of an "abstract attitude" (Goldstein, 1939). Finally, if one can predict possible behaviors, then one can predict, anticipate, and evaluate the behaviors of others as well, enabling the individual to engage in complex social interactions (Stone, Baron-Cohen, & Knight, 1998).

There have been several attempts to remediate executive function deficits through the prediction and self-monitoring of behaviors, with the implicit objective of establishing an expectation that enables the patients to compare the predicted and actual results of their behavior. Cicerone and Giacino (1992) described the use of a prediction paradigm in two patients with traumatic brain injuries, both of whom exhibited chronic difficulties in their social functioning over a year after their injuries. Both patients performed well on formal neuropsychological measures of executive functioning and were capable of functioning independently to conduct fundamental activities of daily living, but exhibited poor judgment and difficulties in social functioning due to their apparent inability to anticipate the detrimental effects of their behavior. They were able to function effectively in relatively structured situations in which their actions were constrained, but both patients experienced difficulty when required to anticipate the effects of their behavior in less structured social situations. Thus, they exhibited a disability in adjusting their social behaviors on the basis of their expected consequences.

The need for these patients to develop an ability to predict the results of their behavior and adjust their behavior to different situational demands was recognized, particularly with regard to nonroutine problem-solving demands. During the baseline treatment evaluation, the patients were administered a modified version of the Tower of London (Shallice, 1982). This task was selected because it requires the anticipation of errors in order to achieve a successful solution and also provides a number of problem-solving trials that vary in level of difficulty (i.e., number of moves required to solution). It was noted in both cases that the latencies before the initial move were unrelated to problem difficulty and there was even a slight tendency for the patients to spend *less* time thinking about the more difficult trials. In other words, these patients spent about the same amount of time in attempting both the easy trials of a problem-solving task and the most difficult ones, so that their efforts were unrelated to the task demands. These within-session behaviors appeared to mirror the patients' functional difficulties, reflecting a failure both to anticipate the consequences of their behavior before acting and to adapt their behavior to the vicissitudes of different situations. We subsequently implemented a training procedure that simply involved having the patients predict the required steps to solution on each trial of the problem-solving task. Patients were provided verbal feedback for incorrect predictions, and subjects again predicted the required steps to a solution. The various problem-solving trials were then presented in random order of complexity, and the patients were again asked to predict the number of moves required, to carry out each trial, and to compare the predicted and actual number of moves required. There was a significant overall increase in response latencies when the patients were required to predict their results, with increased response latencies most apparent for the more complex trials, and a strong relationship between response latency and number of required moves with the intervention, suggesting that the amount of cognitive processing was now proportionate to problem difficulty. There was also a marked decrease in errors with the intervention, and both patients' performances actually became error free, so that the act of predicting appeared to induce a set to self-monitor and to self-correct as well. Following this training, the patients were provided (and were themselves asked to provide) multiple examples of daily situations in which the same cognitive processes of predicting their behavior might apply. One of the patients was subsequently able spontaneously to apply the strategy to his time management of daily

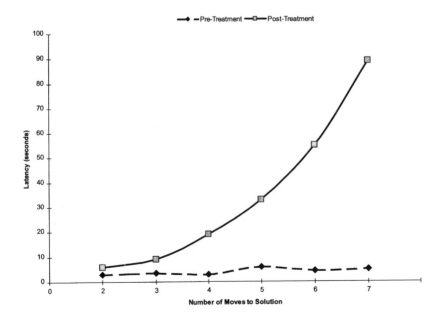

FIGURE 11.1. Average response latencies (number of seconds prior to first move as an index of time spent planning) pretreatment and posttreatment for two patients. The treatment used a prediction paradigm with the Tower of London, as described in the text.

activities and interpersonal communications, both of which had been areas of difficulty. The other patient remained able to use the strategy effectively when given explicit instructions to do so but never spontaneously applied it either within or outside treatment. In that case, a family member was educated as to the nature of the patient's deficits and the need to assume responsibility for cueing strategy use.

Two additional studies of patients with traumatic brain injury suggest that having subjects predict their task performance and providing them with tangible feedback may reduce discrepancies between their predicted and actual performance (Rebmann & Hannon, 1995; Youngjohn & Altman, 1989). In both of these studies, the primary effect of the intervention was related to modification of patients' predictions rather than a change in actual task performance, suggesting an impact on their self-monitoring and appraisal skills.

Several interventions directed at improving patients' ability to self-monitor their behavior have been described. Sohlberg, Sprunk, and Metzelaar (1988) treated a patient with traumatic frontal lobe damage, who exhibited decreased initiation and range of affect. The therapist provided the patient with intermittent external cues (such as placing an index card in front of the subject, with an instruction to initiate conversation) that placed little demand on internal self-monitoring, in order to increase verbal initiation and response acknowledgments. Both behaviors increased during application of the external cueing procedure; the patient's verbal initiation decreased when the external cueing procedure was withdrawn, although the level remained above baseline. Cicerone and Giacino (1992) utilized a formal self-monitoring and reinstatement procedure with another patient who had sustained bilateral frontal traumatic brain injury 3 years prior to entering rehabilitation. During the initial course of rehabilitation, the therapist frequently observed that this man was unable to recognize or correct his errors, either within treatment sessions (e.g., on a proofreading task) or in the course of his daily activities (e.g., taking the wrong lunch from the refrigerator). Upon making an error during subsequent tasks, the patient was stopped immediately; his attention was directed to the error, and he was required to keep a record of his errors and systematically to compare his responses on subsequent trials to his record of prior errors. This procedure assumed that the prerequisite initial step in remediating deficits in self-monitoring is the provision of adequate external feedback. In this patient, the structured error-monitoring system was effective in improving performance on treatment tasks, although withdrawal of the structured error-monitoring procedure resulted in a return to the baseline error rate. This patient was also able to apply an error-monitoring routine to perform successfully a vocational (clerical) task, although he required direct instruction and prompts in that situation as well. In both of these reported interventions, treatment effectiveness was related to the modification of specific behaviors rather than to the internal mediating cognitive processes, and there was limited evidence that the patients were able to apply the strategies independently or in novel situations.

Alderman, Fry, and Youngson (1995) utilized a program of prompts and rewards to enable a patient to exert control over inappropriate behaviors through increased self-monitoring. This was effective in reducing the frequency of inappropriate behaviors within both treatment and community environments. Of interest is the fact that the greatest effect of treatment occurred when external prompts and rewards were withdrawn and the patient was responsible for independent self-monitoring.

Although the interventions discussed in this section utilized different specific procedures, they have all emphasized the need for patients to anticipate and monitor the outcomes of their behavior. It is essential to remember, of course, that the goal of remediation is not the training of task-specific performance but the training and internalization of regulatory cognitive processes. It is also interesting to note that the cognitive process of predicting the potential outcomes of different courses of behavior may be a fundamental aspect of persons' perceived self-efficacy, which in turn influences more generally the exercise of self-regulatory cognitive processes and behavioral control (Bandura, 1997).

LURIA'S VERBAL SELF-REGULATION
AND SHALLICE'S SUPERVISORY SYSTEM

Luria (1966) viewed the effects of frontal lobe injury as a disturbance in the conscious and volitional self-regulation of behavior, while leaving intact or even enhancing the more primitive or reflexive forms of behavior. Disruption of the capacity for self-regulation after neurologic injury is likely to result in two basic symptoms: a loss of intentionality, manifested by decreased spontaneity or initiative, and a loss of critical attitude toward one's own behavior, manifested as a deficiency in matching one's actions with the original intention. According to Luria, the formulation of an internalized plan of action and subsequent self-regulation of behavior is accomplished through the verbal mediation of purposeful activity. This "inner speech," while distinct from the communicative speech function, acquires its directive function through the act of progressive speech internalization. Though normal development, the initially overt, expanded form of speech becomes abbreviated, evolving into self-directed "whispered speech." Gradually, this speech becomes covert and internalized, and takes on a planning and self-regulatory role "between the general intention to solve a problem and its concrete solution" (Luria, 1981, p. 107).

The processes of programming, regulation, and verification of activity have also been characterized by Shallice (1981) in terms of the operation of a supervisory (attentional) system. Cognitive and behavioral processes are considered to be organized into relatively invariant and overlearned routines, or schemas. There are two levels of neuropsychological control over behavioral schemas. *Routine* control, the first level, can be accomplished through contention scheduling, based on the habitual activation of schemas in response to overlearned environmental contingencies. The supervisory–executive system represents a second level of voluntary, strategic control that is necessary when planning and correction of unexpected errors are required, when the appropriate responses are novel or not well learned, or when habitual responses and schemas need to be inhibited. Impairments of the supervisory system result in heightened expression of lower level, habitual schemas, while reducing the ability to initiate more highly adaptive responses. An improvement in executive functioning due to facilitation of the supervisory–executive control process would be expected to result in two types of changes. First, patients should show enhanced performance on tasks requiring novel problem solving and error correction. Second, patients should show improved ability to inhibit the release of inappropriate responses.

Luria and Homskaya (1964) noted that simply having the patient repeat the task instruction is insufficient to reestablish self-regulation. Meichenbaum and Goodman (1971) developed a self-instructional training procedure that recapitulated the progressive internalization of the verbal act, which should facilitate the training and development of verbal self-regulation. Cicerone and Wood (1987) used a modification of Meichenbaum's self-instructional training procedure for the treatment of a patient's executive function deficits after frontal lobe trauma. Three years following his injury, the patient exhibited marked impulsivity, inappropriateness in social situations, and lack of realistic planning for his future. He frequently interrupted conversations of other family members and friends, his own speech became expansive and circumstantial, and it often appeared that "he doesn't think before he does something." Neuropsychological evaluation 4 years after injury was most notable for the patient's marked impairment of planning ability and difficulty evaluating the results of his own actions. For example, he exhibited marked impulsivity and disinhibition on choice reactions and conditional motor responses. On a test of imitation of postures, he made numerous, random responses before reaching a final position and showed marked impairment on motor tasks when the stimulus and response were not isomorphic (e.g., "conflict" and go/no-go reactions). Although he showed no evidence of a primary visuospatial or constructional impairment, his ability to copy a complex figure was poorly organized.

A self-instructional training procedure was implemented to teach the patient to plan ahead and monitor step-by-step performance while inhibiting inappropriate behaviors. The training task was again the Tower of London, selected to simulate the nonroutine cognitive selection processes required of the supervisory–executive system. It is worth noting that while the specific task was the same as that used with other, previously discussed, patients, the nature of the therapeutic intervention was modified and adapted in accordance with the conceptual formulation of the nature of the patient's deficits. In this case, the pretreatment baseline performance was characterized by the patient's frequent errors on the initial trial of a problem and inability to independently correct his errors with repetition of the same problem situation. In addition to his unplanned and incorrect moves on performance of the training task, he also demonstrated a large number of off-task verbalizations and behaviors (which were recorded and analyzed separately from his incorrect moves). Three stages of training were subsequently implemented. In the first stage, the patient was required to verbalize aloud his moves on the training task before and during actual performance. In the second stage, training was identical except that the patient was instructed to whisper rather than to verbalize aloud. Finally, in the third stage, the training task was repeated and the patient was instructed to "talk to himself" silently before and during actual task performance. During the first stage of training, a dramatic reduction in his incorrect moves remained stable over the remaining course of treatment. There was also a more gradual reduction and eventual cessation of off-task behaviors over the course of treatment. At the completion of the 8-week treatment program, evidence for transfer of training was also observed on neuropsychological measures of planning ability, and the patient's performance remained improved at 4-month follow-up. Measures of generalization to his functional, real-life behaviors were monitored throughout treatment. In addition, following the initial self-instructional training, he received an additional 12 weeks of instruction in applying and self-monitoring the verbal mediation strategy to his everyday behaviors. Generalization was not observed during the initial treatment period, but the patient demonstrated a progressive, systematic increase in the application of principles of planning and self-regulation over the ensuing period of extended generalization training. A somewhat ironic, and amusing, illustration of his independent use of a self-control strategy occurred during the discharge conference, when he appropriately stopped his mother from interrupting.

Cicerone and Giacino (1992) subsequently evaluated the same self-instructional protocol with 6 patients in a multiple baseline across subjects design. Five of the patients had sustained traumatic brain injury

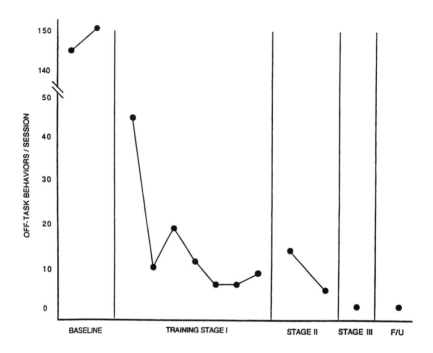

FIGURE 11.2. Frequency of off-task behaviors during baseline and training stages for one participant receiving self-instructional treatment. Copyright 1992 by IOS Press B.U. Reprinted with permission.

and 1 patient had a falx meningioma, all were at least 1-year postonset of their injury or illness, and all evidenced damage to the frontal lobes (although this anatomic information was not a criterion for inclusion in the treatment study). The patients were selected for the intervention because they exhibited both impaired planning and self-monitoring on the basis of family observations and therapist reports, and evidence of impaired performance on the Wisconsin Card Sorting Test (WCST), the Tinker Toy Test, or Wechsler Intelligence Scale for Children—Revised mazes. Treatment was again delivered in three stages to promote the progressive internalization of verbal self-regulation, as described earlier. Five of the 6 patients showed marked reduction of errors as a result of the initial self-instructional training. Evaluation of pre- and posttraining changes on the psychometric measures indicated significant improvements on mazes errors and WCST perseverative responses, again suggesting that the effectiveness of training was related to the patients' improved ability to inhibit impulsive or perseverative responses. The improvement in problem-solving errors and reduction of inappropriate responses with the intervention are consistent with the predictions derived from Shallice's (1981) model of supervisory control and support the potential effectiveness of verbal mediation in establishing effective self-regulation and improving executive function deficits. Additional behavioral observation in some patients indicated that the reduction in errors was accompanied by reductions in various disinhibited, off-task behaviors during task performance, so that it is unlikely that the effect of training was restricted to learning task-specific behaviors.

The principles and techniques of self-instructional training are based on a sound framework of neurolopsychological function and behavioral therapy, and appear to be applicable to a wide range of problem behaviors. The intervention is directed explicitly toward the internalization of self-regulatory processes, and therefore is by its nature accessible in a variety of situations. The use of verbal self-regulation as a treatment strategy should also have relevance in the treatment of emotional disorders after neurological illness or injury, for example, in patients who exhibit increased emotional lability.

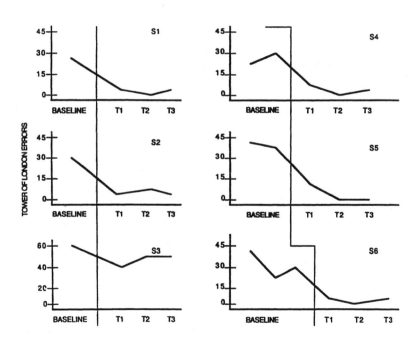

FIGURE 11.3. Multiple baseline across six subjects showing Tower of London errors during baseline and self-instructional training stages. Copyright 1992 by IOS Press B.U. Reprinted with permission.

DUNCAN'S GOAL NEGLECT

Duncan (1986) noted that a fundamental aspect of executive dysfunction is the loss of control of action by its desired results. He suggested that most behavior is under the control of a particular set of goals, and that these goals elicit the relevant actions from a large, potential store of (covert and overt) actions. Through a process of means–end analysis, the result of each action is evaluated in order to detect differences between the current state and goal state, and this process continues to elicit actions until the mismatch between the current state and the goal state is reduced to zero. As a consequence of frontal lobe damage, this typical structure of goal-directed behavior is disrupted, and behavior therefore loses its purposeful character. This formulation relied explicitly on the work of Luria (1966; Luria, Pribram, & Homskaya, 1964) and Shallice (1981), and implicitly resembled Teuber's (1964) concept of error detection and correction through the process of corollary discharge. Duncan (Duncan, Emslie, Williams, Johnson, & Freer, 1996) also noted that patients with frontal lobe damage may exhibit a dissociation between the relative preservation of verbal knowledge, and the failure of this knowledge to guide behavior through the activation of the appropriate goals and actions (Luria, 1966; Milner, 1963). This tendency to disregard the requirements of a given task, even when these are verbally appreciated, represents a fundamental aspect of executive dysfunction, referred to as *goal neglect*.

Levine and his colleagues (Levine, Robertson, et al., 2000) developed a formalized intervention for executive dysfunction, referred to as goal management training (GMT), based on Duncan's (1986; Duncan et al., 1996) theory of goal neglect. The process of GMT involves five discrete stages of what is essentially a general purpose, problem solving algorithm (e.g., D'Zurilla & Goldfried, 1971). In stage 1, participants are trained to evaluate the current state of affairs and relevant goals ("What am I doing?"). The relevant goals are selected in stage 2 (the "main task"), and further partitioned into subgoals in the stage 3 (the "steps"). In stage 4, participants are assisted with the learning and retention of goals and subgoals ("Do I know the steps?"). In the stage 5, participants are taught to self-monitor the results of their actions with the intended goal state ("Am I doing what I planned to do?"), and in the event of a mismatch the entire process is repeated. Levine, Robertson, et al. (2000) described two applications of GMT to patients with neurological injury, each of whom demonstrated impairment on a task considered sensitive to impairments of self-regulation and goal achievement. In the first example, 30 patients were randomly assigned to receive either a brief trial of GMT or an alternative treatment of motor skills training. The GMT consisted of a single session in which participants were instructed to apply the problem-solving algorithm to two functional tasks (proofreading and room layout), which involved keeping goals in mind, analysis of subgoals, and monitoring outcomes. Patients in the motor skills training condition practiced reading and tracing mirror-reversed text and designs; a trainer provided general instruction and encouragement, but the treatment procedure did not include any processes related to GMT. Treatment effectiveness was assessed on several paper-and-pencil tasks that resembled the training tasks and were intended to simulate the kind of unstructured, everyday situations that might elicit goal management deficits. Participants who received GMT demonstrated significant reduction in errors and prolonged time to task completion (presumably reflecting increased care and attention to the tasks) on two of the three outcome measures following the intervention.

In the second example of GMT (Levine, Robertson, et al., 2000), a single patient with attention and executive deficits secondary to encephalitis was taught to perform meal preparation (involving management of multiple subgoals) using the GMT procedure. Meal preparation was assessed through direct observation of problematic behaviors (e.g., failure to assemble the necessary ingredients, repeated checking of instructions, and sequencing errors) and a self-report diary. The patient demonstrated a significant reduction in observed problematic behaviors and self-reported difficulties following the training.

Levine, Robertson, et al. (2000) noted that the GMT was similar to a procedure described by von Cramon, Mathes-von Cramon, and Mai (1991), who also utilized a problem-solving intervention intended to facilitate patients' ability to reduce the complexity of a multistage problem by breaking it down into manageable subgoals. Training was provided to 37 subjects, who, with various etiologies of brain damage, were identified as poor problem solvers on formal tests of planning and response regulation. The intervention was based on five aspects of problem solving (D'Zurilla & Goldfried, 1971) and included training in problem orientation, problem definition and formulation, generation of alternatives, decision making, and solution verification. When compared with an alternative treatment directed at memory training, the patients who received the problem-solving training demonstrated both significant gains on measures of planning ability and improvement on behavioral ratings of executive dysfunction, such as awareness of cognitive deficits, goal-directed ideas, and problem-solving ability.

DAMASIO'S "SOMATIC MARKERS"
AND DISTURBANCE OF SOCIAL COGNITION

Patients with orbitofrontal damage may represent a particular challenge to management and rehabilitation. These patients may exhibit profound disturbances of emotional regulation and everyday social cognition, although they demonstrate intact performance on formal neuropsychological testing and preserved ability to describe verbally the appropriate responses to situations (Eslinger & Damasio, 1985). Animals with orbitofrontal lesions demonstrate an alteration in emotional reactivity and regulation (Butter & Snyder, 1972) that may result in marked disruption of socially appropriate responding and social adaptation (Kling & Steklis, 1976; Mesulam, 1986). In patients with orbitofrontal lesions, the loss of emotional and social mediation results in behavior that is rigidly dictated by patients' immediate environment. Lhermitte (1986) described an environmental dependency syndrome in which patients' behaviors in complex social situations are based primarily upon the salient characteristics of the immediate environment, with loss of the flexibility and adaptability required to behave effectively in those situations. These patients also exhibited apathy, indifference to social rules, and lack of self-criticism. Lhermitte reported that environmental dependence was particularly apparent in patients with lesions of the orbitofrontal lobes, due to the loss of the normal frontal functions of modulation and inhibition that allow the unmediated activation of parietal lobe systems and a direct response to environmental stimuli.

Eslinger and Damasio (1985) provided a seminal description of a patient with bilateral orbitofrontal damage who did not exhibit deficits on formal tests of executive functioning but did exhibit a marked impairment of interpersonal functioning, judgment, and decision making in everyday social functioning. They attributed the disturbance of social cognition following orbitofrontal lesions to the inability to analyze and integrate the premises of real-life situations in order to select the appropriate response from among many options. According to Damasio, Tranel, and Damasio (1991), the process of response selection in social cognition requires the integration of environmental, sensory information projected from parietal cortices and the autonomic, visceral information projected from limbic cortices. This confluence of external and internal information in the orbitofrontal cortex allows patients to assign emotional and motivational significance to the representation of events in the environment. The investigators propose that the fundamental mechanism by which the orbitofrontal cortex guides social behavior is therefore through the activation of "somatic markers" in conjunction with the cognitive representations of the environment to mark the "implied meaning" of a situation (i.e., the value and anticipated consequences of possible responses). It has subsequently been shown that orbitofrontal damage may result in a failure of autonomic processes to trigger both the appropriate behavioral response (Damasio, Tranel, & Damasio, 1991), and insensitivity to future consequences (Bechara, Damasio, Damasio, & Anderson, 1994).

Cicerone and Tanenbaum's (1997) reported case of a woman with impaired social cognition following traumatic orbitofrontal injury included a description of their efforts to rehabilitate her neuropsychological functioning. The patient exhibited episodes of abrupt crying and laughing, rigidity and "obsessive" behaviors during the course of her daily homemaking activities, and increased sensitivity to feedback or criticism that had resulted in increasingly frequent arguments and interpersonal conflicts with her four children. When seen for neuropsychological consultation 6 months after her injury, she demonstrated inconsistent and superficial awareness of her neurologic deficits. She had a complete anosmia, but other sensory and motor functions were intact. Basic attention functions, memory, perceptual and constructional abilities, and language were intact. She exhibited impaired performance on language and memory tests that required her to overcome the "direct connotations" of verbal statements (Luria, 1981). On formal measures of executive functioning, she exhibited significant disinhibition on tests of motor regulation, and reduced verbal and behavioral fluency, but other measures were generally within normal limits. The patient was also administered several tests of "social cognition" intended to reflect the kind of disturbances described by Damasio (Saver & Damasio, 1991). On these measures, she demonstrated significant impairments in her ability to interpret nonverbal interpersonal interactions and the meanings of social exchanges in different contexts, and to predict the most likely consequences of social situations.

During the course of her treatment, the therapist attempted to increase her awareness of problem areas and their impact on her performance of daily living and social functioning. Initially, she exhibited an inability to inhibit socially inappropriate behaviors and to appreciate an alternative perspective, for example, interrupting salespeople and becoming argumentative when her needs were not addressed immediately. She was able to acknowledge these behaviors when she viewed them on the videotape and fairly quickly appeared to modify her behavior when external cues were present in the community (e.g., the overt presence of the therapist and video camera). However, she continued to have difficulty internalizing these constraints in order to guide her behavior. Videotaped feedback from her individual and group treatment sessions was also provided to facilitate her recognition of any discrepancies between her spontaneous evaluation of her performance and her "objective" evaluation of the videotaped sessions. She had particular difficulty utilizing complex or subtle forms of information arising from social interactions, so that her social judgment was particularly affected. Over the course of this treatment, she developed intellectual awareness of the nature of these problems; however, for the most part, she remained unable to monitor her behavior in the context of her real-life interactions. Although she benefited from tangible cues to signal her behavior (such as direct instruction or a prompt from the therapist), she was unable to utilize her own emotional states or feelings of cognitive dissonance to guide her behavior. Her attempts to control her behavior (e.g., her pathological laughing and her verbal tangentiality), were often accomplished through the suppression of nearly all spontaneous behavior.

Following nearly 9 months of treatment, she demonstrated improvement in her capacity for basic behavioral regulation as well as continued evidence of intact planning, self-monitoring, and self-regulation on formal neuropsychological testing. Despite this, she exhibited continued difficulty and functional impairments in monitoring and controlling her emotional responses, and particularly her complex social interactions. Her husband continued to report that she was unable to benefit from feedback or to accept constructive criticism from others, and he described substantial problems due to his wife's inflexibility, rigidity, egocentricity, poor empathy, and nonreinforcing social behaviors. When presented with a single, well-structured situation, with well-defined response requirements, she was able to define the appropriate response, However, she continued to have difficulty when she needed to analyze social situations containing multiple priorities and to guide her own behavior according to the appropriate responses. Thus, the failure to appreciate the relationship between her actions and goals *in the relevant social context* characterized her impairment. While she was able to resume many of the basic, instrumental activities of daily living that she performed before her injury, she continued to exhibit a profound impairment in her social functioning.

Evaluation of this patient's treatment suggests that she was able to benefit from explicit feedback concerning her social and emotional behavior in specific situations, and this enabled her to correct her mistakes and produce the appropriate response within those situations. However, in novel, real-life situations, she remained unable to appreciate the subtle social cues required to guide her behavior effectively and she appeared unable to monitor her own emotional responses or to acknowledge the socially inappropriate aspects of her behavior.

Von Cramon and Mathes-von Cramon (1994) have also described the treatment of a 33-year-old physician whose bilateral traumatic frontal lobe injury resulted in decreased social behavior that they related to an inability to use both subtle social signals to monitor the effect of his behavior on others his preserved knowledge to organize his behavior. Treatment consisted of providing the patient with a formal (written) problem-solving algorithm, which included problem identification and analysis, generation of hypotheses and decision making, and evaluation of solutions. This algorithm was applied to the patient's ability to make accurate histopathological diagnoses. Initially, these rules were guided externally by the therapist, who provided the patient with an invariant set of questions to guide his behavior. External guidance was gradually substituted by overt self-instruction and internal guidance until the patient could work alone. He was also required to predict his expected performance and to rate his actual performance. These self-predictions also allowed use of the method of goal attainment scaling to evaluate his performance, specifically, the accuracy of diagnoses and coherence of reports. Following treatment, von Cramon and Matthes-von Cramon noted that the patient was able to utilize a routinized, external structure to improve *specific behaviors in the situations in which they had been trained*, but this improvement was not apparent in novel situations, and the patient continued generally to overestimate his level of intellectual competence.

It appears that patients with disturbances of social cognition after orbitofrontal lesions may improve their functioning through the establishment of specific competencies, but there is little evidence for the effectiveness of treatments that allow them to regain the ability to integrate and respond fully to the subtle complexities and nuances of the social environment. In some cases, it may be possible to teach patients to "mind read," that is, to recognize the specific verbal and nonverbal behaviors that signal other people's social and emotional intentions and meanings. As emphasized by the theory of somatic markers, however, more effective treatment of these impairments is likely to require increased emphasis on the instigation of patients' emotional (and perhaps visceral) experience. Although this area has not really been explored in the context of neuropsychological rehabilitation, it is interesting to note the proposed role of orbitofrontal cortex in the process of affective regulation and the "restorative" functions of the self (Schore, 1994).

CONCLUSIONS

Despite subtle differences, there are striking commonalities among the theoretical perspectives I have discussed. All of the theories reflect the role of anticipatory processes, the regulation of behavior through the correspondence of actions and their intended effects, and the role of error detection and utilization in adaptive behavior. Interventions for executive dysfunction also appear to reflect these processes, through the use of overt predictions, verbal mediation and adaptive problem solving, and formal self-monitoring strategies. It is likely that these procedures are related to the establishment of an internal cognitive representation or expectancy of an action and its intended consequences, to the active comparison of the internal cognitive representation and information about the actual results produced by behavior, and to the salience of feedback that allows for error recognition and evaluation. In all of the intervention procedures, it is necessary to make overt (i.e., conscious and deliberate) a cognitive process that may compensate for the disrupted neurological function.

Continued refinements in the concept of executive functioning will clearly have an impact on clinical and methodological issues in rehabilitation. For example, the efforts to "fractionate" the functioning of the frontal lobes at both neurophysiological and neuropsychological levels are likely to result in more precise formulations as to the nature and subtypes of executive dysfunction. Even with our present knowledge, it is critical to tailor the intervention to the nature of the deficit. For example, at a basic level, disturbances of executive function can be characterized as both negative (e.g., apathy, adynamia, loss of abstract attitude) and excessive behaviors (e.g., disinhibition, lability, perseveration), and there is little evidence to indicate which interventions are more appropriate for specific deficit areas. The need to target interventions to specific problem behaviors will become more pronounced as we are better able to refine the nature of executive impairments, and it is likely to be a critical factor in determining the efficacy of different interventions.

In addition to these questions of "how to treat," there are questions regarding "whom to treat." While it is commonly assumed that executive function deficits are common in certain types of neurological illness, such as traumatic brain injury, our ability to demonstrate the effectiveness of interventions will undoubtedly be diluted if we attempt to provide the same treatment to all persons with acquired brain injury, without some basis for selection. In the case of the executive functions, this may be especially complicated by the observation that some patients can exhibit profound impairments in their real-life social and interpersonal functioning but appear relatively intact on formal measures of executive ability. We will need to develop measures that allow for more precise determination of the presence and severity of deficits, as well as the impact of comorbid deficits, on treatment effectiveness. For example, what impact does expressive language impairment have on the use of verbal self-regulation, or comorbid memory impairments on the ability to learn problem-solving strategies? Finally, there is a need for continued development of appropriate outcome measures. This is, again, particularly salient in the area of executive functioning given the potential discrepancy between performance on laboratory measures and indices of real-life performance. Fortunately, there appears to be continued development of both laboratory (e.g., Levine, Dawson, Boutet, Schwartz, & Stuss, 2000) and clinical (e.g., Ownsworth, McFarland, & Young, 2000) assessment procedures.

Each of the theories suggest that disturbances of executive functioning produce a loss of functional and social autonomy, reflected in decreased volitional behavior (Teuber), aspontaneity and loss of intentionality (Luria), emergence of habitual reactions (Shallice), passivity (Duncan), and environmental dependence (Lhermitte, Damasio). Thus, effective interactions for executive impairments will have to incorporate not only the cognitive aspects but also emotional, motivational, and social aspects as central features of executive dysfunction. In many instances, the training of relatively stable and invariant behavioral routines will allow patients to function in specific situations in the absence of higher order executive functioning. It remains both more difficult and potentially more rewarding to restore the more flexible, self-directed, supervisory processes that represent the highest level of social adaptation and human autonomy.

REFERENCES

Alderman, N., Fry, R. K., & Youngson, H. A. (1995). Improvement of self monitoring skills, reduction of behaviour disturbance and the dysexecutive syndrome. *Neuropsychological Rehabilitation 5*, 193–222.

Bandura, A. (1997). *Self-efficacy: The exercise of control.* New York: Freeman.

Bechara, A., Damasio, A. R., Damasio, H., & Anderson, S. W. (1994). Insensitivity to future consequences following damage to human prefrontal cortex. *Cognition, 50*, 7–15.

Butter, C. M., & Snyder, D. R. (1972). Alterations in aversive and aggressive behaviors following orbital frontal lesions in rhesus monkeys. *Acta Neurobiologica Experimental, 32*, 525–565.

Cicerone, K. D., & Giacino, J. T. (1992). Remediation of executive function deficits after traumatic brain injury. *NeuroRehabilitation, 2*(3), 12–22.

Cicerone, K. D., & Wood, J. C. (1987). Planning disorder after closed head injury: A case study. *Archives of Physical Medicine and Rehabilitation, 68*, 111–115.

Cicerone, K. D., & Tanenbaum, L. N. (1997). Disturbance of social cognition after traumatic orbitofrontal brain injury. *Archives of Clinical Neuropsychology, 12*, 173–188.

Damasio, A. R., Tranel, D., & Damasio, H. C. (1991). Somatic markers and the guidance of behavior: Theory and preliminary testing. In H. S. Levin, H. M. Eisenberg, & A. L. Benton (Eds.), *Frontal lobe function and dysfunction* (pp. 217–229). New York: Oxford University Press.

Duncan, J. (1986). Disorganization of behaviour after frontal lobe damage. *Cognitive Neuropsychology, 3,* 271–290.

Duncan, J., Emslie, H., Williams, P., Johnson, R., & Freer, C. (1996). Intelligence and the frontal lobe: The organisation of goal-directed behaviour. *Cognitive Psychology, 30,* 2257–2303.

D'Zurilla, T. J., & Goldfried, M. R. (1971). Problem solving and behavior modification. *Journal of Abnormal Psychology, 78,* 107–126.

Eslinger, P. J., & Damasio, A. R. (1985). Severe disturbance of higher cognition after bilateral frontal ablation: Patient EVR. *Neurology 35,* 1731–1741.

Fink, G. R., Marshall, J. C., Halligan, P. W., Frith, C. D., Driver, J., Frackowiak, R. S. J., & Dolan, R. J. (1999). The neural consequences of conflict between intention and the senses. *Brain, 122,* 497–512.

Goldman-Rakic, P. S. (1988). Topography of cognition: Parallel distributed networks in primate association cortex. *Annual Review of Neuroscience, 11,* 137–156.

Goldstein, K. (1939). *The organism.* New York: American Book Company.

Godefrey, O., & Rousseaux, M. (1997). Novel decision making in patients with prefrontal or posterior brain damage. *Neurology, 49,* 695–701.

Karnath, H. O., Wallesch, C. W., & Zimmermann, P. (1991). Mental planning and anticipatory process with acute and chronic frontal lobe lesions: A comparison of maze performance in routine and non-routine situations. *Neuropsychologia, 29,* 271–290.

Kling, A., & Steklis, H. D. (1976). A neural substrate for affiliative behavior in non-human primates. *Brain, Behavior and Evolution, 13,* 216–238.

Levine, B., Dawson, D., Boutet, I., Schwartz, M., & Stuss, D. T. (2000). Assessment of strategic self-regulation in traumatic brain injury: Its relationship to injury severity and psychosocial outcome. *Neuropsychology, 14,* 491–500.

Levine, B., Robertson, I. A., Clare, L., Carter, G., Hong, J., Wilson, B. A., Duncan, J., & Stuss, D. T. (2000). Rehabilitation of executive functioning: An experimental–clinical validation of goal management training. *Journal of the International Neuropsychological Society, 6,* 299–312.

Lhermitte, F. (1986). Human autonomy and the frontal lobes: Part II. Patient behavior in complex and social situations: The "environmental dependency syndrome." *Annals of Neurology, 19,* 335–343.

Luria, A. R. (1966). *Higher cortical functions in man.* New York: Basic Books.

Luria, A. R. (1981). *Language and cognition.* Washington, DC: Winston.

Luria, A. R., & Homskaya, E. D. (1964). Disturbance in the regulative role of speech with frontal lobe lesions. In J. M. Warren & K. Akert (Eds.), *The frontal granular cortex and behavior* (pp. 353–371). New York: McGraw-Hill.

Luria, A. R., Pribram, K. H., & Homskaya, E. D. (1964). An experimental analysis of the behavioral disturbance produced by a left frontal arachnoidal endothelioma. *Neuropsychologia. 2,* 257–280.

Meichenbaum, D., & Goodman, J. (1971). Training impulsive children to talk to themselves: A means of developing self-control. *Journal of Abnormal Psychology, 77,* 115–126.

Mesulam, M.-M. (1986). Frontal cortex and behavior. *Annals of Neurology, 19,* 320–325.

Milner, B. (1963). Effects of different brain lesions on card sorting. *Archives of Neurology, 9,* 100–110.

Ownsworth, T. L., McFarland, K., & Young, R. M. (2000). Development and standardization of the Self-Regulation Skills Interview (SRSI): A new clinical assessment tool for acquired brain injury. *Clinical Neuropsychologist, 14,* 76–92.

Rebmann, M. J., & Hannon, R. (1995). Treatment of unawareness deficits in adults with brain injury: Three case studies. *Rehabilitation Psychology 40,* 279–287.

Saver, J. L., & Damasio, A. R. (1991). Preserved access and processing of social knowledge in a patient with acquired sociopathy due to ventromedial frontal damage. *Neuropsychologia, 12,* 1241–1249.

Schore, A. N. (1994). *Affect regulation and the origin of the self: The neurobiology of emotional development.* Hillsdale, NJ: Erlbaum.

Shallice, T. (1981). Neurologic impairment of cognitive processes. *British Medical Bulletin, 37,* 187–192.

Shallice, T. (1982). Specific impairments of planning. *Philosophic Transactions of the Royal Society of London [Biology], 298,* 199–209.

Shallice, T., & Burgess, P. (1991). Deficits in strategy application following frontal lobe damage in man. *Brain, 114,* 727–741.

Sohlberg, M. M., Sprunk, H., & Metzelaar, K. (1988). Efficacy of an external cueing system in an individual with severe frontal lobe damage. *Cognitive Rehabilitation, 6,* 36–41.

Stone, V. E., Baron-Cohen, S., & Knight, R. T. (1998). Frontal lobe contributions to theory of mind. *Journal of Cognitive Neuroscience, 10,* 640–656.

Teuber, H.-L. (1964). The riddle of frontal lobe function in man. In J. M. Warren & K. Akert (Eds.), *The frontal granular cortex and behavior* (pp. 410–444). New York: McGraw-Hill.

Van Hoesen, G. W., Vogt, B. A., Pandya, D. N., & McKenna, T. M. (1980). Compound stimulus differentiation behavior in the rhesus monkey following periarcuate ablation, *Brain Research, 186,* 365–378.

von Cramon, D. Y., & Mathes-von Cramon, G. (1994). Back to work with a chronic dysexecutive syndrome? (a case report). *Neuropsychological Rehabilitation, 4,* 399–417.

von Cramon, D. Y., Mathes-von Cramon, G., & Mai, N. (1991). Problem solving deficits in brain injured patients. A therapeutic approach. *Neuropsychological Rehabilitation, 1,* 45–64.

Youngjohn, J. F., & Altman, I. M. (1989). A performance-based group approach to the treatment of anosognosia and denial. *Rehabilitation Psychology 34,* 217–222.

CHAPTER 12

The Rehabilitation of Neurologically Based Social Disturbances

LYNN M. GRATTAN
MARJAN GHAHRAMANLOU

For more than a century, disturbances in social behavior or functioning have been reported as troublesome sequelae of neurologically related accidents, illnesses, and disease. These social disturbances include a broad spectrum of awkward, aberrant, uncooperative, or contextually inappropriate behaviors that disrupt interpersonal relationships. In neurological and neurosurgical patients, the disruptive social behavior may be attributed to diverse personality, affective, or cognitive alterations associated with the primary cerebral damage, or a reaction to the illness or injury and its sequelae.

Regardless of cause, the convergence of data suggests that these social difficulties often present a more serious barrier to adjustment, adaptation, and rehabilitation than physical, sensory, or cognitive disturbances (Eslinger, Grattan, & Geler, 1995). They disrupt family life, friendships, vocational readjustment, and relationships with caregivers and treatment providers. Additionally, they limit the patient's ability to benefit from social support or to resume previously enjoyed social and leisure activities. Subsequently, social dysfunction represents an important target for rehabilitation or intervention services.

Despite its importance, the rehabilitation of social disturbances in patients with cerebral impairment is an exceedingly challenging task. Most clinicians and researchers agree that personality, affective, and interpersonal processes are inherently complex. Similarly, human social behavior in and of itself is a multivariate and complicated phenomenon. Individual patients bring unique psychosocial histories, premorbid lifestyles, and patterns of social interaction to the treatment setting that influence their psychosocial readjustment. The relationships between cerebral dysfunction and acquired social disturbances are poorly understood, and coexisting disturbances of attention, language, memory, awareness, and perceptual and executive functions confound the psychotherapeutic treatment process.

Subsequently, models for conceptualizing social disturbances and directing the treatment process are necessarily multidimensional; based upon a combination of theoretical, rational, and empirical foundations; and continue in the process of development. The model we find most useful for understanding the nature of psychosocial disturbances, their contributory factors, and treatment alternatives may be found in Figure 12.1. The model, and subsequent interventions discussed in this chapter, is organized around the primary social disturbances associated with acquired cerebral damage, including disturbances of *social self-regulation, social self-awareness, social sensitivity,* and *social problem solving.* The range of potential interventions is broadly classified as psychoeducational, supportive, behavioral, psychotherapeutic, and pharmacological. The effectiveness of a particular intervention is strongly influenced by the nature of individuals' neurological illness, disease, or injury; their premorbid psychosocial status; and comorbidities and postinjury environmental demands. Hence, multiple factors must be considered when designing, selecting, modifying, or implementing a social intervention.

An important assumption made in this chapter is that the reader has some knowledge and background in psychology, psychiatry, or clinical social work. The successful application of the rehabilitation methods and techniques discussed in this chapter necessitates familiarity with basic principles of neurobehavioral or neuropsychological assessment, psychotherapeutic intervention, and behavioral change. Moreover, most of the psychosocial interventions discussed in this chapter need to be implemented by a mental health professional. The treatment provider needs to be able to establish a trusting, caring, and empathic relationship with the patient; to administer feedback in a nonthreatening way; to anticipate adverse psychological reactions; and to apply flexibly different methods and models of psychotherapy and rehabilitation where appropriate.

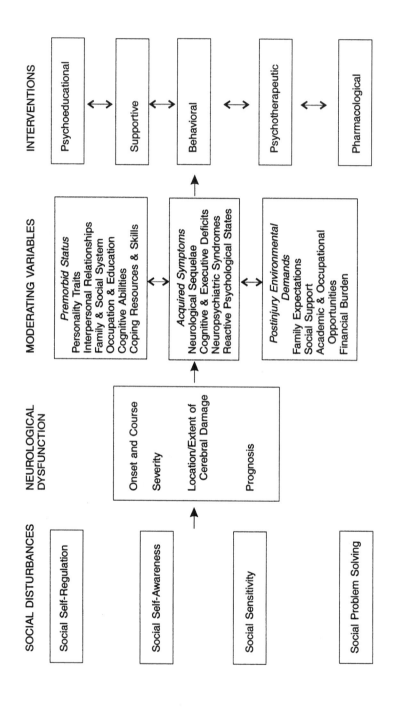

FIGURE 12.1. A Neuropsychological Model for Psychosocial Interventions.

NEUROLOGICALLY BASED PSYCHOSOCIAL
DISTURBANCES AND THEIR MANAGEMENT

The wide range of social disturbances that accompany cerebral damage are classified into four broad areas: disturbances of *self-regulatory processes*, disturbances of *social sensitivity*, disturbances of *social problem solving*, and *disturbances in social self-awareness*. One or more of these psychosocial disturbances may coexist in a patient. The emergent psychosocial disturbance(s) is (are) largely dependent on the nature and severity of the cerebral damage, the patient's premorbid status, associated cognitive or neurologic difficulties, and postinjury environmental demands. Some of the most dramatic social disturbances can be seen in patients with traumatic brain injuries, frontal lobe strokes or tumors, early-stage frontal lobe dementias or Pick's disease, or advanced stages of Alzheimer's, Huntington's or Parkinson's dementias. However, they can also be associated with seizure disorders, moderate to advanced stages of multiple sclerosis, alcohol-related dementias, some neurotoxic syndromes, or herpes simplex encephalitis. Essentially, any pathological condition that disrupts frontal–limbic systems, including the prefrontal cortex, anterior cingulate, insula and amygdala, could place persons at risk of social disturbances (Bechara, Damasio, Tranel, & Damasio, 1997; Cahill, Babinsky, Markowitsch, & McGaugh, 1995; Fuster, 1989; Lane, Reiman, Ahern, Schwartz, & Davidson, 1997; Reiman et al., 1997; Vogt, Finch, & Olson, 1992).

Table 12.1 summarizes many of the empirically based behavioral/cognitive-behavioral intervention studies to date that have resulted in some success managing acquired social disturbances. These methods have been generally most effective in managing disturbances in *self-regulatory processes*. It is noteworthy that in the vast majority of cases, single-case designs were used. In some instances, standard techniques and methods were modified to suit better the neurologic participant. When reported, generalization and maintenance of the behavioral changes have been included in Table 12.1.

Disturbances in Self-Regulatory Processes

These social difficulties have as their basis an inability to manage effectively the initiation, inhibition, rate, intensity, and duration of social interactions (Eslinger et al., 1995). At one end of the continuum, social disinhibition and impulsivity dominate the clinical picture, whereas at the other end, varying degrees of pathological inertia (abulia, bradykinesia, pseudodepression) or loss of social interest underlie the troublesome social interactions. Viscosity, or "stickiness," in social discourse

TABLE 12.1. Summary of Behavioral and Cognitive-Behavioral Research Studies That Target Social Disturbances

Study	Population	N	Target problems	Interventions	Outcome
Taylor & Persons (1970)	Multiple sclerosis	1	Disruptive complaining	Social reinforcement	Improvement
Taylor & Persons (1970)	Traumatic brain injury	1	Psychotic verbalization	Behavior modification	Improvement
Hollon (1973)	Traumatic brain injury	1	Loud persistent howling, hitting, scratching, and use of profanity	Behavior modification	Improvement
Hollon (1973)	Traumatic brain injury	1	Wailing, frantic pleading	Behavior modification	Improvement
Kushner & Knox (1973)	Traumatic brain injury	1	Uncooperative behavior	"Utilization technique" Encouraging a patient to resist in order to give up an undesirable behavior	Improvement
Horton (1979)	Traumatic brain injury	1	Inappropriate touching	Behavior management	Dramatic decline in touching behavior
Waye (1980)	Huntington's chorea	1	Poor compliance Temper outbursts Disrobing in public	Behavior modification	Decrease in presenting problems
Horton & Howe (1981)	Traumatic brain injury	1	Foul language and biting staff	Behavior modification (Report card system and response cost procedure)	Dramatic improvement; findings replicated in two additional settings
Heffenstein & Wechsler (1982)	Nonprogressive brain injury	16	Interpersonal and communication skills	Interpersonal process recall	1. Decrease in trait anxiety 2. Increase in self-concept 3. Increase in interpersonal and communication skills 4. Greater frequency of specific behaviors related to interpersonal and communication skills

Study	Population	N	Target behaviors	Treatment	Results
Welden & Yesavage (1982)	Senile dementia	48	1. Psychiatric symptoms 2. Eating and dining problems 3. Dressing and grooming problems 4. Bathing problems 5. Toileting problems 6. Responsibility 7. Communication 8. Social interaction 9. Independent living	Relaxation training	Significant improvement on all subscales of Geropsychiatric Profiles
Lira, Carne, & Masri (1983)	Severe brain injury	1	Violent physical temper outbursts and impulsivity	Stress inoculation program	Major gains in anger reduction and significant improvement in overall functioning 5 months postdischarge
Prigatano, Fordyce, Zeiner, Roueche, Pepping, & Wood (1984)	Traumatic brain injury with control group	18	1. Acceptance of cognitive deficits 2. Personality disturbances	Individual and group awareness with intensive cognitive training	1. Increased speed of information processing 2. Improvement in interpersonal skills 3. Reduction of emotional distress
Gajar, Schloss, Schloss, & Thompson (1984)	Traumatic brain injury	2	Inappropriate conversational behaviors	Feedback and self-monitoring	Substantial improvement
Schloss, Thompson, Gajar, & Schloss (1985)	Traumatic brain injury	2	Deficient heterosexual social skills	Self-monitoring	Improvement
Eames & Wood (1985)	Traumatic brain injury	24	Behavioral disorders	Behavior modification (token economy)	High proportion achieved dramatic and lasting improvements in behavior, personal social independence
Burke & Lewis (1986)	Traumatic brain injury	1	Surplus maladaptive social behaviors: 1. Loud verbal outbursts 2. Interruptions 3. Nonsensical talk	Individualized behavior point system	Improvement in all of the target behaviors; loud verbal outbursts and interruptions were most responsive to treatment

(continued)

TABLE 12.1. (*continued*)

Study	Population	N	Target problems	Interventions	Outcome
Braunling-McMorrow, Lloyd, & Fralish (1986)	Traumatic brain injury	3	Social skills	Six social skills component areas: 1. Compliments 2. Social interaction 3. Politeness 4. Criticism 5. Social confrontation 6. Questions/answers	Improvement in social skills in all targeted areas
Crawford & McIvor (1986)	Multiple sclerosis	23	Emotional and mood disturbance	Stress management group using relaxation, cognitive and behavioral strategies	Reduction in psychological distress
Cicerone & Wood (1997)	Closed head injury	1	Impaired planning ability and poor self-control	Individualized cognitive training	Significant improvement
Whaley, Stanford, Pollack, & Lehrer (1986)	Frontal lobe damage	1	Six types of inappropriate behaviors: 1. Touching others 2. Picking at any particles on clothing 3. Picking particles from tables or the floor 4. Playing with elevator buttons, light switches, doorknobs, etc. 5. Blowing particles from the tabletops 6. Verbal interruptions and requests of an inappropriate nature	1. Behavior modification 2. Lithium therapy	Significant decline in inappropriate behaviors after treatment with token economy, no additional change with lithium; evidence of generalization and maintenance of treatment
Johnson & Newton (1987)	Severe traumatic brain injury	11	Social interaction	Group Social Skills Training Program HIPSIG (Head Injured Persons Social Interaction Group)	Some improvement, did not meet statistical significance

Study	Subject type	N	Target behavior(s)	Treatment	Outcome
Johnson & Newton (1987)	Severe traumatic brain injury	10	Social adjustment and interaction	Group treatment	Group changes not significant but some trend toward improvement
Goldberg, Hoss, & Chesna (1988)	Brain injury	1	Depression and emotional lability	Guided imagery and music	Short-term gains with no evidence of long-term maintenance
Hegel (1988)	Closed head injury	1	Verbal outbursts	Operant conditioning and token economy	Improvement in both compliance and disruptive vocalizations
Brotherton, Thomas, Wisotzek, & Milan (1988)	Severe head injury	4	Six target behaviors: 1. Self-manipulation 2. Posture 3. Speech dysfluencies 4. Personal attention 5. Reinforcing feedback 6. Positive statements	Traditional social skills training program	Three patients showed treatment effects with evidence of generalization across situations and maintenance at 1-year follow-up
Guiles, Fussey, & Burgess (1988)	Severe head injury	1	Verbal interaction skills	Combined cognitive-behavioral methods	Significant clinical change in and out of session and at follow-up
Burke, Wesolowski, & Lane (1988)	Brain injury	5	Physical aggression	Behavior therapy: 1. High-density reinforcement 2. Reinforcer sampling 3. Environmental control 4. Selection of appropriate responses 5. Inconvenience review 6. Self-control training 7. Self-monitoring	Significant decline in aggression immediately after program for all 5 patients
Lewis, Nelson, Nelson, & Reusink (1988)	Brain injury	1	Socially inappropriate talk	Three types of feedback contingencies: 1. Attention and interest 2. Systematic ignoring 3. Correction	1. Correction contingency was more effective than systematic ignoring in decreasing inappropriate remarks 2. Attention and interest greatly increased the frequency of target behavior
Wood (1988)	Traumatic brain injury	1	1. Poor cooperation 2. Argumentative manner	Behavior program (interval-based token reinforcement procedure)	Considerable decrease in argumentative behavior and refusals to cooperate

(continued)

TABLE 12.1. (*continued*)

Study	Population	N	Target problems	Interventions	Outcome
Wood (1988)	Traumatic brain injury	1	Inappropriate sexual behaviors	Behavior program and token economy	Decrease frequency of target behavior
Foxx, Martella, & Marchand-Martella (1989)	Closed head injury	3	Four areas: 1. Community awareness and transportation 2. Medication 3. Alcohol and drugs 4. Stating one's rights 5. Emergencies, injuries, and safety	Problem-solving program: 1. Cue cards 2. Response practice 3. Self-correction 4. Response specific feedback 5. Modeling 6. Self-monitoring 7. Positive reinforcement 8. Individualized performance criterion levels	Six-month follow-up indicated generalization of problem-solving skills comparable to normal individuals
Zencius, Wesolowski, Burke, & McQuade (1989)	Traumatic brain injury	1	Problematic work behaviors	Antecedent stimulus control	Improvement
Zencius, Wesolowski, Burke, & McQuade (1989)	Traumatic brain injury	1	Noncompliance	Antecedent stimulus control	Improvement
Andrewes (1989)	Traumatic brain injury	1	Aggression and screaming	Behavioral management Time-Out on the Spot (TOOTS)	Improvement
Zencius & Wesolowski (1990)	Traumatic brain injury	1	Impatience and agitation	Behavioral management	Improvement
Zencius, Wesolowski, & Burke (1990)	Traumatic brain injury	1	Dysfunctional verbal and physical behaviors	Behavioral differential reinforcement	Reduction to near zero rates

Study	N	Population	Target problem	Intervention	Outcome
Lysaght & Bodenhamer (1990)	4	Severe head injury	Functional adaptation (poor management of environmental stressors)	Relaxation training program	All 4 patients achieved lower levels of physiological arousal and demonstrated some generalization
Crane & Joyce (1991)	2	Traumatic Brain Injury	Verbal and physical aggression	"Cool down" training procedure	Effective in reducing both verbal and physical aggression
Zencius & Wesolowski (1991)	2	Traumatic brain injury	Verbal aggression	Behavioral strategies: 1. Contracts 2. Reinforcement 3. Response cost 4. Restitution (apology)	Improvement
Crane & Joyce (1991)	1	Traumatic brain injury	Aggression	Behavioral management "Cool down" procedure	Improvement
Rolider, Williams, Cummings, & Van Houten (1991)	1	Traumatic brain injury	Aggressive outbursts	Behavioral management	Improvement
Wesolowski & Zencius (1992)	1	Traumatic brain injury	Aggression	Behavioral management	Improvement
Fluharty, Sellon, & Glassman (1994)	1	Traumatic brain injury	Lack of initiation Impaired problem-solving	Cognitive therapy and "advocacy"	Improvement
Youngson & Alderman (1994)	1	Traumatic brain injury	Fear of incontinence resulting in psychosocial difficulties Avoidance and escape behaviors	Cognitive-behavioral therapy Graded exposure and differential reinforcement	Improvement
Mittenberg, Tremont, Zeilinski, Fichera, & Rayls (1996)	58	Mild head trauma	General distressing symptoms (e.g., memory problems, anxiety, depression, dizziness)	Cognitive-behavioral therapy	Improvement
Johnson & Davis (1998)	3	Traumatic brain injury	Isolation and lack of social support	Supported relationships intervention: To increase social contacts between persons with TBI and nondisabled community. Consisted of matching and introducing each subject with a community participant, brief training, and weekly phone calls	Improvement in social integration

(continued)

TABLE 12.1. (*continued*)

Study	Population	N	Target problems	Interventions	Outcome
Schlund & Pace (1999)	Traumatic brain injury	3	Maladaptive behaviors	Weekly feedback to support adaptive behavior	Improvement in the variability and frequency of maladaptive behaviors
Ducharme (2000)	Traumatic brain injury	1	Maladaptive behaviors (e.g., aggression)	Remedial behavior therapy	Improvement
Raskin (2000)	Traumatic brain injury	1	Poor impulse control Poor problem-solving skills	Cognitive remediation	Significant improvement
Sohlberg (2000)	Traumatic brain injury	1	Irritability and anger outbursts	Behavioral management	Improvement
Hovland & Mateer (2000)	Traumatic brain injury	1	Abrupt yelling	Behavioral management: Compensatory strategies included relaxation techniques, cognitive/ self-talk techniques, logistical approaches, and prearranged response/cues from significant others	Improvement
Hovland & Mateer (2000)	Traumatic brain injury	1	Agitation and anger	Anger management techniques	Improvement
O'Leary (2000)	Traumatic brain injury	5	Aggressive verbal and physical outbursts	Anger management: training Coping Skills Groups Maintained written "hassle" logs	Reduction in number of angry outbursts, which was successfully generalized and maintained for 10-week follow-up

and limited appreciation for interpersonal boundaries are additional examples of the disruption of self-regulatory processes.

Some of the most troublesome behaviors in this regard are related to disinhibition and poor impulse control, including, but not limited to, disinhibited verbalizations, inappropriate sexual conduct, aggression, and ritualistic behavior (Burke, Weslowski, & Lane, 1988; Ducharme, 2000; Goldstein, 1952; Hegel, 1988; Hollon, 1973; Horton, 1979; Hovland & Mateer, 2000; Taylor & Persons, 1970; Waye, 1980; Wood, 1988). Although disturbances in self-regulatory processes may have serious adverse effects on family life and rehabilitation efforts, extant data suggest that they are potentially amenable to cognitive restructuring and behavioral management methods.

The primary goals of cognitive-behavioral interventions are twofold: (1) to increase self-awareness and monitoring, and (2) to bring a maladaptive behavior initially under control, then either restore or shape the specific behavioral problems into responses that are more socially acceptable within the treatment setting (Wood, 1984). Maintenance and generalization of these gains are then dependent on the reinforcements made by the brain-injured patients' "receiving environment," which includes their family and community (Hogan, 1988). As illustrated in Table 12.1, observable improvements in social inhibition, frustration tolerance, and emotional self-regulation have been reported using diverse cognitive and behavioral methods. Stress inoculation training, behavioral management, and cognitive restructuring are among the methodologies that have been used effectively to manage or treat persons with self-regulatory disturbances.

STRESS INOCULATION TRAINING

Stress inoculation training (SIT) is potentially useful for cerebrally compromised patients who have impulse control, anger management, and frustration tolerance difficulties. Pioneering work using SIT on a client with a traumatic brain injury (TBI) was conducted by Lira, Carne, and Masri (1983). The results were dramatic in an individual who, post-TBI, had poor impulse control, reduced frustration tolerance, and episodes of aggression toward person and property. A significant reduction in the patient's anger outbursts was reported, as well as an eventual return to part-time employment and independent living. The intervention was based on Novaco's (1976) three-phase model of SIT. In the first phase of this model, the brain-injured individuals learn about anger, its role in their lives, and the rationale for developing alternative methods of anger expression. Specific anger-evoking situations are identified and reactions to each scenario are discussed within the appropriate range. The second phase focuses on cognitive and behavioral skills acquisition. Brain-injured individuals are asked to evaluate anger-evoking triggers, practice positive self-verbalizations, and think of alternative ways to approach the problem. Finally, within the application training phase, a hierarchy of "real-life" anger situations, and responses to each, is role-played.

More recently, the potential utility of SIT was systematically evaluated within a small sample of adults with TBI (Aeschleman & Imes, 1999). Findings supported the potential utility of this method in managing impulsive behaviors within the treatment setting. However, as with many cognitive-behavioral methods, the intervention did not readily generalize into the real-life setting. In summarizing their results within the context of other studies, the authors concluded that (1) the SIT method is probably most useful for less severely injured persons, and (2) the effectiveness of the intervention would be maximized with the frequent application of consistent and meaningful cues in the social setting.

BEHAVIORAL MANAGEMENT

Behavioral management programs have also been employed with some success in an effort to address angry outbursts, irritability, and interruptions in social settings (cf. Burke & Lewis, 1986; Burke et al., 1988; Ducharme, 2000; Hovland & Mateer, 2000; Ruff, Camenzuli, & Mueller, 1996; Sohlberg, 2000). Behavioral management models used in most rehabilitative settings attempt to modify maladaptive behaviors through a systematic functional analysis plan (i.e., stepwise progression from simple to complex) targeted at the antecedents and/or consequences of any given behavior. In patients with dementia, for example, the antecedent for many problem behaviors is a lack of appropriate stimulation. Hence, an effort either to increase or decrease the frequency and nature of the patient's perceived stimulation might actually result in more adaptive social behaviors (Weiner, Teri, & Williams, 1996). Reinforcement, an important component of many of these management programs, is often effectively used in conjunction with feedback, multiple cueing, repetition, and modeling, in order to enhance the learning process experienced by individuals with brain injury. Differential reinforcement of other behavior, time-out on the spot, and cool down training are some examples of successful behavioral management programs aimed at decreasing verbal and physical aggression in such patients (Andrewes, 1989; Crane & Joyce, 1991; Hegel & Ferguson, 2000). Interval-based token economies, individualized behavior point systems, and feedback contingencies (i.e., attention and interest, systematic ignoring, and correction) have also been reported to be effective behavioral strategies in reducing loud verbal outbursts, interruptions, nonsensical or socially inappropriate talk, sexual disinhibition, and argumentative mannerisms within this population (Burke & Lewis, 1986; Eames & Wood, 1985; Lewis, Nelson, Nelson, & Reusink, 1988; Wood, 1988). Although the scientific foundation of behavioral management is rapidly growing, it is noteworthy that the empirical validation of clinical methods used in many behavior management programs has been limited to case studies, a few of which incorporated multiple-baseline designs (Hegel, 1988; Hegel & Ferguson, 2000; Page, Luce, & Willis, 1989).

Pharmacological interventions have also been effective in treating disorders of aggression; however, such a review is outside the scope of this chapter. The reader may find further information in the reviews by Mintzer, Hoernig, and Mirski (1998), Pabis and Stanislav (1996), Rapp, Flint, Herrmann, and Proulx (1992), and Yehuda (1999) of interest. Further research is needed to explore the efficacy of combining behavioral techniques with pharmacological interventions for the management of aggressive behavior in neurological patients.

COGNITIVE RESTRUCTURING

Patients' neurologically based self-regulatory disturbances, such as poor self-control, have also improved with cognitive training programs (cf. Fluharty, Sellon, & Glassman, 1994; Mittenberg, Tremont, Zeilinski, Fichera, & Rayls, 1996; Youngson & Alderman, 1994). However, these approaches are most successful when applied to persons with otherwise-intact cognitive and emotional capacities, including reasonably intact memory, language, abstraction, and interpretive abilities, as well as the ability to understand and apply in real life the principles learned in the therapeutic setting.

Cognitive restructuring consists of a heterogeneous set of procedures that target the individual's own cognitive mediation in better understanding his or her specific behavioral responses within various environmental contexts. Strong emphasis is placed on monitoring patients' thoughts, beliefs, and emotional as well as behavioral reactions, in order to enhance or regain abilities to make correct predictions about future actions and potential environmental consequences. Such interventions, when combined with environmental cues, may be particularly useful for helping patients manage their viscosity, or stickiness, in social discourse. In the same vein, these interventions may also prove useful in helping patients to manage difficulties with interpersonal boundaries. These and other self-regulatory processes can be managed as patients increase self-monitoring skills, learn compensatory strategies, and practice these relearned skills during and following rehabilitation.

Raskin (2000) reported a case of a 43-year-old woman with TBI, for whom cognitive remediation was used to address impulse control problems. In one instance, Raskin's patient noticed some furniture on the street, misread the situation, and began collecting the pieces she liked. She did not consider the possibility that the furniture belonged to people in the process of moving. In treatment, she was presented with a variety of ambiguous situations and asked to provide three plausible interpretations for the facts of the situation. Ongoing practice of these skills led to her increased accuracy in sizing up a situation. Moreover, significant improvement was also noted in her ability to evaluate a situation adequately and generate alternative hypotheses, prior to acting on these beliefs.

INTERVENTION METHODS FOR STIMULATING SOCIAL INTEREST

When self-regulatory disturbance involves patients' difficulty in initiating and maintaining interest in social interactions, researchers have applied other methods. Dopamine agonist treatments, that is, bromocriptine, are among the most successful interventions for increasing interest, responsiveness, and appreciation of social activity (cf. Eslinger et al., 1995). We have found these treatments particularly useful with younger and/or socially active and gregarious patients prior to sustaining mesial, frontal, and prefrontal lobe damage as a result of head injury or surgical correction of anterior communicating artery aneurysms. For further information on the use of bromocriptine with disorders of initiation, see Imamura et al. (1998), Marin, Fogel, Hawkins, Duffy, and Krupp (1995), or Catsman-Berrevoets and von Harskamp (1988).

Another intervention that demonstrates some promise in stimulating social activity is pet therapies. When a wine bottle, a plant, and a puppy were introduced to a group of withdrawn males on an inpatient geriatric unit, the presence of the puppy stimulated the most dramatic increase in social behavior (Robb, Boyd, & Pristask, 1980). Similarly, Draper, Gerber, and Layng (1990) examined the effects of using pets in group psychotherapy with neurological patients, who were withdrawn and demonstrated little spontaneous speech as a result of dementia, closed head injury, or mental retardation. Findings indicated that the presence of the animals stimulated and facilitated communication between the therapist and the withdrawn patients. Adams (1997) worked with a 72-year-old female stroke patient using two sheepdogs, Charlie and Josh. The patient's verbalizations reportedly increased as a result of the intervention. Although the curative factors of pet therapy are the topic of ongoing discussion, the use of pets may be one way to gain access to spontaneous or withdrawn rehabilitation patients. The reader is referred to Fine (2000) for further discussion on the selection and use of animals for pet-assisted therapy programs.

Finally, reminiscence therapies can facilitate social stimulation. Predicated on the geriatric patient's natural tendency to gain satisfaction and pride from reviewing the past, this supportive intervention can be applied to stimulate interpersonal communication within dementia groups or among family members. Old photographs of local scenes or historical events, personal photographs, books, magazines, and newspapers can be used to stimulate interaction with isolated dementia patients. Through the process, all members of a rehabilitation team can learn more about their patient. Patients with mild- to moderate-stage dementia appear to benefit most, gaining or maintaining interpersonal connectiveness with others through the process (Kasl-Godley & Gatz, 2000). With some withdrawn neurological patients, we have used this method as a starting point, not as an end, in the psychosocial intervention.

In summary, cognitive and behavioral methods, when applied systematically and repetitively, can help patients to remain socially active and behave appropriately. As patients learn better to identify and manage the strong reactions associated with some social situations, their internal sense of self-control is heightened and reinforced, in and of itself. Methods for improving the initiation and social engagement process are less well developed. The use of dopamine agonist therapies may be useful in stimulating biologically based disorders of initiative. Pet and reminiscence therapies, and other novel approaches to psychotherapy, such as music or art therapies, may also help the process of social engagement.

Disturbances in Social Sensitivity

Social sensitivity refers to the inability to understand another person's perspective, point of view, or emotional state. Self-centeredness, insensitivity and reduced empathy have all been associated with cerebral damage in a variety of etiologies (Eslinger et al., 1995; Grattan, Bloomer, Archambault, & Eslinger, 1994; Prigatano, 1999). The therapeutic journey for these patients generally involves three important components: (1) learning that they are important to others, (2) learning that their interpersonal behaviors have an impact on others, and (3) relearning social skills. Combined role-playing and perspective-taking exercises in conjunction with constructive feedback and social skills retraining are among the most widely recommended intervention techniques. Seemingly simple interventions such as teaching effective listening skills or improving accuracy in communicating empathetic understanding can be particularly effective in helping patients' social sensitivity. Interventions that encourage exploration and reference to the thoughts and feelings of others also enhance interpersonal sensitivity. Involving family members in this therapeutic effort can be useful, especially in a supportive family environment.

Group therapy is often recommended as a suitable method for managing difficulties with interpersonal sensitivity. Although there are strong theoretical reasons for this approach, few empirical data link specific group interventions to specific social difficulties and specific outcomes. Nevertheless, some researchers and clinicians are beginning to provide some helpful direction in this regard. For instance, Sohlberg (2000) compared the outcomes of two groups' methods for treating the emotional sequelae of mild TBI. The first group, considered a traditional support group, comprised 15–20 members, who came to monthly meetings at their discretion, discussed topics of general interest to the members, and had an open enrollment over the 2-year treatment period. The second, smaller group (5–7 members) maintained the same membership, encouraged members to make attendance commitments, discussed issues of personal relevance to each individual (e.g., improving listening skills), and used an insight-oriented approach. Although interpersonal sensitivity was not measured per se, one noteworthy outcome was that members of the smaller, closed, insight-oriented group reported lasting improvement in the ability to receive feedback. Because the ability to receive feedback is an indicator of the ability to listen and to attend to another person's perception of the member, this ability may indeed reflect a heightened sensitivity and appreciation for another's point of view. The larger, open-ended group also reported some general improvements; however, these gains were not maintained over time.

The group intervention study by Sohlberg (2000) highlights the importance of small, closed, cohesive, individually focused groups for dealing with the social–emotional problems of persons with mild cerebral injuries or diseases. Membership selection is also an important factor when developing or implementing psychosocial interventions for cerebrally compromised patients. Prospective members need to be pre-screened for their capacity to tolerate the group situation at both a cognitive and emotional level and in terms of their ability to manage strong emotions. Each member should also have a postmorbid history of being able to relate to at least one person in the family or community. To facilitate a common ground and understanding, it is recommended that therapy groups comprise persons with similar etiology (e.g., stroke, head trauma, multiple sclerosis) and age range.

Interpersonal process recall (IPR) can facilitate improvement of a variety of patients' interpersonal skills and is potentially applicable to increasing their interpersonal sensitivity (Heffenstein & Weschler, 1982). Essentially, the method involves videotaping the patient during interaction with another person and using this tape as the basis for therapeutic intervention. The therapist reviews the tape with the patients and encourages them to recall their thoughts and feelings during the interaction. The process is used to facilitate patients' awareness and insight into their interpersonal styles and to provide a foundation for improvement.

More recently, Benedict et al. (2001) compared the efficacy of a specific skills-based psychosocial intervention to standard supportive psychotherapy in a group of patients with multiple sclerosis and social difficulties. The experimental intervention, part of a larger neuropsychological compensatory training (NCT) program, focused on teaching, rehearsal, reflection, and self-monitoring of specific prosocial behaviors. These included active and attentive listening, perspective taking, and facilitative communication. At posttreatment, significant differences were found between the experimental and comparison groups in scores of a modified Social Aggression Scale. Although both intervention groups demonstrated a general reduction of inappropriate social behaviors, a significant decline in excessive speech and social aggression was specific to the experimental intervention. The reduction of excessive speech was accompanied by a concomitant reduction in egocentric speech, a surrogate measure of empathy. This study highlights the importance of targeting specific social competencies in psychosocial interventions.

In summary, a growing body of literature indicates that social sensitivity skills can be improved in cerebrally compromised patients. Role playing, perspective-taking exercises, and IPR can be used within the context of individual, insight-oriented, or supportive psychotherapies. Group therapy can also be useful if participants are carefully selected for participation. Moreover, small, stable, structured groups seem to contribute to better outcome. Finally, a developed NCT program appears to show some promise in reducing inappropriate social behavior.

Disturbances in Social Problem Solving

Disturbances in social problem solving that accompany neurological injury are often the product of a variety of higher level cognitive and behavioral difficulties, including difficulties with judgment, reasoning, or the ability to take into consideration multiple pieces of interpersonal or environmental information in a social situation. Effective social problem solving can also be limited by mental inflexibility, or the inability to respond to new or changing social circumstances (Grattan, Bloomer, et al., 1994). Finally, some patients have considerable difficulty applying social knowledge in the real-world setting (see also Cicerone & Wood, 1987, Chapter 12). Social problem solving is a complex process. From a neuropsychological perspective, case studies in our laboratory suggest that social problem solving involves six basic skills:

1. The ability to perceive, understand, and interpret accurately the social situation and its context.
2. The ability to define the social problem and its relevance to the individual and the goals he or she wishes to attain.
3. The ability to generate alternative solutions.
4. The ability to review each plausible solution, to anticipate and evaluate the potential consequences or outcomes, and to select the most appropriate action for the circumstances.
5. The ability to implement the chosen solution and to evaluate its effectiveness.
6. The ability to seek and apply alternative solutions if the original plan is ineffective.

All of this needs to happen in a dynamic social environment, where the cerebrally compromised patient may either be required to generate rapid solutions or challenged to maintain emotional control.

Most social problem-solving interventions include social skills training and address one or more aspects of this complex process. To date, the model of D'Zurilla and Goldfried (1971; D'Zurilla & Nezu, 1982) has been popular in guiding social problem-solving interventions and studies of neuropsychological patients. It focuses on four basic problem-solving skills: (1) problem definition and formulation of goals, (2) generation of alternative solutions, (3) selection of an appropriate solution, and (4) implementation and verification of the solution. Although the model provides a useful heuristic, in most cases, it needs to be adapted for use with neurological patients. The use of the self-report inventory to assess these skills may not be appropriate for all cerebrally compromised individuals. Additionally, the model assumes normal cognitive, information-processing, and emotional capacities—a faulty assumption with regard to most neuropsychological patients. Finally, D'Zurilla and Goldfried's model was developed for general problem-solving difficulties in daily living. Hence, it may not suitably address the specific social challenges that confront patients with head injuries, stroke, or dementia.

Several investigations have focused on identifying the specific social problem-solving skills that are deficient in persons with acquired cerebral damage. Most researchers agree that these patients have difficulty generating alternative solutions in social problem-solving situations (cf. Kendall, Shum, Halson, Bunning, & Teb, 1997; Warschausky, Cohen Parker, Levendosky, & Okun, 1997). Hence, social problem-solving training programs in the neurorehabilitation setting place a high priority on brainstorming or tasks that generate actions. Interestingly, when Kendall et al. (1997) complemented the use of the traditional self-report problem-solving inventory with a video task, they observed another important aspect of the social problem-solving process. Based upon video data, Kendall and her colleagues found that adult TBI patients also demonstrated significantly poorer performance than matched community controls in *identifying* or *defining social problems*. These findings are supported by data from our laboratory, which suggest that difficulties in social judgment associated with orbitofrontal lobe damage may be at least partially related to problems in distinguishing between positive and negative social interactions (LeDuc, Herron, Greenberg, Eslinger, & Grattan, 1999). Accordingly, attention to earlier stages of the social problem-solving process needs to be incorporated into social skills training. This includes increasing the accuracy of social perceptions, making judgments about what is or what is not a social problem, and defining the problem. For the cerebrally compromised individual, this may necessitate attention to the rehabilitation of more rudimentary cognitive processes and skills (e.g., language, paralinguistic, abstraction, working memory, executive abilities).

In summary, social problem solving, a complex, multistage process, is potentially modifiable with neuropsychological patients. Further research is needed to identify both the critical stages of the problem-solving process in various neurological populations and the critical elements of a comprehensive social problem-solving training program.

Disturbances in Social Self-Awareness

Social self-awareness refers to a specialized form of knowledge and insight about oneself in social situations (Grattan, Eslinger, Mattson, Rigamonti, & Price, 1994; Eslinger et al., 1995). Its deficits represent a specialized form of neurologically based unawareness. The more general category of deficit unawareness has been reviewed elsewhere and may be of interest to the reader (Bisiach, Valler, Perani, et al., 1986; Blonder & Ranseen, 1994; McGlynn & Schacter, 1989; Prigatano & Schacter, 1991).

Accurate social self-awareness involves a realistic appraisal of processes such as how one affects others or how well one manages strong emotions in interpersonal situations. It is important for executing interpersonal behaviors that are contextually and socially appropriate, and for facilitating the maintenance of positive relationships over time. Alterations in social self-awareness may result in both tactless comments and other inappropriate social behaviors. Moreover, inaccurate social self-awareness can lead to difficulty identifying social problems or the individual's contributions to them. Subsequently, the patient may have reduced motivation for social interventions, may fail to implement appropriate compensatory strategies, or may maintain unrealistic expectations

in interpersonal relationships. Disturbances in social self-awareness have
been reported following head trauma (Prigatano, 1996) and frontal lobe
strokes and tumors (Grattan, Eslinger, et al., 1994; LeDuc et al., 1999).
Furthermore, research from our laboratory suggests that disturbances in
social self-awareness may be dissociated from other knowledge-based
deficits following orbital or orbital–polar frontal lobe damage (LeDuc et
al., 1999). This finding lends support to a neuropsychological model of
awareness. Accordingly, identifiable neural systems operate in parallel or
hierarchical fashion and guide the cognitive subsystems that process deficit awareness in general and social self-awareness in particular. General
neuropsychological models have been previously proposed by Bisiach,
Valler, Perani, Papagno, and Berti (1986) and McGlynn and Schacter
(1989), and the reader may find these reviews of interest. It is noteworthy, however, that such biological explanations do not preclude the fact
that psychological factors, most notably the defense mechanism of denial, also contribute to the clinical picture. An important contemporary
challenge for clinicians and researchers alike is determining which elements of unawareness are neurologically mediated, and which are more
psychological in nature. This has important implications for the nature
of the intervention. Regardless of etiology, however, most authors agree
that interventions need to be attempted. The development of intervention programs for raising social self-awareness lags far behind interventions for improving other social capacities. Nevertheless, some general
principles usually facilitate clinical interventions with these patients, including the following:

1. The therapist needs to recognize that despite the presence of social unawareness, most persons with acquired neurological illness, diseases, or injuries are not happy with their altered, limited social lives. Hence, the treatment provider can potentially
   connect with and motivate patients despite their disturbance in
   social self-awareness.
2. The therapist needs to determine if patients' social unawareness
   is contributing to social problems.
3. The awareness intervention strategy needs to have an educational component that is specifically tailored to patients' neurological conditions and difficulties.
4. Increasing patients' knowledge of their deficits may require con-
   frontations, which are probably most useful if done gradually,
   with mildly impaired persons who can tolerate some degree of
   psychological discomfort.
5. The therapist or caregiver needs to develop an appreciation for
   the role of denial and resistance in the life of patients.

The last principle requires some elaboration, clarification, and direction, because it is often the most challenging aspect of the treatment. The psychologically based defense mechanisms of "denial" and "resistance to change" serve very useful and important functions. They protect the cerebrally compromised patient from catastrophic anxiety, depression, helplessness, and despair. To give up these defenses, regardless of their maladaptive nature, exposes patients to more discomfort than they already feel. To patients, facing the reality of losing their cherished relationships with family, friends, classmates, or coworkers far outweighs the inconveniences they suffer as a result of the denial. Helping patients to establish a comfortable continuity between their premorbid social life and current social activities can facilitate the process of acceptance. If a therapist is faced with resistance, he or she slowly brings the resistance to patients' attention. This can be done by demonstrating its presence, its purpose, its ramifications, and how it operates in the therapy. It is also useful to point out possible reasons for the resistance (by demonstrating that it protects patients from the threat of facing their social fears) and to reassure patients that they will be able to handle the situation through the course of therapeutic involvement (if this is the case). The reality of patients' social situations must be *gradually* brought to awareness, within the context of a positive therapeutic relationship. This usually takes time and requires considerable patience from both the patient and the therapist.

In summary, the mechanisms for disturbances of social self-awareness include a combination of neurological and cognitive alterations, combined with psychologically mediated defense mechanisms. Of all of the social difficulties associated with cerebral disruption, we know least about effective interventions for improving disturbances in social self-awareness. What we do know is that the therapies need to be highly individualized; they need to progress slowly and cautiously, and to balance both educational and psychotherapeutic components. Significant challenges lie ahead to determine the essential factors of a social self-awareness intervention and those who would benefit from it.

CONCLUSIONS

Historically, the majority of research efforts have focused on describing the nature and extent of social disturbances associated with a variety of neurological illnesses, accidents, or diseases. Admittedly, some were conducted at a time when brain damage and its social consequences were thought to be permanent and recalcitrant to change. However, most of these studies were driven by the assumption that identifying the patterns, issues, and mechanisms associated with social readjustment would provide a rational basis for developing interventions. More recently, pioneering efforts have been made to integrate what we know about the social disturbances of cerebrally compromised patients with the methods, models, and instruments of psychology, psychotherapy, and behavioral change. This chapter has reviewed many of the creative, novel, and persistent efforts in this regard.

Currently, interventions for neurologically mediated social disturbances are in their early stages of development. Most of the intervention studies reviewed involve single- or multiple-case studies, or very small samples that demonstrate their effectiveness but limit their generalizability. The use of control groups or comparative treatments has increased in recent years, and it is important that these efforts continue. Potential confounding factors such as cognitive status, premorbid personality, affective and coping styles, or other stressors are often taken into consideration but not formally measured or evaluated. Finally, the models and measures underlying many of the studies would benefit from further validation. Despite these methodological challenges, the accumulated studies suggest that disturbances in *self-regulatory*, *social sensitivity*, *social problem-solving*, and *social self-awareness* processes are potentially treatable or manageable. These early studies provide an important foundation for future development in this field.

ACKNOWLEDGMENTS

We gratefully acknowledge the assistance of Amy Brazil for her assistance with library research and manuscript preparation. Preparation of this chapter was partly supported by Grant No. NIH/NINDS 1R29NS33608-01A1, "Favorable Outcome in Ischemic Stroke Survivors," awarded to Lynn M. Grattan.

REFERENCES

Adams, D. L. (1997). Animal assisted enhancement of speech therapy: A case study. *Anthrozooes, 10,* 53–56.

Aeschleman, S. R., & Imes, C. (1999). Stress inoculation training for impulsive behaviors in adults with traumatic brain injury. *Journal of Rational-Emotive and Cognitive-Behavior Therapy, 17,* 51–65.

Andrewes, D. G. (1989). Management of disruptive behavior in the brain-damaged patient using selective reinforcement. *Journal of Behavior Therapy and Experimental Psychiatry, 20,* 261–264.

Bechara, A., Damasio, H., Tranel, D., & Damasio, A. R. (1997, February 28). Deciding advantageously before knowing the advantageous strategy. *Science,* pp. 1293–1295.

Benedict, R. H. B., Sapire, A., Priore, R. L., Miller, C., Munschauer, F. E., & Jacobs, L. D. (2001). Neuropsychological counseling improves social behavior in cognitively impaired multiple sclerosis patients. *Multiple Sclerosis, 6*, 391–396.

Bisiach, E., Valler, G., Perani, D., Papagno, C., & Berti, A. (1986). Unawareness of disease following lesions of the right hemisphere: Anosagnosia for hemiplegia and anosagnosia for hemianopia. *Neuropsychologia, 24*, 471–482.

Blonder, L. X., & Ranseen, J. D. (1994). Awareness of deficit following right hemisphere stroke. *Neuropsychiatry, Neuropsychology and Behavioral Neurology, 7*, 260–266.

Braunling-McMorrow, D., Lloyd, K., & Fralish, K. (1986). Teaching social skills to head injured adults. *Journal of Rehabilitation, 52*, 39–44.

Brotherton, F. A., Thomas, L. L., Wisotzek, I. E., & Milan, M. A. (1988). Social skills training in the rehabilitation of patients with traumatic closed head injury. *Archives of Physical Medicine and Rehabilitation, 69*, 827–832.

Burke, W. H., & Lewis, F. D. (1986). Management of maladaptive social behavior of a brain injured adult. *International Journal of Rehabilitation Research, 9*, 335–342.

Burke, W. H., Weslowski, M. D., & Lane, I. (1988). A positive approach to the treatment of aggressive brain injured clients. *International Journal of Rehabilitation Research, 11*, 235–241.

Cahill, L., Babinsky, R., Markowitsch, H. J., & McGaugh, J. L. (1995, September 28). The amygdala and emotional memory. *Nature, 377*, 295–296.

Catsman-Berrevoets, C. E., & von Harskamp, F. (1988). Compulsive pre-sleep behavior and apathy due to bilateral thalamic stroke: Response to bromocriptine. *Neurology, 38*, 647–649.

Cicerone, K. D., & Wood, J. C. (1987). Planning disorder after closed head injury: A case study. *Archives of Physical Medicine Rehabilitation, 68*, 111–115.

Crane, A. A., & Joyce, B. G. (1991). Brief report: Cool down: A procedure for decreasing aggression in adults with traumatic head injury. *Behavioral Residential Treatment, 6*, 65–75.

Crawford, J. D., & McIvor, G. P. (1986). Stress management for multiple sclerosis patients. *Psychological Reports, 61*, 423–429.

Draper, R. J., Gerber, G. J., & Layng, E. M. (1990). Defining the role of pets and animals in psychotherapy. *Psychiatric Journal of the University of Ottawa, 15*, 169–172.

Ducharme, J. M. (2000). Treatment of maladaptive behavior in acquired brain injury: Remedial approaches in postacute settings. *Clinical Psychology Review, 20*, 405–426.

D'Zurilla, T. J., & Goldfried, M. R. (1971). Problem solving and behavior modification. *Journal of Abnormal Psychology, 78*, 107–126.

D'Zurilla, T. J., & Nezu, A. (1982). Social problem solving. In P. C. Kendall (Ed.), *Advances in cognitive-behavioral research and therapy* (Vol. 1, pp. 201–274). New York: Academic Press.

Eames, P., & Wood, R. (1985). Rehabilitation after severe brain injury: A follow-up study of behaviour modification approach. *Journal of Neurology, Neurosurgery and Psychiatry, 48*, 613–619.

Eslinger, P. J., Grattan, L. M., & Geder, L. (1995). Implications of frontal lobe lesions on rehabilitation and recovery from acute brain injury. *NeuroRehabilitation, 5*, 161–182.

Fine, A. H. (Ed.). (2000). *Handbook on animal assisted therapies: Theoretical foundations and guidelines for practice.* San Diego: Academic Press.

Fluharty, G., Sellon, C., & Glassman, N. (1994). Optimizing outcome through cognitive therapy and advocacy: A case study. *Brain Injury, 8,* 729–734.

Foxx, R. M., Martella, R. C., & Marchand-Martella, N. E. (1989). The acquisition, maintenance, and generalization of problem solving skills by closed head-injured adults. *Behavior Therapy, 20,* 61–76.

Fuster, J. M. (1989). *The prefrontal cortex: Anatomy, physiology and neuropsychology of the frontal lobe* (2nd ed.). New York: Raven Press.

Gajar, A., Schloss, P. J., Schloss, C. N., & Thompson, C. (1984). Effects of feedback and self-monitoring on head trauma youths' conversation skills. *Journal of Applied Behavior Analysis, 17,* 353–358.

Giles, G. M., Fussey, I., & Burgess, P. (1988). The behavioral treatment of verbal interaction skills following severe head injury: A single case study. *Brain Injury, 2,* 75–79.

Goldberg, F. S., Hoss, T. M., & Chesna, T. (1988). Music and imagery as psychotherapy with a brain damaged patient: A case study. *Music Therapy Perspectives, 5,* 41–45.

Goldstein, K. (1952). The effect of brain damage on the personality. *Psychiatry: Journal for the Study of Interpersonal Processes, 15,* 245–260.

Grattan, L. M., Bloomer, R. H., Archambault, F. X., & Eslinger, P. J. (1994). Cognitive flexibility and empathy after frontal lobe lesion. *Neuropsychiatry, Neuropsychology and Behavioral Neurology, 7,* 251–259.

Grattan, L. M., Eslinger, P. J., Mattson, K., Rigamonti, D., & Price, T. (1994). Evidence for a specialized role of the frontal lobes: Social self awareness. *INS Program and Abstracts, 1,* 106.

Hegel, M. T. (1988). Application of a token economy with a non-compliant closed head-injured male. *Brain Injury, 2,* 333–338.

Hegel, M. T., & Ferguson, R. J. (2000). Differential reinforcement of other behavior (DRO) to reduce aggressive behavior following traumatic brain injury. *Behavior Modification, 24,* 94–101.

Heffenstein, D. A., & Wechsler, F. S. (1982). The use of interpersonal process recall (IPR) in the remediation of interpersonal and communication skill deficits in the newly brain-injured. *Clinical Neuropsychology, 4,* 139–143.

Hogan, R. (1988). Behavior management for community reintegration. *Journal of Head Trauma Rehabilitation, 3,* 62–71.

Hollon, T. H. (1973). Behavior modification in a community hospital rehabilitation unit. *Archives of Physical Medicine Rehabilitation, 54,* 65–68.

Horton, A. M. (1979). Behavioral neuropsychology: A clinical case study. *International Journal of Clinical Neuropsychology, 1,* 44–47.

Horton, A. M., & Howe, N. R. (1981). Behavioral treatment of the traumatically brain-injured: A case study. *Perceptual and Motor Skills, 53,* 349–350.

Hovland, D., & Mateer, C. A. (2000). Irritability and anger. In S. R. Raskin & C. A. Mateer (Eds.), *Neuropsychological management of mild traumatic brain injury* (pp. 187–212). New York: Oxford University Press.

Imamura, T., Takanashi, M., Hattori, N., Fujimori, M., Yamashita, H., Ishhi, K., & Yamadori, A. (1998). Bromocriptine treatment for perseveration in demented patients. *Alzheimer's Disease and Associated Disorders, 12,* 109–113.

Johnson, K., & Davis, P. K. (1998). A supported relationship intervention to increase social integration of persons with traumatic brain injuries. *Behavior Modification, 22,* 502–528.

Johnson, D. A., & Newton, A. (1987). HIPSIG: A basis for social adjustment after head injury. *British Journal of Occupational Therapy, 50,* 47–52.

Kasl-Godley, J., & Gatz, M. (2000). Psychosocial interventions for individuals with dementia: An integration of theory, therapy and a clinical understanding of dementia. *Clinical Psychology Review, 20,* 755–782.

Kendall, E., Shum, D., Halson, D., Bunning, S., & Teb, M. (1997). The assessment of social problem-solving ability following traumatic brain injury. *Journal of Head Trauma Rehabilitation, 12,* 68–78.

Kushner, H., & Knox, A. W. (1973). Application of the utilization technique to the behavior of a brain-injured patient. *Journal of Communication Disorders, 6,* 151–154.

Lane, R. D., Reiman, E. M., Ahern, G. L., Schwartz, G. E., & Davidson, R. J. (1997). Neuroanatomical correlates of happiness, sadness and disgust. *American Journal of Psychiatry, 154,* 926–933.

LeDuc, M., Herron, J. E., Greenberg, D., Eslinger, P. J., & Grattan, L. M. (1999). Impaired awareness of social and emotional competencies following orbital frontal lobe damage. *Brain and Cognition, 40,* 174–177.

Lewis, F. D., Nelson, J., Nelson, C., & Reusink, P. (1988). Effects of three feedback contingencies on the socially inappropriate talk of a brain-injured adult. *Behavior Therapy, 19,* 203–211.

Lira, F. T., Carne, W., & Masri, A. M. (1983). Treatment of anger and impulsivity in a brain damaged patient: A case study applying stress inoculation. *Clinical Neuropsychology, 5,* 159–160.

Lysaght, R., & Bodenhamer, E. (1990). The use of relaxation training to enhance functional outcomes in adults with traumatic head injuries. *American Journal of Occupational Therapy, 44,* 797–802.

Marin, R. S., Fogel, B. S., Hawkins, J., Duffy, J., Krupp, B. (1995). Apathy: A treatable syndrome. *Journal of Neuropsychiatry and Clinical Neurosciences, 7,* 23–30.

McGlynn, S. M., & Schacter, D. L. (1989). Unawareness of deficits in neuropsychological syndromes. *Journal of Clinical and Experimental Neuropsychology, 11,* 143–205.

Mintzer, J. E., Hoernig, K. S., & Mirski, D. F. (1998). Treatment of agitation in patients with dementia. *Clinics in Geriatric Medicine, 14,* 147–175.

Mittenberg, W., Tremont, G., Zeilinski, R. E., Fichera, S., & Rayls, K. R. (1996). Cognitive-behavioral prevention of post-concussive syndrome. *Archives of Clinical Neuropsychology, 11,* 139–145.

Novaco, R. W. (1976). The cognitive regulation of anger and stress. In P. C. Kendall & S. E. Hollon (Eds.), *Cognitive-behavioral interventions: Theory, research and practice* (pp. 241–285). New York: Academic Press.

O'Leary, C. (2000). Reducing aggression in adults with brain injuries. *Behavioral Interventions, 15,* 205–216.

Pabis, D. J., & Stanislav, S. W. (1996). Pharmacotherapy of aggressive behavior. *Annals of Pharmacotherapy, 30,* 278–287.

Page, T. J., Luce, S. C., & Willis, K. (1989). Rehabilitation of adults with brain injury. *Behavioral Residential Treatment, 7,* 169–179.

Prigatano, G., Fordyce, D. J., Zeiner, H. K., Roueche, J. R., Pepping, M., & Wood, B. C. (1984). Neuropsychological rehabilitation after closed head injury in young adults. *Journal of Neurology, Neurosurgery and Psychiatry, 47,* 505–513.

Prigatano, G. P. (1996). Behavioral limitations TBI patients tend to underestimate: A replication and extension to patients with lateralized cerebral dysfunction. *Clinical Neuropsychologist, 10,* 191–201.

Prigatano, G. P. (1999). *Principles of neuropsychological rehabilitation,* New York: Oxford Press.

Prigatano, G. P., & Schacter, D. L. (Eds). (1991). *Awareness of deficit after brain injury.* New York: Oxford University Press.

Rapp, M. S., Flint, A. J., Herrmann, N., & Proulx, G. B. (1992). Behavioral disturbances in the demented elderly: Phenomenology, pharmacotherapy and behavioral management. *Canadian Journal of Psychiatry, 37,* 651–657.

Raskin, S. A. (2000). Executive functions. In S. A. Raskin & C. A. Mateer (Eds.), *Neuropsychological management of mild traumatic brain injury* (pp. 113–133). New York: Oxford University Press.

Reiman, E. M., Lane, R. D., Ahern, G. L., Schwartz, G. E., Davidson, R. J., Friston, K. J., Yun, L.-S., & Chen, K. (1997). Neuroanatomical correlates of externally and internally generated human emotion. *American Journal of Psychiatry, 154,* 918–925.

Robb, S., Boyd, M., & Pristash, C. L. (1980). A wine bottle, a plant, and a puppy, catalysts for social behavior. *Journal of Gerontological Nursing, 6,* 721–728.

Rolider, A., Williams, L., Cummings, A., & Van Houten, R. (1991). The use of a brief movement restriction procedure to eliminate severe inappropriate behavior. *Journal of Behavior Therapy and Experimental Psychiatry, 22,* 23–30.

Ruff, R. M., Camenzuli, L., & Mueller, J. (1996). Miserable minority: Emotional risk factors that influence the outcome of mild traumatic brain injury. *Brain Injury, 10*(8), 551–565.

Schloss, P. J., Thompson, C. K., Gazar, A. H., & Schloss, C. N. (1985). Influence of self-monitoring on heterosexual conversational behaviors of head trauma youth. *Applied Research in Mental Retardation, 6,* 269–282.

Schlund, M. W., & Pace, G. (1999). Relations between traumatic brain injury and the environment: Feedback reduces maladaptive behavior exhibited by three persons with traumatic brain injury. *Brain Injury, 13,* 889–897.

Sohlberg, M. M. (1998). Awareness intervention: Who needs it? *Journal of Head Trauma Rehabilitation, 13,* 62–78.

Sohlberg, M. M. (2000). Psychotherapy approaches. In S. R. Raskin & C. A. Mateer (Eds.), *Neuropsychological management of mild traumatic brain injury* (pp. 137–156). New York: Oxford University Press.

Taylor, G. P., & Persons, R. W. (1970). Behavior modification techniques in a physical medicine and rehabilitation center. *Journal of Psychology, 74*(1), 117–124.

Vogt, B. A., Finch, D. M., & Olson, C. R. (1992). Functional heterogeneity in cingulate cortex: The anterior executive and posterior evaluative regions. *Cerebral Cortex, 2,* 435–443.

Warschausky, S., Cohen, E. H., Parker, J. G., Levendosky, A. A., & Okun, A. (1997). Social problem solving skills of children with traumatic brain injury. *Pediatric Rehabilitation, 1,* 77–81.

Waye, M. F. (1980). Treatment of an adolescent behaviour disorder with a diagnosis of Huntington's chorea. *Journal of Behavior Therapy and Experimental Research, 11,* 239–242.

Weiner, M. F., Teri, L., & Williams, B. T. (1996). Psychological and behavioral management. In M. F. Weiner (Ed.), *The dementias: Diagnosis, management, and research* (2nd ed., pp. 138–173). Washington, DC: American Psychiatric Press.

Wesolowski, M. D., & Zercius, A. H. (1992). Treatment of aggression in a brain injured adolescent. *Behavioral Residential Treatment, 7,* 205–210.

Whaley, A. L., Stanford, C. B., Pollack, I. W., & Lehrer, P. M. (1986). The effects of behavior modification vs. lithium therapy on frontal lobe syndrome. *Journal of Behavioral Therapy and Experimental Psychiatry, 17,* 111–115.

Wood, R. (1988). Management of behavior disorders in a day treatment setting. *Journal of Head Trauma Rehabilitation, 3*(3), 553–561.

Wood, R. L. (1984). Behavior disorders following severe brain injury: Their presentation and psychological management. In N. Brooks (Ed.), *Closed head injury: Psychological, social and family consequences* (pp. 195–219). Oxford, UK: Oxford University Press.

Yehuda, R. (1999). Managing anger and aggression in patients with post-traumatic stress disorder. *Journal of Clinical Psychiatry, 60,* 33–37.

Youngson, H. A., & Alderman, N. (1994). Fear of incontinence and its effects on a community based rehabilitation programme after severe brain injury: Successful remediation of escape behavior using behavior modification. *Brain Injury, 8,* 23–36.

Zencius, A. H., & Wesolowski, M. D. (1991). Reducing verbal aggression in adults with brain injury. *Behavioral Residential Treatment, 6*(3), 155–164.

Zencius, A. H., Wesolowski, M. D., Burke, W. H., & McQuade, P. (1989). Antecedent control in the treatment of brain-injured clients. *Brain Injury, 3,* 199–205.

CHAPTER 13

Emotion-Related Processing Impairments

CLAIRE V. FLAHERTY-CRAIG
ANNA M. BARRETT
PAUL J. ESLINGER

In recent years, there has been a renewed interest in the neurobiology and neuropsychology of emotions, particularly as more refined experimental measures and theoretical ideas have emerged. Especially important is the idea that emotional processing is intertwined with educational, motivational, and prosocial aspects of behavior, and vital for adaptation and decision making in many circumstances. The perception of other people, ourselves, objects, and actions as "rewarding" or "revolting" entails emotional processes that can greatly influence behavior. The convergence of cognitive and emotional streams of processing, possibly in prefrontal and paralimbic cortices, provides a necessary foundation for psychological development and continuing adaptation. Acquired brain injury may disrupt this foundation and more specific emotion-related processes in clinically problematic ways, ranging from profound akinetic mutism to hypomania and disinhibition. Therefore, understanding current models and conceptions about emotion and the brain is increasingly important for the recognition of emotion-related neurobehavioral disorders, their management, and overall neurorehabilitation success.

In the earlier part of the 20th century, brain physiology research associated emotional processing with the limbic system, including structures of the hippocampus, the diencephalon, and the cingulate gyrus (e.g., Papez, 1937). By the latter half of the century, however, a growing body of literature supported the additional involvement of neocortical systems in emotional regulation and experience (e.g., Heilman & Satz, 1985). Neurobehavioral studies identified a number of brain structures and processes subserving emotion and emotion-related behaviors. Important areas included the autonomic centers of the brainstem, the diencephalon, the limbic system (including the amygdala, septal nuclei, cingulate gyrus, and paralimbic cortices), and the cortical association regions of, particularly, the right hemisphere. While certain structures appeared to be involved in primary emotional states, others were thought to mediate the perception and expression of emotion, the associative emotional value of stimuli, motivation, and the regulation of emotion.

In the last 25 years, research into the brain mechanisms of emotion has become interdisciplinary, representing a broadening of perspectives from numerous scientific fields. Interdisciplinarity has allowed for more complementarity between the realms of psychology and physiology. Modern approaches to emotion research incorporate the tenets of clinical psychology, cognitive psychology, neuroanatomy, neuropsychology, neuroimmunology, neuroendocrinology, neuropharmacology, neurophysiology, and psychiatry. From this complex juxtaposition of disciplines, a broader and more refined understanding of the processes of human emotion is emerging, with applications to many clinical disciplines and, particularly, to the neuropsychological rehabilitation of emotional disorders following brain injury.

The aim of this chapter is to present an overview of emotion-related processing disorders for the purposes of identifying potential applications to neurorehabilitation and advancing the scientific study of interventions for emotion-related processing disorders. In comparison to disorders such as amnesia, aphasia, and hemispatial neglect, emotion-related processing disorders have been less articulated and less studied. Yet they are tremendously important to recognize and treat. Family members, clinicians, and many patients themselves attest to the fundamental role of adaptive emotional processing in neurorehabilitation, transition to home, and quality of life after brain injury. In this chapter, we hope to identify the major trends in description, assessment, and management of emotion-related processing disorders after brain injury. Emotion-related processing disorders are not to be confused with psychiatric disorders, which are beyond the scope of this chapter. Emotion-related processing disorders refer to the altered perception, expression, and use of emotional information conveyed through social interactions and utilized in everyday functioning for organizing, prioritizing, and accomplishing social and instrumental tasks. We organize the chapter to summarize first the current ideas about emotion and brain systems. Then, we describe measurement approaches, along with findings that pertain to emotional perception, expression, memory, and responsivity following brain injury. Finally, we discuss applications to rehabilitation.

EMOTION AND THE BRAIN

General Observations

From a neuropsychological standpoint, "emotion" may be defined as reactions to an appropriately evocative stimulus involving cognitive appraisal/perception, subjectively experienced feeling, autonomic and neural arousal, expressive behavior, and goal-directed activity (Plutchik, 1984). Currently, two general theories of emotion predominate in the literature. One is a cognitive approach, emphasizing the role of cognitive processes in mediating emotional experiences. The other is more biologically oriented, proposing distinct systems for cognition and emotion, while allowing for interaction and reciprocity between the two systems. Rolls (1990) has adopted an empirical approach to the neural basis of emotion. He suggests that "emotions can usefully be defined as states produced by instrumental reinforcing stimuli" (p. 162). A primary reinforcer is unlearned, whereas a secondary reinforcer operates as part of stimulus–reinforcement associations in which expressions of reward and nonreward alter behaviors through contingency consequences. Such associations are thought to have motivational significance. Rolls argues that key portions of the brain mediate adaptive responding that is based on such stimulus–reinforcement associations. Furthermore, structures such as the orbitofrontal cortex appear to be critical for adjusting responding according to changing environmental contingencies, allowing for more flexible and optimal responses in complex settings.

Evolution has resulted in a progressive elaboration of neural circuitry encircling the brainstem core, the most primitive of which regulates the autonomic, endocrine, and motor activities of the body. These primitive structures remain vital to the fundamental mechanisms underlying both emotional receptivity and expression. Further advances in human brain cytoarchitecture saw the emergence of the limbic system, allowing for greater sensitivity to emotional stimuli from the environment, greater flexibility in emotional responsiveness, and enhanced capacity to learn from the positive and negative consequences of stimuli and actions. Most recently, cortical structures began to differentiate, beginning with paralimbic circuitry surrounding the limbic system and progressing into neocortical processes. Characterized by an unprecedented elaboration of architecture and neural networking, this most advanced cortex permitted more refined emotional perception, sophisticated anticipation and planning capacities, and allowed for greater regulation of emotional responsivity (MacLean, 1990). Current models posit these systems as interrelated though distinct, emerging developmentally at different points in time, with perception not a prerequisite for expression (Borod et al., 1990).

The elaboration that characterized neocortical development was also accompanied by integration with the more primitive brainstem structures via descending and ascending projections. Descending connections underlie the capacity for the neocortex to regulate the emotion-related functions of the limbic system and brainstem. This is referred to as top-down hierarchical organization, exemplified by evidence that human emotion often depends on cognitive processes such as attribution and evaluation. Descending control also allows for greater elegance of peripheral response, incorporating autonomic, endocrine, and motor system effector functions. In a complementary fashion, ascending connections project from the lower brainstem diencephalon and limbic regions to the neocortex, with bottom-up influence on cortical processing during different emotional and motivational states. Interoceptive information from the musculature and viscera is also transmitted via ascending connections.

Recent Animal Models of Emotion-Related Frontal Networks

The limbic system and prefrontal cortex share a multitude of connections and, possibly, developmental trends that may mediate certain aspects of cognitive–emotional integration. Barbas has described *basolateral* and *mediodorsal* trends in prefrontal development that appear to emanate from frontal limbic moieties (1995; Barbas & Pandya, 1989, 1991). The basoventral trend emerges from the limbic cortex of the posterior orbitofrontal region, increasing in cell layers and architectonic definition as it spreads rostrally and laterally to the inferior bank of the arcuate sulcus (ventral areas 46 and 8 on the lateral prefrontal surface). In contrast, the mediodorsal trend arises from the medial limbic cortex located near the genu of the corpus callosum. This trend spreads rostromedially to the region of the frontal pole, then dorsally to the upper bank of the arcuate sulcus (dorsal areas 46 and 8). Both trends arise from the limbic cortex, become progressively elaborated in cytoarchitecture, and interconnect with a variety of similarly developed cortical tissue of the temporal and parietal lobes in parallel pathways.

A different approach to understanding prefrontal–limbic anatomy has been described by Price, Darmichael, and Drevets (1996). These investigators have used tract-tracing techniques in the nonhuman primate model to identify distinctive *orbital* and *medial–orbital* prefrontal networks. The orbital network is organized to provide convergent analysis of diverse unimodal sensory processing such as olfaction, taste, somesthesis, vision and visceral functions. Although initial projections arrive in posterior and lateral orbitofrontal cortex (areas 13, 12, and adjacent rostral-inferior insula), there is multimodal convergence of these diverse projections in more central orbitofrontal cortex (areas 13 and 11). This arrangement may permit the reception and integration of sensory processing with more emotion-related limbic processing, such as reinforcement contingencies and associative value. The medial–orbitofrontal network is thought to be organized differently. It encompasses intense projections among medial–prefrontal regions (particularly areas 24, 32, 10, 25, and 14), but also interconnections with multimodal integration areas such as the superior temporal sulcus and the cingulate gyrus. Despite these differences, both networks receive intense projections from the amygdala and appear to have linkages with structures that mediate limbic and neocortical influences on behavior, such as the dorsomedial nucleus of the thalamus, the ventral striatum, and the ventral pallidum.

An interesting and important extension to structural models of prefrontal–limbic interactions is physiological recording and behavioral data. Rolls and colleagues have examined several parameters of single-cell activity in relationship to behavioral responses in the alert monkey (e.g., Thorpe, Rolls, & Maddison, 1983; Wilson & Rolls, 1990; Rolls, 1990). They reported that two-thirds of recorded orbitofrontal neurons were selectively responsive to food as well as to aversive tastes. Certain cells showed selective bimodal responding; that is, the same cell was activated independently by the sight of a banana and the taste of banana. In addition to cross-modal responding, orbitofrontal cells also appeared capable of representing the motivational significance of stimuli, such as their reward value. In this paradigm, cells were identified that initially responded to the reward of a flavorful liquid in a go–no-go discrimination task, with the reward signaled by one of two stimuli. However, as the reward contingency was reversed (i.e., the previously rewarded stimulus now signaled nonreward), these neurons shifted their activation pattern to the new reward-signaling stimulus. These were termed "conditional" orbitofrontal neurons, since the sensory aspects of processing were always the same but the neurons appeared to encode the current reward value or motivational significance of the stimuli, such as a type of emotion-related working memory system.

Rolls (1990) also provided a comparison of orbitofrontal activity to the amygdala and hypothalamus in similar tasks. Neurophysiological recordings in the hypothalamus indicated that cells fired under specific states, such as hunger and thirst, and activated autonomic as well as cortical regions. Cells in the amygdala showed frequent firing but not with the high degree of specificity and flexibility shown by orbitofrontal neurons. Hence, comparison of diencephalic, limbic, and cortical patterns of activity illustrate both bottom-up and top-down types of neural encoding and transmission.

Current Human Models of Emotion and Brain: The Emotional Motor System

The study of human emotion and its alterations with neurological disease and trauma has grown steadily in recent decades. Several new constructs and extensions to the animal model literature have emerged. One construct introduced to represent the neural organization of human emotion is the emotional motor system (EMS) (Ross, 1996). Anatomically, the EMS is comprised of the limbic system and various descending connections with the hypothalamus, periaqueductal grey, and related brainstem nuclei. Conceptually, the EMS differentiates between emotional and volitional behavior, the latter predominantly organized by the primary sensorimotor and supplementary motor neocortices. In contrast, the EMS refers to a set of neural networks rather than to a distinct anatomical entity. Researchers seeking to verify its existence have agreed upon two necessary criteria:

1. Motor behaviors associated with the EMS must be considered predominantly emotional.
2. Emotional behaviors are organized predominantly through the EMS.

Leventhal (1984) acknowledged the subjective, private nature of human emotional experience, while operationalizing the observable, often quantifiable behaviors associated with it. His construct of "emotional indicators" refers to behaviors organized primarily through the endocrine, visceral, and somatic effector systems. Emotional indicators can include verbal and paralinguistic forms of communication, as well as certain cognitive capacities that are recognized as emotional indicators. Ross's (1996) recent review of the emotional processing literature revealed continuing debate about whether a particular indicator, or group of indicators, was necessary or sufficient to identify an emotional experience. He argued that the pivotal theory remains that of James and Lange (James, 1890), which proposed that an emotion is experienced when the organism becomes aware of visceral and somatic changes induced by some event. Thus, emotions are the interactive result of distinct visceral changes. This view is contradicted by studies in sympathectomized patients who nonetheless report the ability to feel emotions. Heilman (1997) considered the facial feedback hypothesis of emotion and rejected it in part because patients with facial paralysis do not report changes in emotional experience (Keillor, Barrett, Crucian, Kortenkamp, & Heilman, 1999). However, a body of literature in support of an association between different physiological changes and different emotions also exists. A compromise position suggests that the presence of visceral feedback may enhance emotional experience and possibly provide a stronger influence on decision making and behavior.

Evidence for impairment of the EMS comes from studies of distinct patient groups with pathological affect. Patients with pathological display of affect exhibit emotional behaviors in a digital (on–off) fashion, in response to trivial external stimuli. Emotional displays are often intense and stereotypical, involuntary, and discordant with the patient's emotional state, which often is normal. Three documented conditions have been identified:

1. Pseudobulbar palsy, due to bilateral lesions affecting the neocortical motor system and its descending connections. This necessitates disruption of the pyramidal motor cortex or subcortical tracts comprised of fibers from the motor, premotor, and primary sensory cortices descending through the posterior limb of the internal capsule. Lesions may also involve the premotor cortex or its descending pathways that course through the genu and anterior limb of the internal capsule.
2. Unilateral or bilateral lesions (or more rarely, epileptic activity) involving the basal forebrain, medial temporal lobe, diencephalon, or brainstem tegmentum.
3. Unilateral brain lesions involving primarily the right frontal operculum, when combined with a major depressive disorder. Presentation involves emotional displays, such as weeping, that are out of proportion to perceived inner emotional state. Displays terminate as acutely as they commence, upon pharmacological management with antidepressants, weeks before resolution of depressed mood.

Such clinical observations, in combination with animal experiments elucidating the role of the posterior hypothalamus and periaqueductal grey in the production of emotional display behavior, lend support to the concept of the EMS. However, as an emotional indicator, pathological display of affect is neither necessary nor sufficient for an emotional experience to occur. In summary, the EMS model does not represent a single emotional process that is anatomically localizable or physiologically distinct. Rather, it recognizes a hierarchical level of organization to emotion and homeostasis among a number of motor systems delegated to modulate different levels of emotional behavior.

Cortical and Subcortical Regulation of Emotional Behavior

In humans, neuroanatomical localization of emotional experience began with the pioneering work of Penfield and Jasper (1954) who stimulated cortical and ganglionic structures in awake surgical patients. They first identified the temporal limbic system and the anterior temporal and inferior frontal cortices as vital to the capacity for emotional experience. More recent work has suggested that human emotional response is manifested only if the amygdala or hippocampus is stimulated directly, or if stimulation of the temporal and frontal neocortices is propagated into the amygdala and hippocampus. The amygdala is postulated to endow sensory information with affective tone via strong connections with the neocortex and insula.

In addition to experiential phenomena, the frontotemporal limbic system has a strong influence on regulation of noncognitive emotional display, autonomic and neuroendocrine functions, and drive behaviors via extensive amygdalar–hypothalamic–orbitofrontal neural circuitry (see Aggleton, 1992, for summary). Stimulation of the orbitofrontal cortex, for example, causes transient changes in autonomic processes such as respiration, heart rate, blood pressure, and gastric motility (Eslinger, 1999). In primates and other mammals, these indicators are interconnected at the level of the hypothalamus, diverging through various descending multisynaptic pathways. Physiologically, many of these connections to alpha motor and interneurons in the spinal cord and brainstem are modulated via norepinephrine or serotonergic receptors.

Hemispheric Specialization and Emotion-Related Processing

Hemispheric specialization refers to the phenomenon whereby certain higher functions are differentially represented in the two cerebral hemispheres and are significantly affected by damage to one hemisphere. Early work based on clinical case studies proposed a special role for the right hemisphere in human emotional behaviors including facial, limb, and body gestures, affective prosody of speech, as well as a spectrum of paralinguistic functions, (e.g., connotation, inference, irony, and metaphor) in propositional speech (see Ross, 1996, for review). If a statement contains an affective–prosodic message at variance with its verbal–linguistic meaning, the prosodic message takes precedence in normal controls, but not in subjects following right-hemisphere brain injury (Wolfe & Ross, 1987).

Critchley (1939) was one of the first to apply the term "kinesics" to the study of nonverbal communication, including movements of the limbs, body, and face. He distinguished pantomime from gestures:

- Pantomime—movements that convey specific semantic information (e.g., thumbs up for "yes"). These skilled movements are mediated via the praxis system associated with the left hemisphere.
- Gesture—movements used to highlight, emphasize, and embellish the emotional meaning of speech, usually associated with the right hemisphere.

Over the past 30 years, more systematic studies have shifted the focus away from the concept of right-hemisphere dominance for emotional behavior. Newer models have emphasized intrahemispheric specialization, with frontal neocortical modulation of emotional expression and an anterior–posterior differentiation of emotional expression and comprehension, respectively (e.g., Heilman, 1997; Heilman, Bowers, & Valenstein, 1993; Borod, 1992; Gainotti, 1972; Robinson & Benson, 1981; Ross, 1985; Denes, Caldognetto, Semenza, Vagges, & Zetten, 1984; Etcott, 1981; Adolphs, Damasio, Tranel, & Damasio, 1996; Bowers, Coslett, Bauer, Speedit, & Heilman, 1987); Tucker, Watson, & Heilman, 1977).

Currently, there are four hypotheses regarding cortical specialization of human emotion (Erhan, Borod, Tenke, & Bruder, 1998; Heilman, 1997; Heilman, Bowers, & Valenstein, 1993; Heilman, Blonder, Bowers, & Crucian, 2000):

1. The right-hemisphere hypothesis: The right hemisphere is specialized for the expression and experience of emotion.
2. The valence hypothesis: The left hemisphere is specialized for the expression and experience of positive emotions. The right hemisphere is specialized for the expression and experience of negative conditions.
3. The anterior/valence posterior right/perception hypothesis: Posterior regions of the right hemisphere are specialized for the perception of both positively and negatively valenced emotions. Frontal regions of the left hemisphere are specialized for the expression and experience of positive emotions. Frontal regions of the right hemisphere are specialized for expression and experience of negative emotions.
4. Modular hypothesis: This hypothesis combines aspects of the va-

lence model with neuroanatomical areas associated with arousal control and mediation of motor activation (e.g., approach and avoidance).

Borod (1992) recently reviewed the literature on intra- and inter-hemispheric regulation of emotion. Studies involved evaluation of normals, covering a broad spectrum of methodologies, and demonstrated a right-hemisphere advantage for the perception of emotional information. These studies used dichotic presentation of affectively toned auditory material (natural speech, nonverbal vocalizations, and musical passages), as well as tachistoscopic presentation of words and facial expressions (see also Bryden & Ley, 1983; Erhan et al., 1998).

Studies involving evaluation of subjects with brain damage have also included the auditory, lexical, and facial channels. For both facial and lexical channels, right-hemisphere brain damage was associated with more impairment than left-hemisphere damage. For the auditory channels, findings have been more equivocal, with little support for the valence hypothesis. However, findings suggest a role for the right posterior regions in the processing of both facial and auditory emotional stimuli (see Borod, 1992; Adolphs et al., 1996).

Although a number of paradigms have been applied to test these hypotheses, it is fair to say that the role of the two hemispheres in emotional processing has yet to be completely elucidated.

A Central Emotion Processor or Distributed Processors?

The distinction between emotional expression and perception is one of vital importance to the study of human emotion. From a theoretical standpoint, it remains of fundamental importance to clarify whether emotional processing is regulated by one central system, two or more interrelated subsystems, or distinct neural networks responsible for expression and perception, respectively.

Recent investigations of normal subjects have reported associations between facial and vocal channels of emotional communication (Borod et al., 1990; LoCastro, 1972). Consistent with this, research on patients with brain damage has generally supported an association between facial and vocal channels for both expression and perception (Ross & Mesulam, 1979; Benowitz et al., 1983; Borod et al., 1990). Although, some evidence in normals supports the existence of two distinct and independent processing systems (Izard, 1977; Borod, 1992), the more common clinical finding is some degree of both perceptual and expressive impairment.

ASSESSING DISORDERS OF EMOTIONAL PROCESSING: MEASUREMENT APPROACHES

Paradigms of Emotional Arousal

Crucian et al. (1999) developed a paradigm to test emotional arousal in controls and stroke patients. They showed these subjects emotionally provocative slides (pinups) paired with tones resembling a heartbeat. The investigators hypothesized that physiological reactivity to the false-heartbeat feedback and to the stimulus slide would differ between left- and right-brain injured subjects. Subjects' heart rates were recorded with a voltage monitor while they viewed the stimulus slides and listened to the tones. Patients with left-hemisphere damage rated the slides as more emotional when they thought the tones were their own heartbeat. These patients also showed more cardiac reactivity to the false-heartbeat tone (their heartbeat would parallel the tone beat). Findings were interpreted within a framework positing that the left hemisphere modulates or inhibits emotional reactivity to visceral feedback.

In a quite different approach, Slomine, Bowers, and Heilman (1999) used a shock-anticipation paradigm on subjects with right-hemisphere damage and matched controls. Subjects received electric shocks. During the period before they received the shocks, changes in their galvanic skin response were recorded as a measure of autonomic arousal. Subjects also verbally reported their feelings during the period preceding the shock. Results demonstrated that although subjects with right-hemisphere damage demonstrated less autonomic change when receiving electric shocks (and thus had decreased autonomic reactivity), they had comparable levels of anticipatory anxiety when compared with controls. Thus, reduced visceral feedback did not clearly cause changes in the emotional experience of the patients with right-hemisphere damage.

The interplay of emotional processing and attention has been investigated with two techniques by Lang, Bradley, and colleagues (see Bradley & Lang, 2000; Lang, Bradley, & Cuthbert, 1998). These techniques have been used in combination to define the relationship between physiological markers of emotional arousal and subjective reports of affective state. Subjects view, listen to, or otherwise experience standardized pictures (Lang, Bradley, & Cuthbert, 1999) or sound (Bradley & Lang, 1999) stimuli. The investigators not only measured a number of physiological parameters while showing subjects the stimuli (e.g., skin conductance responses, motor unit activity in facial muscles, heart rate) but also examined the magnitude of the eyeblink startle reflex. Subjects subjectively rated the stimuli using a mannikin-based graphic scale depicting different levels of arousal and valence (Bradley & Lang, 1994; Lang, 1980). Findings indicated that the eyeblink response was potentiated for negative stimuli and increased with arousal. The opposite was true for positive stimuli. Based on this work, the researchers have suggested mechanisms for abnormal emotional processing in anxiety disorders and antisocial personality disorder, but the method has not yet been used extensively on neurological patients with emotional processing disorders or to plan treatment for these patients.

Measures of Emotional Perception and Expression

One of the earliest experimental measures of hemispatial differences in the processing of emotional expression was the chimeric face task of Levy, Heller, Banich, and Burton (1983). Another important source of standardized emotion-related stimuli has been the facial pictures devised by Ekman and Friesen (Ekman & Friesen, 1976, 1978). Standardized pictures include males and females demonstrating neutral facial expressions, in addition to six types of emotional expressions: happiness, surprise, sadness, fear, anger, and disgust. These have been used in neuropsychological studies (e.g., Adolphs et al., 1996; Borod et al., 1990).

Borod et al. (1990) undertook to develop and refine a battery of emotional processing tests, applying them to research on neurological and psychiatric clinical populations as well as normals. The parameters included *communication channel* (facial, vocal), *processing mode* (expression, perception), and *emotional valence* (positive, negative). For their perception tasks, the facial pictures devised by Ekman and Friesen (1976) were applied in both discrimination and identification formats. For the vocal channel, discrimination and identification were explored utilizing tasks designed by Tucker et al. (1977), whose vocal identification discrimination stimuli consisted of four sentences with neutral content (e.g., "Fish can jump out of the water") spoken by a male actor in one of three emotional tones (happiness, sadness, anger) and in a neutral tone. On the identification task, subjects presented with tape recordings of emotionally intoned sentences were required to identify the emotion in each. Ability to discriminate is evaluated by presenting subjects with two sentences spoken by the same actor, in either the same or a different emotional expression. Responses are indicated with reference to a 5-by-8-inch card, on which the names of the four possible expressions are printed in a vertical array.

Borod and her colleagues (1990) also explored emotional expression in clinical populations by applying standardized measures they had developed over the previous 10 years. For the facial channel, subjects were videotaped while deliberately producing a range of emotional expressions in response to oral commands: happiness, pleasant surprise, interest/excitement, sadness, anger, fear, disgust, and neutrality. For the vocal channel, subjects were audiotaped while producing the same eight expressions.

The Florida Affect Battery (FAB) is an instrument developed at the University of Florida for assessment of neurological patients with emotional processing disorders (Bowers, Blonder, Feinberg, & Heilman, 1991). In subtests of this battery, subjects are first asked to identify and match pictures of emotional facial expressions. Because disorders of facial recognition may affect recognition of emotional facial expression, a control task for facial pattern perception is included. Subjects must match a face to one of an array of emotional faces *by identity* rather than by the emotion expressed. As a test of emotional prosodic comprehension, subjects name the affective intonation of taped sentences, then match the sentences for affective intonation. Taped stimuli are both prosodically incongruent (the meaning of the sentence and the affective intonation differ, e.g., "The children laughed at the clown," expressed in an angry tone) and congruent (the sentence meaning matches the affective intonation). In cross-modal matching, the last part of the battery, subjects match emotional faces to emotional prosodic stimuli and vice versa. No affective expressions or representations are assessed directly.

Bowers et al. (1991) designed a questionnaire with a gesture response set to operationalize emotional facial imagery as an internal visual representation (e.g., If someone is angry, are his or her eyebrows lowered?). Notably, other investigators (see Jacobs, Shuren, Bowers, & Heilman, 1995) who have applied the measure have suggested that the representation of emotional faces may rely on both motor and visual imagery. More recently, Nelson, Drebin, Uchiyama, and Uchiyama (1998) completed a validity study of the Neuropsychology Behavior and Affect Profile (NBAP) to evaluate personality change in patients with head trauma. Concurrent validity was confirmed on two closed head injury (CHI) samples. Greatest postinjury predictive validity in terms of classifying individuals by CHI severity was found for prognosia (socially defective communication) and depression.

Measures of Affective State and Empathy

One standardized approach to measurement of affective state following brain injury has been administration of various personality inventories (Table 13.1). Personality self-report questionnaires have long been recognized as valuable tools in the evaluation of emotion-processing deficits following brain injury. Factors in overall personality, depression, anxiety, paranoia, and mania are examined by the Minnesota Multiphasic Personality Inventory (MMPI; Hathaway & McKinley, 1942) and its recent revision (MMPI-2). In their use of the MMPI with trauma patients,

TABLE 13.1. Personality Inventories

Reference(s)	Inventory of personality	Affective construct indicators	Standardized population sample
		Projective tests	
Baker (1956); Beck et al. (1961); Exner (1986)	Rorschach Technique	Emotional constriction, catastrophic reaction	Psychiatric inpatients
Murray (1938); Bellak (1986);	Thematic Apperception Test	Catastrophic reaction, depression	Psychiatric inpatients
Lanyon (1972); Lanyon & Lanyon (1980)	Incomplete Sentence Task	Hostility, anxiety, depression	Adolescent normals
		Objective tests	
Hathaway & McKinlay (1951); Butcher, Dahlstrom, et al. (1989); Greene (1991)	Minnesota Multiphasic Personality Inventory	Depression, hypomania, anxiety (via hysteria, hypochondriasis, psychasthenia)	Psychiatric inpatients
Costa & McCrae (1978)	Neuroticism–Extraversion–Openness Personality Inventory	Anxiety, anger (via hostility)	Adult normals
Brooks, Campsie, et al. (1986); Brooks & McKinlay (1983)	Current Personality Profile	Irritability, anger, anxiety, depression	Adult brain trauma patients

for example, Dikmen and Reitan (1977) identified patterns of change in emotional regulation and personality associated with time since brain injury.

Objective inventories of personality include the Neuroticism–Extraversion–Openness personality profile (NEO; Costa & McCrae, 1978) and Personality Assessment Inventory. Projective tests include the thematic apperception test (TAT; Bellak, 1986) and the Incomplete Sentences Task (Lanyon, 1972; Lanyon & Lanyon, 1980). Affective state can be evaluated by the Beck self-report inventories of depression (Beck & Steer, 1993a), anxiety (Beck & Steer, 1993a), and hopelessness (Beck & Steer, 1993c). Inventories for empathy can be evaluated with emphasis on both cognitive and affective domains, by the self-report/family-report inventories modified from Hogan (1969), Mehrabian and Epstein (1972), and Davis (1994).

EMOTION PERCEPTION STUDIES

Perception of Emotion in Faces

Borod et al. (1990) conducted clinical studies of emotional perception of the facial channel, involving patients with schizophrenia, unipolar depression, right-brain damage, and Parkinson's disease, in addition to normal controls. Subjects were required to discriminate and identify photographs portraying facial emotion. Emotional stimuli comprised a set of slides (Ekman & Friesen, 1978) depicting 12 different posers (six males, six females), as described in the measurements section.

Findings for the emotion discrimination task included a significant correlation by gender, with females performing better than males. Patients with right-hemisphere brain injury were found to be significantly less accurate in emotional facial discrimination than most of the other clinical groups and the normal control sample. The exception was the sample with schizophrenia, from which they did not significantly differ. Overall, subjects discriminated positive emotions more accurately than negative emotions, consistent with the findings of others (Borod et al., 1990; Zuckerman, Lipets, Koivumaki, & Rosenthal, 1975). Findings for the facial emotion identification task did not differ by gender, while patients with right-hemisphere brain injury were again found to be significantly less accurate than those with Parkinson's disease and normal controls. Patients with right-hemisphere brain damage and controls identified neutral faces more accurately than positive faces, identifying negative emotions with the least accuracy. Again, overall indications were that positive emotions were discriminated more accurately than negative emotions.

Blonder, Gur, and Gur (1989), using the FAB, showed that individuals with Parkinson's disease also may have perceptual deficits for emotional facial expressions. Subjects made more errors in matching faces by emotion than by identity. Bowers et al. (1991) showed that patients with right-hemisphere damage had defective recognition of prosodic and facial emotion, and deficient ability to match prosody to emotional facial expressions. When subjects listened to computer-generated auditory sentences describing emotional gestures (such as facial expression), those with right-hemisphere damage did poorly at naming the emotions associated with these descriptions, but not with descriptions of a situation that should provoke an emotion (e.g., "The children tracked mud all over the new white carpet"). Findings were interpreted as indicating that these subjects had defective internal representations of emotional gestures (Blonder et al., 1991).

Bowers et al. (1991) demonstrated a specific deficit in emotional facial imagery in patients with right-hemisphere damage, using a yes/no questionnaire of their own design ("If someone is angry, are his or her eyebrows lowered?"). Jacobs et al. (1995) applied this emotional facial imagery questionnaire in a study of patients with Parkinson's disease but free of any right-hemisphere dysfunction. Deficits were demonstrated in emotional facial imagery but not in object imagery. From these data, Jacobs and his colleagues concluded that the representation of emotional faces may rely on both motor and visual imagery, presumably due to decreased activity in the premotor cortex, supporting both emotional facial movements and a motor representation of these movements.

In work with normal subjects, Borod and Koff (1989) examined the hemispatial biases for emotional chimeric faces, using the chimeric face task of Levy, Heller, Banich, and Burton (1983). The normal subjects demonstrated a significant left-sided bias for judging chimeric faces, associated with the production of lateral eye movements in response to emotional instructions. Asymmetries for chimeric facial production were significantly correlated with asymmetries for the location of self-generated emotional images in space. Overall findings supported the contention of right-hemisphere dominance in the processing of emotional facial expression.

Perception of Emotional Intonation of Speech

Borod et al. (1990) conducted clinical studies of perception of vocal emotion, in which subjects were required to discriminate and identify recordings of emotionally intoned sentences. No significant differences were found in capacity to discriminate vocal emotion intonations between normals and subjects with right-hemisphere brain injury. Interestingly, among other clinical groups, patients with unipolar depression were found to be more accurate in the discrimination task than patients with right-hemisphere injury. For the vocal emotion identification task, normal controls were found to be significantly more accurate than the sample with right-brain injury. There was no significant difference for valence for any group. In a later study, Borod et al. (1992) also suggested right-hemisphere specialization for the identification of emotional words in written format, on both the sentence and single-word levels. The valence of the stimuli did not affect results.

A summary of research findings for brain regions pivotal to emotional perception is provided in Table 13.2.

Case Illustration of Emotional Perception Impairment

E, a 65-year-old, right-handed gentleman, developed left-sided weakness and impairments of spatial cognition due to right-hemisphere vascular disease. Acute brain computed tomography (CT) indicated right frontal–temporal–parietal intracerebral hemorrhage with right to left shift. Following surgical evacuation, brain magnetic resonance imaging (MRI) indicated an area of abnormal signal in the right occipital–parietal cortical and subcortical regions, consistent with resolving right-posterior hemorrhage (Figure 13.1). One week following admission, he was noted to be alert and oriented, while emotionally fragile, with bouts of anxiety and confusion. His eyes were conjugately deviated to the right, with loss of leftward saccades but preservation of leftward pursuit movements. Logorrhea was observed, along with socially inappropriate behavior, including sexual disinhibition and jocularity, in this formerly quiet, reserved administrator.

E was improving until, 5 months later, he developed an acute right parietal–occipital hemorrhage, which worsened his residual neurological and neuropsychological difficulties (Figure 13.2). During his 3-week rehabilitation admission, he displayed a moderate anxious depression, with little improvement at the time of discharge despite pharmacological management with Serzone, 100 mg twice a day. Logorrhea remained in evidence from the time of his first admission, but sexually inappropriate verbiage and behavior were no longer observed. Outpatient neuropsychological services were established, focusing on cognitive and emotional issues. E expressed concerns that he had become a burden to his wife, and he appeared unable to appreciate her emotional state beyond overt happiness and anger. Thus, while registering that she was happy, he could no longer differentiate among such positive emotions as pleasant surprise, joy, or excitement. He perceived her expressions of disappointment, sadness, anger, and fear as anger. According to his wife, this

TABLE 13.2. Localization of Brain Regions Requisite for Integrity of Emotional Perception

Reference(s)	Channel(s)	Task requirements	Brain regions[a]	Study sample(s)
Bowers et al. (1981)	Face	Internal mental representation	Right hemisphere	Right-hemisphere brain-injured
Levy et al. (1983)	Face	Discrimination, identification	Right hemisphere	Normal right-handers and left-handers
Borod & Koff (1989)	Face	Discrimination, identification	Right hemisphere	Normal right-handers
Borod et al. (1989)	Face	Judgment of intensity	Right hemisphere	Normal right-handers, right-hemisphere brain-injured
Blonder et al. (1989)	Face	Identification	Basal ganglia	Normal right-handers, Left/right hemi-Parkinson's disease patients
Borod et al. (1990)	Face	Discrimination, identification	Right hemisphere	Normal right-handers, right-hemisphere brain-injured, unipolar depressives, schizophrenics, Parkinson's disease patients
Jacobs et al. (1995)	Face	Internal mental representation (imagery)	Right hemisphere	Right-hemisphere brain-injured
Adolphs et al. (1996)	Face	Recognition of negative emotions, especially fear and sadness	Right-inferior parietal cortex and right-mesial anterior infracaicarine cortex	Right-hemisphere lesion patients
Bowers et al. (1991)	Face, Prosidy	Identification	Right hemisphere	Right-hemisphere brain-injured
	Face and Prosidy	Association	Right hemisphere	Right-hemisphere brain-injured
Borod et al. (1989, 1990)	Prosidy	Perception	Right hemisphere	Normal right-handers, right-hemisphere brain-injured, unipolar depressives, schizophrenics, Parkinson's disease patients
Erhan et al. (1998)	Prosidy	Discrimination, identification	Right hemisphere	Right-hemisphere stroke patients
Borod et al. (1992)	Written expression (sentence and single word level)	Identification	Right hemisphere	Normal right-handers, right-hemisphere brain-injured, left-hemisphere brain-injured

[a]Based on studies of brain lesion patients, emotionally disturbed patients, and normal control subjects.

acquired emotional processing deficit was apparent in his relationships, where he frequently displayed inappropriate reactions and responses without apparent understanding or a sense of empathy. Remediation work was continued with E and his wife for 9 months on a biweekly basis. His deficiencies in proprioception, left inattention, left–right disorientation, and spatial confusion persisted, although he made steady gains to the point that he could return to his hobbies, swimming and golf. However, his emotional processing deficits also persisted, including loss of emotional salience and affective empathy. To compensate, he had learned to apply cognitively mediated approaches to empathy. Spe-

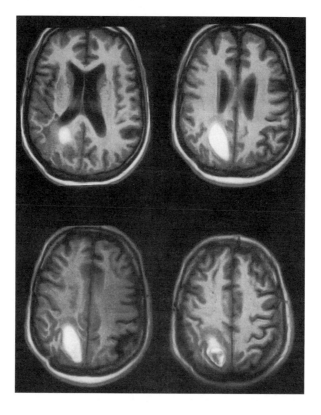

FIGURE 13.1. Brain MRI scan of patient E demonstrating increased signal in the right temporoparietal cortical and subcortical regions following hemorrhage and surgical evacuation of a right arteriovenous malformation (AVM). The images are T-1 axial cuts. Area of hemorrhage ranged from the subcortical border of the occipital–temporal lobe to the occipital–parietal region. The patient exhibited impairments in working memory, attentional processing (with left neglect), proprioception, memory, social salience, and emotional perception.

cifically, he learned to respond more appropriately to others, albeit on a verbal level, and only when he was provided with sufficient verbal information to identify correctly the emotion and emotional state normally associated with the social situation at hand.

The case of E serves to demonstrate the predominant profile of change in emotional processing observed following right-hemisphere disruption. Following this, debilities occurred in E's emotional expression and perception. In the chronic course, E remained limited in his capacity to interpret the emotional state of others, while he could respond appropriately, given sufficient verbal cueing. In this regard, E came to represent an adequate rehabilitation outcome following acquired emotional deficits.

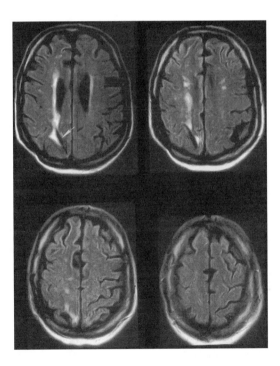

FIGURE 13.2. Second brain MRI scan of patient E showing new onset of right parietal–occipital hemorrhage (increased signal) as well as chronic scarring from earlier right parietal–occipital hemorrhage (arrow). The images are T-1 axial cuts. The patient demonstrated exacerbation in impaired attentional processing (with left neglect), proprioception, memory, and emotional perception.

EMOTIONAL EXPRESSION STUDIES

Emotional Responsivity

By the end of the 19th century, Darwin (1872) had defined the primary emotions as fear, rage, laughter, crying, disgust, and surprise, envisioning them as functional products of evolution. While Darwin assumed that emotional expressions were direct manifestations of physiological conditions, others (Landis, 1924) suggested that some emotional expressions, such as devotion and scorn, were more appropriately viewed as learned behavior emerging from the socialization process. Lynn and Lynn (1938, 1943) conducted the first formal research of facial asymmetry, introducing the term "facedness" to operationalize the relative extent of muscular movements on the left and right sides of the face. Since the 1940s, studies on facial asymmetry have focused on emotional quality, with the quantitative aspects addressed only in the last two decades (Borod & Koff, 1984).

Literature devoted to the analysis of production of emotional expression in response to environmental stimuli comes from studies of patients with neurological impairment, temporal lobe epilepsy (TLE), and psychosomatic disorders, as well as from the psychiatric samples. Borod, Caron, and White (1983) identified characteristic profiles of change in emotional expressiveness for each patient group. Their review of the literature on unilateral brain damage revealed differential effects on emotional behavior as a consequence of laterality of lesion. Overall, the affective expression of patients with right-hemisphere damage is characterized as indifferent (*la belle indifférence*), with euphoria and denial/ minimization of deficits. In contrast, the affective expression of patients following left-hemisphere damage can be more catastrophic, characterized by depression and overexaggeration of deficits. TLE surgical candidates can display either an indifference (right) or catastrophic (left) reaction during a presurgical procedure involving unilateral carotid artery injections of sodium Amytal, which result in temporary inactivation of the hemisphere ipsilateral to the injection site. Furthermore, Bear and Fedio (1977) have proposed a characteristic TLE personality, with distinct styles of emotional expressiveness for those with left- and right-hemisphere epileptic focus. While hypothetical and controversial, the concept has been supported by a number of studies. Patient with right-hemisphere epileptic focus have been characterized as extremely emotive, manifesting interictal symptoms such as anger, sadness, elation, agitation, aggression, and denial/minimization of negative feelings. Patients with left-hemisphere epileptic focus have been characterized as ruminative, socially isolated, obsessive, and humorless, with a propensity for expression of self-deprecating thoughts.

Electroencephalographic (EEG) studies of normals (Davidson, 1985; Sutton & Davidson, 2000) and unipolar depressives (Lindgren et al., 1999; Abercrombie et al., 1998) have evidenced an association between expression of negative affect and decreased functioning of the right hemisphere (see Tucker, 1981, and Davidson, 1998a, 1998b, for reviews). Healthy volunteers undergoing experimental induction of depressive and euphoric moods demonstrated asymmetrical activation over the frontal lobes, with greater activation in the right-frontal region during negative affective responses and relatively greater activation in the left-frontal region during positive affective responses. College students examined solely under the depressive mood induction conditions demonstrated symmetry in bilateral occipital, parietal, and temporal EEG. By contrast, significant asymmetry was evident for the frontal lobes, with relatively greater activation over the right-frontal region during induction of depressed mood.

Sutton and Davidson (2000) found prefrontal brain electrical asymmetry to be a prognostic indicator of reaction to affective stimuli. In their study of right-handed normals, subjects were asked to discriminate type, computer monitor-presented word pairs that differed by affective tone. Relatively greater left-sided anterior frontal resting activity was found to be associated with a greater tendency to select the most pleasant word pair. No such relationship was detected for resting brain activity at central and posterior regions.

Facial Expression of Emotion

A review of the pioneering work on facial asymmetry in emotional processing reveals a controversy in the literature that remains unresolved today (Borod & Koff, 1989; Borod, Koff, & Buck, 1986). Two paradigms permeated the facial asymmetry literature of the 1970s, grounded in theories of lateral dominance on the one hand, and emotional processing on the other. Lateral dominance theory contends that facial asymmetry, akin to handedness and footedness, is a lateralized motoric function controlled by the dominant hemisphere. Alternatively, emotional processing theorists consider facial expression to be controlled by the right hemisphere. While early clinical observers recognized the association between left-sided brain injury and the catastrophic response (Goldstein, 1939), as well as right-sided brain injury and the indifference response (Denny-Brown, Meyer, & Horenstein, 1952), emphasis until the 1960s was placed on the psychological nature of the response (Gainotti, 1972).

Pioneers in emotional processing theory explained these patterns of emotional responses in patients with brain injury by postulating a different functional organization in the two cerebral hemispheres (Gainotti,

1969, 1972). Thus, in the dominant left hemisphere, language allows sensory information to undergo a complex conceptual elaboration (Heilman, Scholes, & Watson, 1975). In the nondominant right hemisphere, sensory data are processed in a more primitive way, retaining their immediateness, affective intensity, and value (Gainotti, 1984).

A comprehensive review of the neuroanatomical substrates of facial expressions is beyond the scope of this chapter. More in-depth treatment of the subjects is available from Borod and Koff (1984), Brodal (1957), and Derryberry and Tucker (1992). Borod, Koff, and Buck (1986) approached the neuropsychology of emotional expression from the standpoint of the face as a primary vehicle of emotional communication. One of the major classifications in the study of facial expression has been the distinction between posed and spontaneous expression, based on evidence in the clinical literature (Borod & Koff, 1984). This dissociation has been suggestive of distinct and potentially independent neuroanatomical pathways for each type of expression. However, elucidation of the distinct pathways has been more successful for posed expression (Borod & Koff, 1984). Thus, posed emotional expression has been associated with right-hemisphere dominance by researchers such as Borod et al. (1986). This relative left-hemiface involvement was found to be independent of handedness.

Volitional movements of the face originate in the lower portion of the precentral gyrus, with fibers traveling to the posterior part of the internal capsule. The seventh cranial nerve, the facial intermediate nerve, provides the major motoric innervation of the muscles in facial expression. The facial nucleus is subdivided such that the ventral portion receives fibers from both motor cortices, while the dorsal portion receives fibers predominantly from the contralateral motor cortex. One important distinction in how these fibers project is the difference between the innervation of the upper and lower face. While the lower face is considered to receive predominantly contralateral projections, the upper face receives predominantly bilateral projections from the motor cortex. The neuroanatomy of involuntary facial expression of emotion is relatively more complex. More structures are implicated, with more involved pathways. Most evidence in the literature suggests that the afferents for spontaneous facial expression originate in the thalamus and/or globus pallidus, and project to the facial nucleus via several synapses (Borod & Koff, 1984).

In their review of the literature concerned with facial emotional expression in normal right-handers, Borod et al. (1981, 1983) found strong evidence for greater intensity of emotional expression or greater extent of muscle movement on the left side of the face for posing emotional expressions, for posing emotional expressions while imagining emotional situations, and for relating emotional experiences. This was especially true for expressions of negative emotion and for positive emotions in males but not females (Borod et al., 1986). Left-hemiface dominance was further evident for nonemotional movement of the facial musculature. The exception was studies of facial asymmetry for posed expressions conducted with composite still photographs, where methodological problems were implicated as underlying the lack of significant findings. Asymmetries in expression were found to be independent of handedness and footedness, while associated with eyedness (Borod et al., 1981; Borod & Koff, 1989; Borod, Koff, Lorch, Nicholas, & Welkowitz, 1988).

In a series of studies relating facial asymmetries during posed and spontaneous expressions to traditional measures of lateral dominance in normal right-handers (Borod & Caron, 1980; Borod et al., 1981; Borod & Koff, 1984; Borod et al., 1983, Borod, Koff, & White, 1983), results were consistent with the idea of cerebral dominance for contralateral facial expression. No relationship was seen between valence of emotion expressed and lateral dominance. In research exploring the effect of hemiface size on facial expression, the right hemiface was found to be significantly larger than the left, suggesting a component of peripheral influence on laterality of facial emotional expression (Borod, 1992).

Blonder, Burns, Bowers, Moore, and Heilman (1993) reported that patients with right-hemisphere damage showed reduced facial expressivity during spontaneous conversation in comparison to both patients with left-hemisphere damage and control subjects. In particular, these patients demonstrated significantly less smiling and laughter. On the other hand, one possible consequence of right frontal lobe injury or bilateral lesions in the neocortical output to brainstem nuclei that control emotional expression is pathological laughter, a condition characterized by emotional responsiveness to environmental stimuli restricted to laughter. In the chronic course, this state of pathological laughter is often dissociated from a relatively preserved range of internal emotional response (Sackheim et al., 1982).

Jacobs et al. (1995) found posed emotional facial expressions to be abnormal and of reduced amplitude in subjects with Parkinson's disease. Richardson, Bowers, Bauer, Heilman, and Leonard (2000) examined video-digitalized images of emotional facial expressions in normal subjects and found that the right upper face was more mobile than the left. The lower face moved differently depending upon the valence of facial expressions, with the right lower face more mobile during fight–flight expressions, and the left lower face more mobile during happy expressions.

A review of findings for brain-injured patients (Borod et al., 1983) included the relative inability of patients with right-hemisphere brain injury to communicate affect spontaneously via facial expression in response to emotionally laden slides. Aspects of emotional expression (responsivity, appropriateness, intensity) in patients with brain damage after left or right cerebrovascular disease were found to be dissociated, with right-hemisphere patients relatively impaired in comparison to left-hemisphere patients or controls (Borod et al., 1988). In this study, performance measures for nonemotional expressions and emotional expressions were uncorrelated, suggestive of a dissociation between these two systems of facial behavior. In addition, single-case studies demonstrated both a lack of variety in facial expression and a paucity of facial movements associated with both speech and fluctuations in mood.

Finally, an interesting area of research that deserves more attention is the hypothesis that patients with frontal lobe lesions produce fewer facial expressions than patients with lesions in the temporal or parietal–occipital regions in either hemisphere.

Expression of Emotional Intonation

Mediation of affective speech by the right cerebral hemisphere was first proposed by Hughlings-Jackson (1880), who noted the preservation of affective speech that often accompanies the loss of propositional speech in aphasic patients following left-hemisphere brain damage. Tucker et al. (1977) reported the corollary for patients with right-hemisphere insult. Deficient in their ability to utilize affective speech, these patients often used propositional speech to express emotions.

In their review of cerebral hemisphere dominance for emotional intonation of speech, Borod et al. (1983) found a limited body of literature comprised primarily of research on the brain-injured population. Findings included two single-case studies involving patients' loss of spontaneous expression of emotion via speech after right-hemisphere injury. Voices were rendered monotonous, dull, and lacking in emotional inflection. Patients' awareness of disability was preserved, with reportedly intact, internal emotional experience and capacity to comprehend the emotional intentions of others.

Additional research includes the findings of Blonder et al. (1989) that subjects with right- and left-hemispheric Parkinsonism were impaired in producing prosodically intoned emotional utterances. Crucian, Preston, Raymer, and Heilman (1997) studied subjects' videotaped body movements and found that subjects acting out emotional expressions would sometimes either approach or move farther away from the camera. These approach–avoidance movements were independent of the positive or negative valence of the emotion expressed, and instead depended on whether the acted-out emotion would be expected to elicit "approach" (anger) or "avoidance" (fear). Table 13.3 provides a summary of research findings for brain regions found to be vital to emotional expression.

Case Illustration of Emotional Expression Impairment

K is a 42-year-old, left-handed male who suffered an industrial accident in which the left orbital frontal cortex and right hypothalamus and thalamus were damaged by penetration of an unspooled wire that penetrated beneath the left eye, through the nasal cavity and cribiform plate, traveling up to graze the left orbital frontal cortex before crossing over and down, to the right hypothalamic and thalamic regions (Figure 13.3).

Two-month follow-up neurological exam indicated left extrapyramidal movements, with involuntary left leg movements in response to left arm movements. A significant dysexecutive syndrome was evident, characterized by personality changes, lack of social inhibition, and decreased attention/concentration. Hypothalamic-associated changes included increased appetite and weight, as well as erectile dysfunction. Electroencephalogram (EEG) was unremarkable. Pharmacological management consisted of bromocriptine 2.5 mg orally, twice a day.

Neuropsychological assessment was notable for impulsivity, distractibility, logorrhea, social disinhibition, lack of empathy, pathological laughter, and a mood characterized as *la belle indifférence*. The patient's facial expression and tone were limited in response to neutrality and mirth. By family report, the patient's personality changes were evident. His premorbid style was described as quietly reserved, with leadership skills that made him a role model both on the job site and in the home. His premorbid sense of humor was described as warm and rich, while appropriate.

Gradually, as K gained more self-awareness, he began to experience a broader range of emotional responses, in particular, anger during times of stress. He developed more instability in his mood state associated with paranoid thoughts. He described fluctuations of mood with no apparent trigger, although he attributed them to changes in his family's behavior since the time of his injury, including their tendencies to question his decisions and no longer acknowledge his authority as head of the household. He was started on risperidone 0.5 mg twice a day and stability of mood improved. Deficits remained essentially unchanged during the next 4 months. Pharmacological management was stabilized at 2 mg risperidone orally, twice a day and with Baclofen tapering. At 5 years posttrauma, K reported a normal range of internal emotional responsiveness to external stimuli and continually improved range of intonation, with continued inability to generate any corresponding facial expression beyond that of laughter. Family reports noted recovery of

TABLE 13.3. Localization of Brain Regions Requisite for Integrity of Emotional Expression

Reference(s)	Channel(s)	Task requirements	Brain region(s)[a]	Study sample(s)
Borod et al. (1981, 1983)	Left hemi-face	Posed expression (to verbal instruction to imagined emotional situations, while relating emotional experience)	Right hemisphere	Normal right-handers, right-brain-injured
Richardson et al. (2000)	Left lower face	Mobility during happy expressions	Right hemisphere	Normal right-handers
	Right lower face	Mobility during fight/flight expressions	Left hemisphere	
Sackeim et al. (1982)	Face	Expressivity (pathological laughter)	Right-frontal cortex, bilateral frontal to brainstem neural networks	Left/right-hemisphere lesion patients, hemispherectomy patients, gelastic epilepsy patients
Blonder et al. (1983)	Face	Expressivity	Right hemisphere	Left/right-hemisphere brain-injured, normal right-handers
Borod et al. (1983, 1988a)	Face	Spontaneous expression	Right hemisphere	Left/right-hemisphere brain-injured, normal right-handers
Borod & Koff (1984, review)	Face	Posed negative expressions	Right hemisphere	Normal right-handers and left-handers, lesion patients
		Spontaneous expression	Thalamus and/or globus pallidus projections to the facial nucleus	
Borod et al. (1990)	Face	Accuracy, intensity	Right hemisphere	Normal right-handers, right-hemisphere brain-injured, unipolar depressives, schizophrenics, Parkinson's disease patients
Jacobs et al. (1995)	Face	Posed expression	Basal ganglia	Parkinson's disease patients
Borod et al. (1985)	Face	Overall expressiveness (i.e., frequency)	Right frontal region	Normal right-handers, right-hemisphere brain-injured, left-hemisphere brain-injured
	Tone		Right hemisphere	

(continued)

TABLE 13.3. (continued)

Reference(s)	Channel(s)	Task requirements	Brain region(s)[a]	Study sample(s)
Hughlings-Jackson (1874) Tucker et al. (1981)	Tone	Spontaneous negative expression (expletives)	Right hemisphere	Left-hemisphere brain-injured
Tucker et al. (1977)	Tone	Spontaneous expression	Right hemisphere (parietal)	Right-hemisphere brain-injured
Ross (1981)	Tone	Posed expression	Right hemisphere	Right-hemisphere lesion-patients
Borod & Koff (1989, review)	Tone	Spontaneous and posed expression	Right hemisphere	Normal right-handers
Blonder et al. (1989)	Tone	Spontaneous expression	Left or right basal ganglia	Normal right-handers, Left/right hemi-Parkinson's disease patients
Gainotti (1972)	Face, Tone, Gesture	Catastrophic depressive response	Left hemisphere	Left-hemisphere lesion-patients
		Indifference response	Right hemisphere	Right-hemisphere lesion-patients
Ross & Mesalum (1979)	Face, Tone, Gesture	Spontaneous expression	Right hemisphere	Right-hemisphere lesion-patients
Tucker (1981)	Ocular	Lateral movements (left-hemispace bias)	Right hemisphere	Normal right-handers
Borod et al. (1988b)	Ocular	Lateral movements (left-hemispace bias)	Right hemisphere	Normal right-handers and left-handers
Davidson (1985, review)	EEG activation	Negative emotion/positive emotion		Right frontal/left frontal regions
Abercrombie et al. (1998)	EEG activation	Negative emotion	Right amygdala	Unipolar depressives
Lindgren et al. (1999)	EEG activation	Negative emotion/positive emotion	Thalamus	Normal right-handers and unipolar depressives

Based on studies of brain lesion patients, emotionally disturbed patients, and normal control subjects.

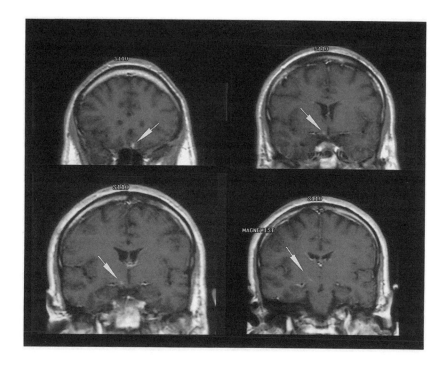

FIGURE 13.3. Brain MRI images of patient K demonstrating abnormal signal in the right hypothalamic and subthalamic regions following penetration by un- spooled steel wire. The upper images are T-1 coronal sections with contrast. Recapitulation of the trajectory suggests that the steel wire penetrated beneath the left orbit, through the nasal cavity and cribiform plate. The wire traveled upward, with initial insult to the left orbital frontal cortex (arrow). It then crossed over to the right orbital frontal cortex (arrow), before penetrating the right hypothalamic and subthalamic regions, completing its course in the area of the right posterior cingulate. The lower images are T-1 coronal sections with contrast. The left image shows lesion in the hypothalamus, while the right image shows lesion in the subthalamic nuclei (arrows). The patient exhibited marked left extrapyramidal movements and a significant dysexecutive syndrome charac- terized by poor attention, disinhibition, and limited emotional expression, with pathological laughter. Bouts of paranoia, initially evident, resolved by the chronic course.

appropriate expression during bouts of anger. However, upon further inquiry, it was clear that during those times, K was displaying a lack of pathological laughter, or a continued neutral expression. He continued to report a sense of *la belle indifférence*, but with burgeoning self-insight. He reported a belief, from a cognitive standpoint, that something was quite different about his interactive style. He indicated that he came to this conclusion gradually, over the years, based on the fact that everyone close to him appeared to think so.

K serves to demonstrate the association between right-hemisphere damage and disruptions in emotional expression, in this case, resulting in pathological laughter. From his accompanying motor and sensory complaints, it was clear that the hypothalamic–cortical neural network disruptions he had experienced involved right anterior cortical networks, including frontal and frontoparietal cortical regions.

K also experienced a significant dysexecutive syndrome subsequent to his left orbital frontal damage, characterized by impulsivity, distractibility, logorrhea, and poor attention/concentration. However, these traits were clearly distinguishable from his emotional processing changes and were largely resolved by 1-year posttrauma. His persistent *la belle indifférence*, accompanied by bouts of paranoia, was likely the result of disruption to frontal–subcortical networks.

From a rehabilitation standpoint, K highlights two concepts: (1) the pivotal role of the family in managing persistent emotional-processing impairments, and (2) Second, the efficacy of cognitive therapeutic approaches in improving communication between the patient and others, particularly those involved in familial or other close relationships. To be more effective, cognitive approaches in such cases must necessarily involve a family therapy approach, working with select family members alone and in conjunction with other family members, and gradually incorporating greater involvement with the patient himself.

Emotional Memory

Cimino, Verfaellie, Bowers, and Heilman (1991) asked subjects to tell stories about autobiographical events based on a cue word. These responses were then assessed by judges for emotional content. Results indicated that subjects with right-hemisphere damage told less emotional stories than did subjects with left-hemisphere injury. Crucian et al. (2000) had subjects with Parkinson's disease and normal controls generate stories based on emotional and nonemotional words. They found that subjects with Parkinson's disease were paradoxically activated compared to controls when given emotional cue words (but only when those cues evoked fight–flight emotions).

Beversdorf et al. (1998) modified questions from Boller, Cole, Vrtunski, Patterson, and Kim (1979) to create sentences with emotional and nonemotional content, and they asked subjects to remember them. Control subjects showed relatively better memory for emotional material, possibly because an internal emotional representation was activated by these sentences and participated in durable instantiation of the material. High-functioning autistic subjects showed no facilitation of memory for emotional stimuli, implying a deficit in emotional semantics available for memory processes.

APPLICATIONS TO REHABILITATION

Overview

The aforementioned studies suggest, first, that patients with right-hemisphere injury, frontal lobe damage, and certain subcortical damage are at highest risk for emotion-related processing disorders. Second, there is variation in the severity and type of emotional processing impairment. Most impairment involves alteration in both expression and perception, and causes some degree of social disability and adjustment difficulty. Third, motor regulation of emotion may be altered separately from the perceptual and experiential aspects of emotion. Fourth, little is known about the process of recovery in emotion-related processing disorders. Finally, specific emotional processing interventions have been examined at a minimal level only. Thus, knowledge of general recovery patterns and formulation of intervention models are at very early stages.

General Intervention Approaches

Neurorehabilitation of acquired emotional processing disorders following brain insult have emphasized a comprehensive, interdisciplinary approach. The program offered nationally by the Brown Schools Rehabilitation Center exemplifies the interdisciplinary treatment approach, integrating the expertise of education, physical therapy, occupational therapy, neuropsychology, psychiatry, substance abuse counseling, vocational rehabilitation, and social work.

Integrated treatment recognizes that each patient with brain injury suffers a unique combination of emotional, behavioral, and cognitive impairments. Team members are cross-trained, to some extent, and dedicated to individualized, interdisciplinary treatment. The integrated approach does not treat the components of a patient's condition separately. Rather, all facets of a patient's condition are viewed within the context of the total rehabilitation program. The goals of integrated treatment are focused on optimizing functional skills, including home and personal management, cognitive skills, interpersonal skills, community skills, avocational pursuits, and vocational potential. Furthermore, integrated treatment considers the patient within the context of the family system. During the inpatient treatment phase, families are encouraged to take an active part in treatment planning meetings. Comprehensive family therapy is available to maximize success following discharge, under the auspices of psychiatry, neuropsychology, or social work, as deemed appropriate. Outpatient follow-up is also available to maximize carryover of individual and family skills gained during the inpatient phase. Intrinsic to its holistic philosophy, the interdisciplinary approach views emotional processing deficits within the context of acquired neurobehavioral change following brain injury. At one end of the spectrum, cross-training among the varied disciplines allows all team members to address core impairments and goals that cut across home and community settings. At the other end of the spectrum, participation in treatment planning by diverse specialists serves to provide a creative atmosphere, conducive to troubleshooting and problem solving. With respect to acquired emotional processing deficits, functionality is generally maximized by a combination of pharmacological intervention and behavior modification approaches drawn from cognitive-behavioral psychology. As recovery proceeds, more emphasis is placed on compensatory techniques. Even cognitive retraining may be more effectively applied if disorders of emotion and psychosocial functioning are similarly addressed (e.g., Mozaux & Richer, 1998). More specific approaches and interventions are considered below.

Management Approaches to Emotion-Related Processing Disorders

In the early recovery stages, left-hemisphere damage can often be associated with a catastrophic depressive response in the absence of any significant deficiencies in emotional perception. Triggs et al. (1999) used transcranial magnetic stimulation, transiently deactivating the left prefrontal lobe, as a treatment for medication-unresponsive depression in patients without neurological disorders. Their subjects improved significantly poststimulation, suggesting that studies of this treatment in neurological patients may be warranted.

When language is expressed emotionally (e.g., emotional prosodic inflection) or has emotional meaning (emotional semantics), it may be better utilized and understood by persons with aphasia (Heilman et al., 1975; Roeltgen et al., 1983) because of relative sparing of right hemisphere emotional processing systems. Similarly, caregivers may initially assume that people with aphasia do not understand anything said around them because of their impaired language. However, these subjects may have relatively spared ability to understand emotional facial expressions and prosodic intonations even in the context of global aphasia (Barrett, Crucian, Raymer, & Heilman, 1999). Not only is sensitivity important when communicating with or around patients with aphasia (as they may well understand pessimistic or pitying remarks), but also more emotionally intoned speech, facial expressions, and gestures may increase communication effectiveness. In contrast, patients with right-hemisphere damage demonstrate decreased emotional expressivity but often normal function in language skills. Restricted emotional expression can be addressed by encouraging such patients to express emotional reactions, states, and intentions semantically. Anderson (1999), who used prosodic imitation to treat emotional prosodic output abnormality in a patient with right-hemisphere stroke, demonstrated improvement of emotional expressivity as evidenced by both formal testing of the patient and by spousal report.

Buccofacial apraxia refers to the inability to perform movements of the face on command or in imitation, in the absence of a comprehension deficit, sensory loss, or motor impairment. Studies examining patients with both left- and right-hemisphere damage report greater impairment of buccofacial praxis following left-hemisphere damage. However, when emotional context is added to the commands or modeling by the examiner, performance improves significantly for both clinical groups. The group with left-hemisphere lesions generally improves to a significantly greater degree than the right-hemisphere group (Borod, Lorch, Koff, & Nicholas, 1987). Thus, emotional cueing has become one mainstay in the remediation of acquired deficiencies in emotional expression following brain injury.

The early stage of acquired emotional processing deficiencies can be associated with anosognosia (disturbed self-awareness) in patients and mood that may vary from indifferent to agitated. Neuropsychological approaches can involve patients in cognitive assessments, therapies related to activities of daily living (ADL), safety precautions, attention training, communication effectiveness, memory remediation, visuospatial problem solving, and efforts at self-monitoring. Until some degree of insight into emotion-related processing changes becomes evident, behavioral approaches are recommended. When confronted prematurely, patients may fail to acknowledge such changes and become highly defensive and guarded. This may have the unwelcome effect of weakening the rapport underlying the therapeutic alliance necessary to progress in the later stages. Written and oral exercises in overall organization of thought are helpful at this stage, particularly if they can be proffered to the patient as relevant to vocational goals.

In contrast to anosognosia on the part of the patient, family members can overreact to perceived changes in the patient's self-awareness, emotional responses, and personality. Family involvement at this stage is focused on intense education and validation with support staff. In addition, whenever possible, it is important to recruit members of the immediate family to take an active role in contributing to remediation of emotional behavioral changes. Such an approach strengthens the patient's psychosocial support network, concomitantly empowering family members. Working with individual family members can be particularly effective in short-circuiting the establishment of a pattern of misunderstanding in their interactions with the patient. Role playing is a useful means of coaching individual family members in developing neutral responses to the patient's indifference. Providing assertiveness training to develop competence can also help family members to handle conflicts with the patient as insight and frustration emerge. One key factor in the determination of remediation approaches is the extent of the patient's cognitively or emotionally based empathetic capacities (Eslinger, 1998). A normal range of empathy can be associated with better social adjustments, supportive relationships, and a prosocial attitude. Low empathy levels can be associated with hostility toward others, family instability, social isolation, and resentment from others. In the affective realm, the hallmark of empathetic capacities is an emotional rapport with others, ranging from a sense of pleasure in response to another's experience of joy to psychic pain in response to another's grief. In the cognitive realm, empathy is a construct delineated by capacity for perspective taking, including the ability to consider different vantage points and the capacity for divergent thinking.

In the transition from acute recovery to an early chronic stage of recovery (3–6 months after cerebral damage), the range of internal emotional responsiveness is approaching baseline, while facial and expressiveness for many patients may remain. For many patients, cognitively based empathetic capacities may be clearly identified but affectively based empathy may be limited by residual anosognosia, reduced arousal, and mood disorder. At this point, patients should receive individual instruction in the use of cognitively based expressive and interactive behaviors. Both family and close friends are of tantamount importance during this stage in providing the emotionally safe environment required for the patient's fledgling attempts to develop expertise in the use of cognitive empathy. Family education remains vital and is focused on active listening and restatement skills, and helping the patient to articulate feelings that cannot be expressed effectively via the face or vocal tone. During this period, it is important that family members validate the patient continually, acknowledging his or her anxiety and confusion in the face of altered family reactions and expectations.

By the chronic recovery stage (1 year and beyond), the patient's emotional intonation and range of internal emotional responsiveness often will have returned to baseline. Cognitive-based emotional communication, empathy and behavior may be showing significantly improved, particularly in patients actively involved in applying these skills to everyday interactions.

FUTURE DIRECTIONS

There are a large number of fundamental questions regarding how to evaluate emotion-related processing disorders, how to conceptualize their diverse components, and how to manage and intervene in an efficacious manner. Considerable progress has been made in the recognition of such disorders, their detrimental effects on recovery and adjustment after brain injury, and the description of prominent component deficits, such as perception of emotional facial expressions and state-congruent emotional expression. The following are important areas of needed research:

1. What are the patterns of recovery from emotion-related processing impairments? The clinical impression is that many persons suffer long-lasting alterations in emotional processing. The impact of these alterations on degree of medical care (acute, postacute and long term), secondary adjustment and psychiatric disorders, speed of recovery, return to home and community-based activities, and return to work remains unclear.

2. Can disorders of emotional expression and/or emotional perception be remediated through neuropsychological or pharmacological interventions? There is some suggestive evidence that dopamine agonists (e.g., bromocriptine), stimulants (e.g., methylphenidate) and serotonin reuptake inhibitors can favorably improve patients' emotional expression after brain injury. However, these studies remain quite limited.

3. Can retraining in emotional face and voice recognition restore accuracy sufficient to improve patients' interpersonal behavior? What is the generalization of such efforts? Does visual imagery training or verbal algorithm training for emotional face recognition provide functional improvement?

4. Is there a role for alternative therapies in remediation of emo-

tional processing disorders, particularly impairments of arousal and expression? Pet-assisted therapies (Fine, 2000) and music therapy (Hauser, Codding, & Eslinger, 2001), and eye movement desensitization and reprocessing (Borod, Vingiano, & Cytryn, 1988; Shapiro, 1995) are three possibilities among others (see Weintraub, 2001).

5. What is the impact of recent findings in the fields of psychoneuroendocrinology and psychoneuroimmunology? One promising bridge between human cognition and affect in the psychoneuroendocrinology literature is seen in the work of Keenan, Ezzat, Ginsburg, and Moore (in press), identifying the prefrontal cortex as a site of estrogen's effect on cognition. Specifically, these researchers identified isolated deficiencies in (a) working memory, (b) sustained attention and preparation for a motor response, and (c) inhibition of appropriate responses in postmenopausal women without estrogen replacement. Some of these capacities are prerequisite for cognitive empathy, currently one of the most powerful prognostic indicators of rehabilitation success following acquired emotion processing impairment.

Continuing research in these and other areas can have a significant impact on potential interventions for emotion processing disorders. It is quite possible that combined pharmacological, psychotherapeutic, and neuropsychological retraining approaches will be formulated to address the diverse levels and facets of these troubling disorders.

REFERENCES

Abercrombie, H. C., Schaefer, S. M., Larson, C. L., Oakes, T. R., Lindgren, K. A., Holden, J. E., Perlman, S. B., Turski, P. A., Krahn, D. D., Benca, R. M., & Davidson, R. J. (1998). Metabolic rate in the right amygdala predicts negative affect in depressed patients. *Neuroreport, 9*(14), 3301–3307.

Adolphs, R., Damasio, H., Tranel, D., & Damasio, A. R. (1996). Cortical systems for the recognition of emotion in facial expressions. *Journal of Neuroscience, 16*, 7678–7687.

Aggleton, J. P. (Ed.). (1992). *The amygdala: Neurobiological aspects of emotion, memory and mental dysfunction.* New York: Wiley–Liss.

Anderson, J. M. (1999). Treatment of expressive aprosodia associated with right hemisphere injury. *Journal of the International Neuropsychological Society, 5*(2), 157.

Barbas, H. (1995). Anatomic basis of cognitive–emotional interactions in the primate prefrontal cortex. *Neuroscience Behavior Review, 19*, 499–510.

Barbas, H., & Pandya, D. N. (1989). Architecture and intrinsic connections of the prefrontal cortex in the rhesus monkey. *Journal of Comprehensive Neurology, 286*, 353–375.

Barbas, H., & Pandya, D. N. (1991). Patterns of correction of the prefrontal cortex in the rhesus monkey associated with cortical architecture. In H. S. Levin, H.

M. Eisenberg, & A. L. Benton (Eds.), *Frontal lobe function and dysfunction* (pp. 35–38). New York: Oxford University Press.

Barrett, A. M., Crucian, G. P., Raymer, A. M., & Heilman, K. M. (1999). Spared comprehension of emotional prosody in a patient with global aphasia. *Neuropsychiatry, Neuropsychology and Behavioral Neurology, 12*(2), 117–120.

Bear, D. M., & Fedio, P. (1977). Quantitative analysis of interictal behavior in temporal lobe epilepsy. *Archives of Neurology, 34,* 454–467.

Beck, A. T., & Steer, R. A. (1993a). *Beck Depression Inventory.* San Antonio, TX: Psychological Corp.

Beck, A. T., & Steer, R. A. (1993b). *Beck Anxiety Inventory.* San Antonio, TX: Psychological Corp.

Beck, A. T., & Steer, R. A. (1993c). *Beck Hopelessness Scale.* San Antonio, TX: Psychological Corp.

Beck, S. J., Beck, A. G., Levitt, E. E., & Molish, H. B. (1961). *Rorschach's test: I. Basic processes* (3rd ed.). New York: Grune & Stratton.

Bellak, L. (1986). *The TAT, CAT and SAT in clinical use* (4th ed.). New York: Psychological Corp.

Benowitz, L. I., Bear, D. M. R., Barrett, A. M., Crucian, G. P., Raymer, A. M., & Heilman, K. M. (1999). Spared comprehension of emotional prosody in a patient with global aphasia. *Neuropsychiatry, Neuropsychology and Behavioural Neurology, 12*(2), 117–120.

Benowitz, L. I., Bear, D. M., Rosenthal, R., Mesulam, M. M., Zaidel, E., & Sperry, R. W. (1983). Hemisphere specialization in non-verbal communication. *Cortex, 19,* 5–11.

Beversdorf, D. Q., Anderson, J. M., Manning, S. E., Anderson, S. L., Nordgren, R. E., Felopulos, G. J., Nadeau, S. E., Heilman, K. M., & Bauman, M. L. (1998). The effect of semantic and emotional context on written recall for verbal language in high functioning adults with autism spectrum disorder. *Journal of Neurology, Neurosurgery and Psychiatry, 65*(5), 685–692.

Blonder, L. X., Bowers, D., & Heilman, K. M. (1991). The role of the right hemisphere in emotional communication. *Brain, 114*(Pt. 3), 1115–1127.

Blonder, L. X., Burns, A. F., Bowers, D., Moore, R. W., & Heilman, K. M. (1993). Right hemisphere facial expressivity during natural conversation. *Brain and Cognition, 21*(1), 44–56.

Blonder, L. X., Gur, R. E., & Gur, R. C. (1989). The effects of right and left hemiparkinsonism on prosody. *Brain and Language, 36,* 193–207.

Boller, F., Cole, M., Vrtunski, P. B., Patterson, M., & Kim, Y. (1979). Paralinguistic aspects of auditory comprehension in aphasia. *Brain and Language, 7*(2), 164–74.

Borod, J. C. (1992). Interhemispheric and intrahemispheric control of emotion: A focus on unilateral brain damage. *Journal of Consulting and Clinical Psychology, 80*(3), 339–348.

Borod, J. C., & Caron, H. (1980). Facedness and emotion related to lateral dominance, sex, and expression type. *Neuropsychologia, 18,* 237–242.

Borod, J. C., Caron, H., & Koff, E. (1981). Asymmetry of facial expression related to handedness, footedness and eyedness: A quantitative study. *Cortex, 17,* 381–390.

Borod, J. C., Caron, H., & White, B. (1983). Facial asymmetry in posed and spontaneous expression of emotion. *Brain and Cognition, 2,* 165–175.

Borod, J. C., & Koff, E. (1984). Asymmetries in affective facial expression. In N. Fox & R. Davidson (Eds.), *The psychobiology of affective development* (pp. 293–323). New York: Erlbaum.

Borod, J. C., & Koff, E. (1989). The neuropsychology of emotion: Evidence from normal, neurological, and psychiatric populations. In E. Perecman (Ed.), *Integrating theory and practice in clinical neuropsychology* (pp. 175–215). New York: Erlbaum.

Borod, J. C., Koff, E., & Buck, R. (1986). The neuropsychology of facial expression. In P. Blanck, R. Buck, & R. Rosenthal (Eds.), *Nonverbal communication in the clinical context* (pp. 196–222). Philadelphia: PSU Press.

Borod, J. C., Koff, E., Lorch, P. M., Nicholas, M., & Welkowitz, J. (1988). Emotional and non-emotional facial behavior in patients with unilateral brain damage. *Journal of Neurology, Neurosurgery and Psychiatry, 51*, 826–832.

Borod, J. C., Koff, E., Perlman-Lorch, M., & Nicholas, M. (1985). Channels of emotional expression in patients with unilateral brain damage. *Archives of Neurology, 42*, 345–348.

Borod, J. C., Lorch, M. P., Koff, E., & Nicholas, M. (1987). Effect of emotional context on bucco-facial apraxia. *Journal of Clinical and Experimental Neuropsychology, 9*(2), 155–161.

Borod, J. C., Virgiaro, W., & Cstryn, F. (1988). The effects of emotion and ocular dominance on lateral eye movement. *Neuropsychologia, 26*(2), 213–220.

Borod, J. C., Welkowitz, J., Alpert, M., Brozgold, A., Martin, C., Peselow, E., & Diller, L. (1990). Parameters of emotional processing in neuropsychiatric disorders: Conceptual issues and a battery of tests. *Journal of Communication Disorders, 23*, 247–270.

Bowers, D., Blonder, L. X., Feinberg, T., & Heilman, K. M. (1991). Differential impact of right and left hemisphere lesions on facial emotion and object imagery. *Brain, 114*(Pt. 6), 2593–609.

Bowers, D., Coslett, H. B., Bauer, R. M., Speedit, L. J., & Heilman, K. H., (1987). Comprehension of emotional prosody following unilateral hemispheric lesions: Processing defect versus distraction defect. *Neuropsychologia, 25*, 317–328.

Bradley, M. M., & Lang, P. J. (1994). Measuring emotion: The Self-Assessment Mannikin and the Semantic Differential. *Journal of Behavior Therapy and Experimental Psychiatry, 25*(1), 49–59.

Bradley, M. M., & Lang, P. J. (1999). *International affective digitized sound system. Technical manual and affective ratings.* Center for Research and Psychological Physiology, University of Florida, Gainesville, FL.

Bradley, M. M., & Lang, P. J. (2000). Measuring emotion: Behavior, feeling and physiology. In R. D. Lane & Nadel, L. (Eds.), *Cognitive neuroscience of emotion* (pp. 242–276). New York: Oxford University Press.

Brodal, A. (1957). *The cranial nerves: Anatomy and anatomical-clinical correlates.* Oxford, UK: Scientific Publications.

Brooks, D. N., & McKinlay, W. (1983). Personality and behavioral change after severe blunt head injury—A relative's view. *Journal of Neurology, Neurosurgery and Psychiatry, 46*, 336–344.

Brooks, N., Campsie, L., Symington, C., Beattie, A., & McKinlay, W. (1986). The five year outcome of severe blunt head injury—a relative's view. *Journal of Neurology, Neurosurgery and Psychiatry, 49*, 764–770.

Bryden, M. P., & Ley, R. G. (1983). Right-hemispheric involvement in the perception and expression of emotion in normal humans. In K. M. Heilman & P. Satz (Eds.), *Neuropsychology of human emotions* (pp. 6–44). New York: Guilford Press.

Butcher, J. N., Dahlstrom, W. G., Graham, J. R., Tellegen, A., Kaemmer, B. (1989). *Manual for the restandardized Minnesota Multiphasic Personality Inventory: MMPI-2.* Minneapolis: University of Minnesota Press.

Cimino, C. R., Verfaellie, M., Bowers, D., & Heilman, K. M. (1991). Autobiographical memory: Influence of right hemisphere damage on emotionality and specificity. *Brain and Cognition, 15*(1), 106–118.

Costa, P. T., & McCrae, R. R. (1978). *The NEO personality inventory.* Odessa, FL: Psychological Assessment Resources.

Critchley, M. (1939). *The language of gesture.* London: Edward Arnold.

Crucian, G. P., Huang, L., Barrett, A. M., Schwartz, R. L., Cibula, J., Anderson, J. M., Friedman, W., & Heilman, K. M (2000). The effect of arousal on affective conversations in Parkinson's disease. *Neurology, 54*(7, Suppl. 3), A204–A205.

Crucian, G. P., Keillor, J. M., Hughes, J. D., Barrett, A. M., Williamson, D. J. G., Bauer, R. M., Bowers, D., & Heilman, K. M. (1999). Hemispheric differences in emotional reactivity to false feedback. *Journal of the International Neuropsychological Society, 5*(2), 110.

Crucian, G. P., Preston, L. M., Raymer, A. M., & Heilman, K. M. (1997). Dissociation of behavioral action and emotional valence in the expression of affect. *Neurology, 48*(Suppl.), A353.

Darwin, C. (1872). *The expression of the emotions in man and animals.* New York: Appleton.

Davidson, R. J. (1985). Affect, cognition and hemispheric specialization. In C. E. Izard, J. Kagan, & R. Zanjone (Eds.), *Emotion, cognition and behavior* (pp. 300–305). New York: Cambridge University Press.

Davidson, R. J. (1988a). Affective style and affective disorders: Perspectives from affective neuroscience. *Cognition and Emotion, 12,* 307–330.

Davidson, R. J. (1988b). Anterior electrophysiological asymmetries, emotion and depression: Conceptual and methodological conundrums. *Psychophysiology, 35*(5), 607–614.

Davis, M. H. (1994). *Empathy: A social psychological approach.* Madison, WI: Brown & Benchmark.

Denes, G., Caldognetto, E., Semenza, C., Vagges, K., & Zetten, M. (1984). Discrimination and identification of emotion in human voice by brain damaged subjects. *Acta Neurologica Scandinavica, 69,* 154–162.

Denny-Brown, D., Meyer, J., & Horenstein, S. (1952). The significance of perceptual rivalry resulting from parietal lesions. *Brain, 75,* 433–471.

Derryberry, D., & Tucker, D. (1992). Neural mechanisms of emotion. *Journal of Consulting and Clinical Psychology, 60*(3), 329–338.

Dikmen, S., & Reitan, R. M. (1977). MMPI correlates of adaptive ability deficits in patients with brain lesions. *Journal of Nervous and Mental Disease, 165*(4), 247–254.

Ehlers, L., & Bratt, N. (1996). The Rorschach Test applied to patients with lesions of the frontal lobe. *Nordisk Psykologi, 48*(1), 57–72.

Ekman, P., & Friesen, W. V. (1976). Measuring facial movement. *Environmental Psychology and Nonverbal Behavior, 1,* 56–75.

Ekman, P., & Friesen, W. V. (1978). *The Facial Action Coding System (FACS): A technique for the measurement of facial action.* Palo Alto, CA: Consulting Psychologists Press.

Erhan, H., Borod, J. C., Tenke, D. E., & Bruder, G. E. (1998). Identification of emotion in a dichotic listening task: Event-related brain potential and behavioral findings. *Brain and Cognition, 37,* 286–307.

Eslinger, P. J. (1998). The neurological and neuropsychological bases of empathy. *European Neurology, 39,* 193–199.

Eslinger, P. J. (1999). Orbital frontal cortex: Historical and contemporary views about its behavioral and physiological significance. *Neurocase, 5,* 225–229.

Etcott, N. (1981). Selective attention to facial identity and facial emotion. *Neuropsychologica, 22,* 281–295.

Exner, J. E. (1986). *The Rorschach: A comprehensive system* (Vol. 1, 2nd ed.). New York: Wiley-Interscience.

Fine, A. H. (Ed.). (2000). *Handbook on animal assisted therapies: Theoretical foundations and guidelines for practice.* San Diego: Academic Press.

Gainotti, G. (1969). Reactions catastrophiques et manifestations dindifference au cours des atteintes cerebrales. *Neuropsychologia, 7,* 195–204.

Gainotti, G. (1972). Emotional behavior and hemispheric side of lesion. *Cortex, 8,* 41–55.

Gainotti, G. (1984). Some methodological problems in the study of the relationships between emotions and cerebral dominance. *Journal of Clinical Neuropsychology, 6*(1), 111–121.

Goldstein, K. (1939). *The organism: A holistic approach to biology derived from pathological data in man.* New York: American Book.

Greene, R. L. (1991). *The MMPI-2/MMPI: An interpretive manual.* Needham Heights, MA: Allyn & Bacon.

Hauser, S., Coddings, P., & Eslinger, P. J. (2001). Music therapy. In M. I. Weintraub (Ed.), *Alternative and complementary treatment in neurological illness* (pp. 255–267). New York: Churchill-Livingstone.

Hathaway, S. R., & McKinley, J. C. (1942). A multiphasic personality schedule (Minnesota): III. The measurement of symptomatic depression. *Journal of Psychology, 14,* 73–84.

Hathaway, S. R., & McKinley, J. C. (1951). *The Minnesota Multiphasic Personality Inventory manual (rev.).* New York: Psychological Corp.

Heilman, K. M. (1997). The neurobiology of emotional experience. *Journal of Neuropsychiatry, 9,* 439–448.

Heilman, K. M., Blonder, L. X., Bowers, D., & Crucian, G. P. (2000). Neurological disorders and emotional dysfunction. In J. C. Borod (Ed.), *The neuropsychology of emotion* (pp. 367–412). New York: Oxford University Press.

Heilman, K. M., Bowers, D., & Valenstein, E. (1993). Emotional disorders associated with neurological diseases. In K. M. Heilman & E. Valenstein (Eds.), *Clinical neuropsychology* (3rd ed., pp. 461–497). New York: Oxford University Press.

Heilman, K. M., & Satz, P. (Eds.). (1985). *The neuropsychology of human emotion.* New York: Guilford Press.

Heilman, K. M., Scholes, R., & Watson, R. T. (1975). Auditory affective agnosia: Disturbed comprehension of affective speech. *Journal of Neurology, Neurosurgery and Psychiatry, 38*(1), 69–72.

Hogan, R. (1969). Development of an empathy scale. *Journal of Consulting and Clinical Psychology, 33*(3), 307–316.

Hughlings-Jackson, J. (1880). On affections of speech from disease of the brain. *Brain, 2,* 323–356.

Izard, C. E. (1977). *Human emotions.* New York: Plenum Press.

Jacobs, D. H., Shuren, J., Bowers, D., & Heilman, K. M. (1995). Emotional facial imagery, perception, and expression in Parkinson's disease. *Neurology, 45*(9), 1696–1702.

James, W. (1890). *The principles of psychology.* New York: Plenum Press.

Keillor, J. M., Barrett, A. M., Crucian, G. P., Kortenkamp, S., & Heilman, K. M. (1999). Emotional experience and perception in a case of facial paralysis: A test of the facial feedback hypothesis. *Journal of the International Neuropsychological Society, 5*(2), 106.

Keenan, P. A., Ezzat, W. H., Ginsburg, K., & Moore, G. J. (in press). Prefrontal cortex as the site of estrogen's effect on cognition. *Psychoneuroimmunology.*

Landis, C. (1924). Studies of emotional reactions: I. A preliminary study of facial expression. *Journal of Experimental Psychology, 7*, 325–341.

Lang, P. J. (1980). Behavioral treatment and bio-behavioral assessment: Computer applications. In J. B. Sidowski, J. H. Johnson, & T. A. Williams (Ed.), *Technology in mental health care delivery systems* (pp. 119–137). Norwood, NJ: Ablex.

Lang, P. J., Bradley, M. M., & Cuthbert, B. N. (1998). Emotion, motivation, and anxiety: Brain mechanisms and psychophysiology [Review, 84 refs.]. *Biological Psychiatry, 44*(12), 1248–1263.

Lang, P. J., Bradley, M. M., & Cuthbert, B. N. (1999). *International Affective Picture System. Technical manual and affective ratings.* Center for research and psychological physiology. University of Florida, Gainesville.

Lanyon, B. P. (1972). Empirical construction and validation of a sentence completion test for hostility, anxiety and dependency. *Journal of Consulting and Clinical Psychology, 39*, 420–428.

Lanyon, B. P., & Lanyon R. I. (1980). *Incomplete Sentences Task: Manual.* Chicago: Stoelting.

Leventhal, H. (1984). A perceptual motor theory of emotion. In K. R. Scherer & P. Ekmon (Eds.), *Approaches to emotion* (pp. 271–292). Hillsdale, NJ: Erlbaum.

Levy, J., Heller, W., Banich, M. T., & Burton, L. A. (1983). Asymmetry of perception in free viewing of chimeric faces. *Brain and Cognition, 2*, 404–419.

Lindgren, K. A., Larson, C. L., Schaefer, S. M., Abercrombie, H. C., Ward, R. T., Oakes, T. R., Holden, J. E., Perlman, S. B., Benca, R. M., & Davidson, R. J. (1999). Thalamic metabolic rate predicts EEG alpha power in healthy control subjects but not in depressed patients. *Biological Psychiatry, 45*(8), 943–952.

LoCastro, J. (1972). Judgment of emotional communication in the facial–vocal–verbal channels. Unpublished doctoral thesis, University of Maryland, Baltimore.

Lynn, J. G., & Lynn, D. R. (1938). Face–hand laterality in relation to personality. *Journal of Abnormal and Social Psychology, 33*, 291–322.

Lynn, J. G., & Lynn, D. R. (1943). Smile and hand dominance in relation to basic modes of adaptation. *Journal of Abnormal and Social Psychology, 38*, 250–276.

MacLean, P. D. (1990). *The triune brain in evolution: Role in paleocerebral functions.* New York: Plenum Press.

Mehrabian, A., & Epstein, N. (1972). A measure of emotional empathy. *Journal of Personality, 40*, 525–543.

Mozaux, J. M., & Richer, E. (1998). Rehabilitation after traumatic brain injury in adults. *Disability and Rehabilitation, 20*(12), 435–447.

Murray, H. A. (1938). *Explorations in personality.* New York: Oxford University Press.

Nelson, L. D., Drebin, C., Uchiyama, P. S., & Uchiyama, C. (1998). Personality change in head trauma: A validity study of the neuropsychology behavior and affect profile. *Archives of Clinical Neuropsychology, 13*(6), 549–560.

Papez, J. W. (1937). A proposed mechanism of emotion. *Archives of Neurology and Psychiatry, 38*, 725–743.

Penfield, W., & Jasper, H. (1954). *Epilepsy and the functional anatomy of the human brain.* Boston: Little, Brown

Plutchik, R. (1984). Emotions: A general psychoevolutionary theory. In K. R. Scherer & P. Ekman (Eds.), *Approaches to emotion* (pp. 197–219). Hillsdale, NJ: Erlbaum.

Price, J. L., Darmichael, S. T., & Drevets, W. C. (1996). Networks related to the orbital and medial prefrontal cortex: A substrate for emotional behavior. *Progress in Brain Research, 107,* 523–536.

Richardson, C. K., Bowers, D., Bauer, R. M., Heilman, K. M., & Leonard, C. M. (2000). Digitizing the moving face during dynamic displays of emotion. *Neuropsychologia, 38*(7), 1028–1039.

Robinson, R. G., & Benson, D. F. (1981). Depression in aphasic patients: Frequency, severity, and clinical pathological correlation. *Brain and Language, 14,* 282–291.

Roeltgen, D. P., Sevush, S., & Heilman, K. M. (1983). Phonological agraphia: Writing by the lexical–semantic route. *Neurology, 33*(6), 755–765.

Rolls, E. T. (1990). A theory of emotion, and its application to understanding the neural basis of emotion. *Cognition and Emotion, 4,* 161–190.

Ross, E. (1981). The Aprospdias. *Archives of Neurology, 38,* 561–569.

Ross, E. (1985). Modulation of affect and nonverbal communication by the right hemisphere. In M. M. Mesulum (Ed.), *Principles of behavioral neurology* (pp. 239–257). Philadelphia: Davis.

Ross, E. (1996). Hemispheric specialization for emotions, affective aspects of language and communication and the cognitive control of display behaviors in humans. In G. Holstege, R. Bandler & C. B Saper (Eds.), *Progress in Brain Research* (Vol. 107, pp. 583–594).

Ross, E., & Mesulam, M. M. (1979). Dominant language functions of the right hemisphere?: Prosody and emotional gesturing. *Archives of Neurology, 36,* 144–148.

Sackheim, H., Greenburg, M., Weisman, A., Gur, R., Hungerbuhler, J., & Geschwind, N. (1982). Hemispheric asymmetry in the expression of positive and negative emotions: Neurologic evidence. *Archives in Neurology, 39,* 210–218.

Shapiro, I. (1995). *Eye movement desensitization and reprocessing.* New York: Guilford Press.

Slomine, B., Bowers, D., & Heilman, K. M. (1999). Dissociation between autonomic responding and verbal report in right and left hemisphere brain damage during anticipatory anxiety. *Neuropsychiatry, Neuropsychology, and Behavioural Neurology, 12*(3), 143–148.

Sutton, S. K., & Davidson, R. J. (2000). Prefrontal brain electrical asymmetry predicts the evaluation of affective stimuli. *Neuropsychologia, 38*(13), 1723–1733.

Thorpe, S. J., Rolls, E. T., & Maddison, S. (1983). Neuronal activity in the orbitofrontal cortex of the rhesus monkey. *Experimental Brain Research, 49,* 93–115.

Triggs, W. J., McCoy, K. J. M., Greer, R., Rossi, F., Bowers, D., Kortenkamp, S., Nadeau, S. E., Heilman, K. M., & Goodman, W. K. (1999). Effects of left frontal transcranial magnetic stimulation on depressed mood, cognition, and corticomotor threshold. *Biological Psychiatry, 45*(11), 1440–1446.

Tucker, D., Watson, R., & Heilman, K. (1977). Discrimination and evocation of affectively intoned speech in patients with right parietal disease. *Neurology, 27,* 947–950.

Tucker, D. M. (1981). Lateral brain function, emotion and conceptualization. *Psychological Bulletin, 89*(1), 19–46.

Tucker, D. M., Steinslie, C. E., Roth, R. S., & Shearer, S. L. (1981). Right frontal lobe activation and right hemisphere performanceL Decrement during a depressed mood. *Archives of General Psychiatry, 38*(2), 169–174.

Weintraub, M. I. (Ed.). (2001). *Alternative and complementary treatment in neurological disease.* New York: Churchill Livingstone.

Wilson, F. A., & Rolls, E. T. (1990). Neuronal responses related to reinforcement in the primate basal forebrain. *Brain Research, 509,* 213–231.

Wolfe, G. I., & Ross, E. D. (1987). Sensory aprosodia with left hemiparesis from subcortical infoartction: Right hemisphere analog of sensory type aphasia with right hemiparesis? *Archives of Neurology, 44,* 661–671.

Zuckerman, M., Lipets, M. S., Koivumaki, J. H., & Rosenthal, R. (1975). Encoding and decoding nonverbal cues of emotion. *Journal of Personality and Social Psychology, 32,* 1068–1076.

PART III

Future Directions

CHAPTER 14

Summary and Analysis of Emerging Intervention Models

PAUL J. ESLINGER

The aim of this volume has been to identify the scientific ideas, models, and data that drive intervention research for neuropsychological impairments. Areas that appear promising have been highlighted alongside those that merit scientific investigation. The prevalence of brain-based disorders are a leading cause of disability worldwide (World Health Organization, 2000). The overriding aim of neuropsychological interventions is to promote maximal adaptive functioning after brain injury through procedures that address impairments, disabilities, and handicaps in multiple areas, including behavioral, cognitive, and social–emotional spheres. Part I, "Foundations of Neuropsychological Interventions," focused on the fundamental principles for neuropsychological intervention research. The theoretical bases for such investigation were described by Barrett and Gonzalez-Rothi (Chapter 2). There is a strong theoretical basis for such research based on expanding knowledge about cerebral plasticity, processes of neural recovery and age, as well as experience-related changes in the central nervous system. There are good scientific reasons to expect both restitutive and compensatory effects of interventions. A critical part of intervention planning is assessment of neuropsychological impairments. In Chapter 3, Bergquist and Malec argued that neuropsychological evaluation must be geared toward not only the *detection of impairment* but also the *characterization of disability*. This represents a shift from the challenge of mainly establishing diagnosis to concomitantly investigating patient functioning in multiple settings, patient capacity to benefit from treatment, and pertinent treatment approaches. Furthermore, they draw attention to growing domains of neuropsychological assessment beyond memory, intellect, visuospatial processing, and other well-established areas with a strong cognitive emphasis. These growing domains are critical to ascertaining disability level and include patient self-awareness, motivation, personality, and mood state. The latter areas have a tremendous impact on interpretation of assessment as well as development of treatment plans and facilitation of real-world outcomes. Thoughtful guidelines are offered for principles of assessment, training, and multidisciplinary collaboration.

The possibilities for direct physiological intervention with medications were addressed by Whyte in Chapter 4. While the possibility of drug treatment breakthroughs for neuropsychological impairments and cognitive disabilities is exciting, the common reality is that a relative degree of benefit can be realized from a limited range of medications, primarily to reduce the level of impairment. There is a large chasm between the action of drugs at the cellular level and the neural mediation of complex behavioral and cognitive processes. Despite these and many methodological obstacles, Whyte outlined conceptual and methodological approaches to this intriguing and embryonic area, drawing upon the enablement–disablement model (Institute of Medicine, 1997). Several research designs are discussed along with subject selection, specification of treatment and measurement of treatment effects. Combined behavioral and pharmacological interventions should also be considered (e.g., Barrett, Crucian, Maddux, & Heilman, 2000). Scientific investigation is a process, not only for medication effects but for all neuropsychological interventions. As Levine and Downey-Lamb argued in Chapter 5, rigorously designed empirical research is fundamental to rehabilitation advances. In particular, the use of randomized control trials with subject and investigator blindness, is becoming possible for some neuropsychological intervention research. But the yield of such research is not assured by that design alone. Selection and description of participants, measurement instruments, moderating psychosocial variables, selection of outcome parameters, timing of assessments, treatment compliance, and theoretical grounding all present important challenges to clinical researchers and funding sources. However, at this stage of development, neuropsychological intervention research should not be limited to large-scale, randomized control trials. In fact, this approach may be unrealistic. Fortunately, Levine and Downey-Lamb also described a number of investigative design options, ranging from quasi-experimental and single-case designs to the rehabilitation probe, among others. Meta-analysis presents another important avenue for evaluation of treatment outcomes.

The following section contains highlighted summaries from Part II, "Models of Intervention for Neuropsychological Impairments." Analyses of the advances in the clinical areas of attention, memory, visual perception, language, praxis, executive function, social behavior, and emotion-related processing are presented, along with thoughts on future directions.

ATTENTION

This is an area of intensive investigation. Disorders of attention, including the hemispatial neglect variety and otherwise, are fundamental stumbling blocks to recovery, functional adaptation, safety, and independence. As Manly, Ward, and Robertson (Chapter 6) conclude, there is a scientific basis for cautious optimism, though rehabilitation research is at an early phase. Two of the most important advances in this area have been (1) the delineation of components and diverse aspects of attention (both theoretical and experimental models), and (2) the assessment of attentional abilities with standardized procedures and techniques.

The construct of attention is increasingly differentiated from perceptual functions (or "data processing systems" as per Posner & Petersen, 1990), yet it is recognized to be a vital, "cohesive glue" that binds multiple perceptual and cognitive processes together. It appears likely that attentional disorders can occur separate and apart from perceptual, memory, and cognitive disorders. Furthermore, there can be different kinds of attentional disorders pertaining to internally and externally oriented systems. These include the following:

- Orienting or spatial attention
- Selective or focused attention ("target selection")
- Vigilance or sustained attention

Disorders of attention are most common after right-hemisphere and prefrontal cortex damage, yet are also prominent with more widespread cerebral dysfunction as well, for example, traumatic brain injury, delirium, and dementia. Hence, their prevalence in neurological disorders is quite high.

Advances in the assessment of attention have been a key influence on rehabilitation research. Manly et al. (Chapter 6) describe several standardized instruments and experimental procedures that are informative and fairly reliable, but validation against "real-world" functioning outside the laboratory and rehabilitation environment is particularly needed.

Interventions for *spatial attentional disorders* (particularly left-hemispatial neglect) emphasize:

- Scanning training that utilizes cues, prompts, and verbally mediated intentional scanning to attend to left-hemispace stimuli.
- Limb activation that intentionally engages patients to use their left-upper extremity to perform motor tasks in left hemispace.
- Sustained attention training aimed at improving voluntary attention to new stimuli ("readiness to respond"), particularly left-sided stimuli.

With each of these approaches, cues and other external aids are gradually reduced in favor of patient self-cueing.

Interventions for *nonspatial attentional disorders* have included:

- Behavioral, goal-based approaches such as reducing attentional slips while reading.
- Behavioral shaping of attention to the problem, in particular, increasing patients' self-monitoring of their problematic behavior.
- General attentional training, now possible through computer-based programs that can be practiced frequently over long time periods.
- Computerized, game-context-type training that emphasizes specific types of attentional processes (e.g., selective attention, sustained attention, etc.).
- Environmental supports such as reminder tones (not unlike the beeping of a wristwatch).

These intervention approaches raise cause not only for optimism but also for caution. Manly, Ward, and Robertson present a succinct and engaging analysis of attention rehabilitation research, clearly pointing out avenues for further research and application. Interventions combining pharmacological and neurobehavioral remediation deserve further investigation as well (e.g., Whyte et al., 1997).

LEARNING AND MEMORY

Perhaps no area of cognitive rehabilitation research generates more discussion than memory disorders, given their prevalent and disabling nature. Furthermore, disorders of learning and memory are among the most common forms of cognitive disability in neurological disease. Thus, Glisky and Glisky (Chapter 7) had to tackle a number of fundamental issues in rehabilitation research. As with other cognitive areas, progress in remediation of memory disorders has been critically dependent on models of normal memory function and the types of alterations that occur with neurological disease. Constructs of memory encoding, storage, and retrieval, short-term versus long-term memory, declarative versus procedural memory, implicit versus explicit memory, and visual versus verbal memory have all signaled contrasting and multiple processes mediating the acquisition, retention, and retrieval of information subsumed under the rubric of memory systems. The neural substrate of these processes has been illuminated in remarkable ways, most recently through functional brain imaging techniques. These findings have reinforced our understanding of how diverse and widespread the acquisition, storage, and retrieval of information is in the brain, and how commonly memory functions are altered by a wide number of neurological diseases. Glisky and Glisky suggest that an integrated approach to rehabilitation may hold the greatest promise for patients' remediation progress spanning cognitive, neurological and functional–behavioral domains pertinent to memory. Four rehabilitation approaches are outlined:

- Restoration of damaged function (restore).
- Optimization of residual function (retrain).
- Compensation for lost function (compensate).
- Substitution with intact function (alternate approach).

Importantly, the authors consider not only the methods employed with each approach but also their limitations, thus pointing out several areas of much needed research. Perhaps most important are questions about cerebral plasticity (restorative, compensatory, substitutive), generalization of training effects, and models of normal memory function.

Four types of specific rehabilitation methods are discussed, including their rationale and application:

- Practice and rehearsal.
- Mnemonic strategies.
- Environmental supports/external aides.
- Domain-specific learning.

These methods span mild to severe memory impairments and task-specific to general functional goals. The more successful applications are those directed at well-defined and specific behavioral goals. Some of the most interesting advances are occurring in the area of environmental supports/external aides where hand-held electronic memory organizers and computers are being adapted to meet the functional goals of individual patients. These aides are likely to be helpful to those with mild to moderate memory impairments and generally intact cognitive functions, but research is clearly needed to evaluate effectiveness. Such aides seem to have tremendous potential for maintaining low costs, application to many functional goals and circumstances, portability, ease of use, and increasing social acceptance in home, community, and vocational settings. Complemented by techniques of spaced retrieval, mnemonic and organizational strategies, and domain-specific memory training (e.g., vanishing aids, errorless learning), the combination of internal and external supports may hold significant promise for a large number of patients with memory disorders. Other possibilities include the use of select pharmacological agents (e.g., acetylcholinesterase inhibitors; Taverni, Seliger, & Lichtman, 1998) alone and particularly in combination with neurobehavioral remediation techniques. Memory rehabilitation research has expanded rapidly and encompasses nearly all of the challenges currently facing the scientific basis of interventions for neuropsychological disorders.

VISUAL PERCEPTION

There are a variety of visual–perceptual impairments that deserve consideration in assessment and rehabilitation domains. The term "visual perception" refers to pattern-, color-, and spatial-related processes that interact with attentional, language, memory, motor, executive and other sensory systems to permit ease of visual recognition, spatial navigation, motion adjustments, and efficiency of many functional activities, ranging from operating vehicles to designing Web sites. Vision–brain research is one of the most advanced areas of cognitive neuroscience, with modeling of multiple pathways, multiple perceptual processes, and even complex interactions between cognitive processes and cell recordings in different vision–brain regions (e.g., Corbetta, 1990; Zeki, 1992; Van Essen, Anderson, & Fellerman, 1992; Leopold & Logothetis, 1996; Motter, 1994; Treue & Maunsell, 1996). Therefore, basic research provides many invigorating ideas regarding fundamental perceptual and attentional processes, and their relationship to more complex visual behaviors. Studies of the spontaneous or natural course of recovery after damage to vision-related structures (cortical and subcortical) are surprisingly limited, even for the disabling hemispatial neglect syndromes. While there is tremendous potential benefit to the practiced application of verbal mediation strategies in visual–perceptual and spatial disorders, formal or standardized guidelines are still underdeveloped. As with other areas of rehabilitation of neuropsychological disorders, formulating specified goals based on assessment as well as patient background, experience, and overall functional goals is key to directing the type of intervention and its particular application. Anderson (Chapter 8) advocates both restorative and compensatory approaches, and supports the general model of selective optimization with compensation (SOC; Freund & Baltes, 1998) as a general rehabilitative framework. Although formulated from the literature on aging, the SOC model specifies selecting priorities and goals, optimizing goal-related abilities through restorative approaches, and compensating through development of alternative approaches, abilities, and techniques. Assessing progress through Goal Attainment Scaling (Malec, 1999) provides a semiquantitative method for feedback and adjustment.

An important aspect of both restorative and compensatory approaches is patient awareness of visual-related changes. Such awareness often is key to patient motivation and adjustment, and essential for improving skills through a variety of therapies. Anderson reported that 85% of patients with right-hemisphere stroke denied visual perceptual difficulties, though assessment indicated otherwise. Depending on the particular nature and extent of deficit, management of visual–perceptual impairments can employ combinations of restorative and compensatory techniques, focused via specified goals and allied deficits, if any. A similar approach can be applied to related visual-processing deficits such as constructional apraxia, optic ataxia, spatial imperception, and motion-related impairments. With the advent of virtual reality techniques, automobile simulators, and computer-related scanning and graphics devices, there are intriguing possibilities for developing more sophisticated visual–perceptual intervention techniques.

LANGUAGE

Interventions for language disorders have drawn from diverse approaches and have been subject perhaps to the most intense scrutiny of their effectiveness. Hinckley (Chapter 9) raises a fundamental point about the relationship between brain–language research and language rehabilitation research; that is, she argues that advances in effective treatments are predicated less on understanding the nature of language deficits and more on understanding the nature of adaptive change in the forms of behavioral and neural plasticity. This argument is not meant to minimize the value of basic research on language and the brain, nor to suggest that such research has no bearing on development of possible interventions. Rather, it suggests that the aims of current intervention research are to identify and develop means for fostering compensatory and adaptive changes for independent, real-world functioning. This may or may not arise from further understanding of clinical deficits and brain–behavior systems, as the aims of these research endeavors are different.

The comprehensive literature review, a type of evidence-based analysis of language rehabilitation from 1990–2000, provided an excellent summary and intriguing overview of the predominant approaches:

- Cognitive neuropsychological
- Cognition and learning
- Compensatory
- Linguistic
- Social
- Neurological

Hinckley further analyzed the goals of each approach, the proposed mechanisms of change through therapy, and related treatment procedures. Importantly, she emphasized that the studies do not necessarily reflect patterns of actual clinical practice, which focus more on functional assessment, goals, and interventions achieved through diverse approaches. Each approach has its strengths and weaknesses. For example, while the cognitive neuropsychological approach can provide a comprehensive, in-depth analysis of certain linguistic processes and consider the results within models of cognition and the brain, the remediation of such localized deficits is less evident. Identifying the patient's impairment as specifically as possible may lead to a more focused intervention approach, but this has yet to be demonstrated clearly. In contrast, compensatory approaches emphasize effective message communication within different settings rather than isolated language or cognitive competencies per se. Yet, compensatory approaches depend upon preserved cognitive abilities of patients and their capacities for learning and employing alternative strategies to improve language effectiveness. In other approaches, there appear to be benefits from linguistically based movement therapy, socially based interventions, learning-based cognitive techniques, and neurologically based approaches, such as melodic intonation therapy. The impact of brain imaging methods such as positron emission tomography (PET) and functional magnetic resonance imaging (fMRI), while intriguing relative to cognitive neuroscience issues, has yet to be realized for intervention research. Applications to language intervention research appear pertinent and feasible within the near future.

Finally, Hinckley suggests that these diverse approaches have many elements in common. Intervention research that focuses on mechanisms underlying adaptive change and skills acquisition might help specify which kinds of interventions result in what types of outcomes for various clinical populations.

PRAXIS

van Heugten (Chapter 10) has provided an interesting and comprehensive analysis of interventions for apraxia. The estimated prevalence of apraxia is considerable among patients with left-hemisphere disease, generally ranging from one-third to one-half of such patients. The chapter emphasized the critical importance of operationalized constructs in defining and differentiating forms of apraxia, as this has been a point of debate in apraxia research. Particularly important is the detection of patients who fail to perform on command but are nonetheless accurate in the natural, spontaneous use of objects and associated actions. van Heugten also emphasizes the interplay of standardized tests and observational techniques in assessing both the clinical occurrence of apraxia and its impact on more ecologically valid, daily activities (e.g., Foundas et al., 1995). Although patients do not complain of praxis deficits per se, it would be misleading to minimize the inability to dress oneself, complete personal hygiene, to prepare meals, and other multistep perceptuomotor skills. In fact, van Heugten argues that "all apraxia variables appeared to be significant predictors of subsequent dependency" (see studies by, among others, Bjorneby & Reinvang, 1985; Sundet, Finset, & Reinvang, 1988; Saeki, Ogata, Okubo, Takahashi, & Hoshuyama, 1993; Goldenberg & Hagman, 1998). Although some recovery of apraxia can generally be expected over a period of at least 5–6 months, certain types of spatial and temporal deficits persist, and many patients may still meet criteria for apraxia. Intervention approaches have focused mainly on compensatory strategies and verbal–visual mediation to generate, guide, and monitor movements. One of the most promising approaches is strategy–training aimed at conferring methods for improving daily functional activities rather than teaching a specific task. Patients improved despite comorbid influences of cognitive impairment, motor impairment, and advanced age. Randomized clinical trials are beginning to be applied in this area and their results are encouraging. Many variables need to be further examined, such as length and frequency of treatment, formal testing versus functional activity effectiveness, differential effects of instructions, assistance and feedback, modalities, time since brain injury, and comorbid cognitive and motor impairments. Generalizability and maintenance of treatment effects also remain areas of concern for further studies to address.

EXECUTIVE FUNCTIONING

Although a plethora of abilities and processes are subserved under the rubric of executive functions, Cicerone (Chapter 11) provides a fresh focus on *regulatory* cognitive processes that potentially promote adaptive behavior in a range of settings. Drawing upon the "corollary discharge" notion of Teuber (1964), he describes intervention approaches that foster patients' *anticipation* and *monitoring* of their own behavior. Problem-solving paradigms that entail the trained prediction of the patient's own behavior, difficulty of the presented problems, and monitoring of actual performance have shown beneficial results. The provision of corrective feedback also appears helpful for reducing errors and encouraging patients to self-monitor and self-correct more accurately. These interventions underscore an important distinction between training of *specific behaviors* and training of *mediating cognitive processes*, such as metacognitive skills. The acts of prediction, self-monitoring, error monitoring, and correction through feedback can potentially trigger activation of neural systems that ready the organism for anticipated change, action, and transition (i.e., a type of "corollary discharge" effect). Such interventions may benefit not only practical problem-solving behaviors but also contribute to patients' perceived self-efficacy.

A related but different approach emanates from the "verbal self-regulatory" and "supervisory attention" constructs of Luria (1996) and Shallice (1981), respectively. Both emphasize the active control or regulation of behavior from internally mediated mechanisms (e.g., action plans, strategic supervision), particularly in novel and nonroutine circumstances. Utilizing a verbally mediated self-instruction approach, trained over three stages, Cicerone suggests that patients with planning and self-monitoring impairments can significantly improve. Benefit was demonstrated not only in standardized executive-function tasks but also real-life skills, the latter requiring specific efforts at generalization and daily application.

Another prominent manifestation of executive impairment is erratic, goal-directed behavior (i.e., goal neglect). The "goal management training" approach of Levine et al. (2000) is a creative intervention that expands upon earlier work of von Cramon, Mathes-von Cramon, and Mai (1991) and D'Zurilla and Goldfried (1971) to foster problem-solving skills. The intervention specifies five discrete training stages that incorporate an extended algorithm or metacognitive strategy for adaptive problem solving in diverse settings. Initial evaluation of results indicated that participants significantly reduced errors and increased time on tasks, particularly with unstructured tasks. This approach capitalized on a cognitive-based training strategy when goals lose their motivational power or patients are too disorganized to accomplish multistep tasks. Further development and application are clearly warranted.

The final area of intervention research Cicerone addresses is the problematic social impairments that arise particularly from orbitofrontal types of cerebral injuries. Studies suggest that such patients can develop compensatory behaviors for the specific social circumstances in which they are trained but cannot effectively utilize their own emotional cues or reactions to self-regulate and guide behavior adaptively. Theory-of-mind capabilities may be quite limited, along with reduced awareness of anticipatory anxiety and other autonomic signals.

Intervention research for executive impairments is leading to demonstrable progress in conceptualizing, evaluating, and managing some of these debilitating impairments that can be difficult for the untrained person to appreciate. Family education and other environmental modifications remain a cornerstone for providing the external supports for executive disorders, though emerging interventions are promising. Most require clearer standardization of procedures and further study of treatment effects.

SOCIAL BEHAVIOR

Far beyond the old labels of organic personality disorder, pseudopsychopathic behavior, and frontal lobe syndrome, research focusing on disturbances of social behavior and their management continues to grow conceptually and scientifically. Disturbances of social behavior are a particular strain for families of affected patients, rehabilitation staff, and patients themselves. Advances have been limited by the fact there are few models of social impairment that have been proposed, and fewer yet subjected to empirical research. Grattan and Gharamanalou (Chapter 12) provide a comprehensive review of both relevant studies and a descriptive model of psychosocial impairments after brain injury. Intervention studies to date have focused mainly on survivors of traumatic brain injury, in whom the physical forces of injury commonly converge on orbitofrontal, anterior temporal, and deep white matter regions. Although behavior management has been a frequent approach, cognitive-behavioral therapies and other skills-based interventions (e.g., relaxation training, social skills, anger management) have also shown promise.

Grattan and Gharamanalou place social disturbances within a larger descriptive model that identifies four main categories of complex social processing:

- Social self-regulation—with core elements: initiate, sustain, inhibit, shift.
- Social self-awareness—the accurate appraisal of oneself in relationship to others.

- Social sensitivity—relating to others within different interpersonal roles.
- Social problem solving—perceiving, comprehending, and working within social circumstances to achieve goals.

Within this classification scheme, it is possible to address more clearly some specific aspects of disturbed social behavior. Examples of stress inoculation training, behavior management, and cognitive restructuring are described for social self-regulatory disorders. Family education and involvement are also quite important. Pharmacological and alternative medicine approaches, such as music therapy, are possible as well (see Weintraub, 2001). Although slow and challenging to modify, alterations of social self-awareness can be addressed through individual- and family-based therapies, balancing the components fostering psychological adjustment in a cautious and steady fashion. Interacting with family members and developing productive ways for them to provide feedback to the patient are important. For impairments of social sensitivity, approaches can include role playing, perspective-taking exercises, interpersonal process recall, and specific skills-based training to promote prosocial behaviors, empathy, and interpersonal communication. Disturbances of social problem solving can be addressed with emphasis on skill-based abilities to perceive and analyze social situations, to identify and implement different response options, and to monitor their effectiveness in a type of metacognitive training approach. This level of remediation requires that patients have some degree of higher cognitive-behavioral abilities that permit reliable perception and communication around social circumstances. An example of such management approaches for social impairments can be found in Gregory and Lough (2000).

Additional areas of investigation and intervention include the mediating roles of "theory-of-mind" processing and social discourse skills in deepening interpersonal communication, comprehension, and problem solving. These more subtle aspects of social interaction may be impaired despite intact perceptual abilities and general language skills.

EMOTION-RELATED PROCESSING

Interest in emotion-related processing has continued to grow in the clinical and basic neurosciences. Flaherty-Craig, Barrett, and Eslinger (Chapter 13) proposed that emotion-related processing has a vital place in rehabilitation–intervention research as well. This view is based on the recognized commonality of these disorders in diverse neurological samples and the importance of emotion processing for social interactions, motivation, psychological adjustment, and recovery of function. Impairments of emotional perception, emotional expression, and emotional responsiveness are the disorders most often described. Studies have generally focused on emotional intonation of speech (prosody), emotional facial expressions, emotional arousal, and the reported experience of emotion after brain injury. These disorders may overlap with psychiatric diagnoses such as depression, apathy, and hypomania but are conceptualized as processing disorders rather than emotional states per se. Patients with frontal lobe and right-hemisphere disease appear to be at highest risk for emotional processing disorders, although subcortical sites of disease can also be implicated.

Rather than being limited to a neural substrate such as the limbic system, emotion processing is thought to be interrelated with visceral–autonomic and cognitive processes throughout subcortical and cortical structures, including the amygdala, the anterior cingulate cortex, the mesial and orbitofrontal cortices, the temporal–parietal–occipital regions, and other limbic–paralimbic areas. Important advances have been made in the recognition and description of these disorders, with formulation of several standardized assessment procedures. Intervention techniques have focused primarily on patient adjustment, patient self-awareness, family education, and *cognitively based* psychological support.

Although intervention approaches for emotion-related processing impairments remain largely descriptive, the expanding interplay of cognitive, social, emotional, and family factors is encouraging. Individualized approaches in single-case studies have drawn upon behavioral, cognitive and social formats to address three problem areas:

- Patient awareness of alterations in emotion-related perception and expression.
- Patient and family knowledge regarding emotion processes and their influence on motivation, social interaction, communication, and community reentry roles.
- Self-regulatory and problem-solving skills pertaining to emotion perception, expression, and experience.

As Prigatano (1999) and others have emphasized, recovery of emotion-related processing impairments takes place within a larger personal context of health concerns, cognitive and motor impairments, social interactions, family dynamics, and psychological adjustment. Providers function largely within a supportive role but increasingly can guide patients and families through stages of recovery and adjustment, drawing upon stronger models and clearer goals for intervention.

Pharmacological approaches have tentatively identified dopamine agonists, low-dosage stimulants, and serotonin reuptake inhibitors as effective agents for certain aspects of emotion-processing disorders, but more comprehensive studies are needed. Moreover, the general course of recovery and outcome with emotion-processing disorders remains unclear. Many patients appear to suffer long-standing alterations. Specific cognitive remediation efforts have been quite limited and require more investigation. A long-term goal is to identify and specify combined pharmacological, psychotherapeutic, and cognitively based remediation approaches.

CONCLUDING COMMENTS

The field of neuropsychological interventions is rapidly growing and combining the interests of both clinicians and researchers in identifying efficacious treatments for more neuropsychological disorders. As the many contributors to this volume emphasize, there is a great need for tighter linkages among the models of normal cognition, emotion, and adaptive change, concise assessment of those diverse processes, and remediation with evolving intervention techniques. Most importantly, this volume has emphasized cross-fertilization of these areas with the ideas and discoveries from each endeavor, arming providers and researchers, we hope, with a broader range of knowledge and methods for advancing the scientific basis for neuropsychological interventions. A growing concern for all clinical fields is the scientific, empirical evidence to support provision of specific interventions and management approaches. For neuropsychological impairments, it is still an early time for such analysis but there is increasing convergence of such evidence from these chapters, recent books, articles, and even an evidence-based analysis of cognitive rehabilitation (Cicerone et al., 2000).

Whether the focus of inquiry is neurobehavioral development and maturation or recovery after brain injury, both draw upon a common neural substrate of cerebral plasticity and adaptation to complex environments. Both draw upon models of neuropsychological functioning, comprehensive assessment, scientific investigation, adaptive change, and outcome over time. Hence, many of the challenges in neuropsychological rehabilitation research are similar to those in other fields, with the emphasis on conceptualizing the nature of adaptive change and identifying ways to promote such change in a positive, ethical, and cost-effective manner. This represents a continuing transition from diagnostic and descriptive analysis of neuropsychological impairments to linking diagnoses with intervention procedures that effect adaptive change in the face of neurological damage and dysfunction. The contribution of brain-based disorders to worldwide disability is increasing, and sound intervention procedures to manage escalating clinical conditions are a major aim of neurorehabilitation research. The particular area of neuropsychological intervention research has the capability to combine neurological, psychological, pharmacological, and functional brain imaging levels of inquiry within scientific and clinical–scientific formats to reduce the levels of disability and handicap that patients suffer and families experience.

REFERENCES

Barrett, A. M., Crucian, G. P., Maddux, C., & Heilman, K. M. (2000). Combined behavioral and cholinergic therapy in neurodegenerative disease using a naming task. *Journal of the International Neuropsychological Society, 6*, 173–174.

Bjorneby, E. R., & Reinvang, I. R. (1985). Acquiring and maintaining self-care skills after stroke: The predictive value of apraxia. *Scandinavian Journal of Rehabilitation Medicine, 17*, 75–80.

Cicerone, K. D., Dahlberg, C., Kalmar, K., Langenbahn, D. M., Malec, J. M., et al. (2000). Evidence-based cognitive rehabilitation: Recommendations for clinical practice. *Archives of Physical Medicine and Rehabilitation, 81*, 1596–1615.

Corbetta, M. (1990). Attentional modulation of neural processing of shape, color and velocity in humans. *Science, 248*, 1556–1559.

D'Zurilla, T. J., & Goldfried, M. R. (1971). Problem solving and behavior modification. *Journal of Abnormal Psychology, 78*, 107–126.

Foundas, A. L., Macauley, B. C., Rayner, A. M., Maher, L. M., Heilman, K. M., & Rothi, L. J. G. (1995). Ecological implications of limb apraxia: Evidence from mealtime behavior. *Journal of the International Neuropsychological Society, 1*, 62–66.

Freund, A. M., & Baltes, P. B. (1998). Selection, optimization, and compensation as strategies of life management: Correlations with subjective indicators of successful aging. *Psychology and Aging, 13*, 531–543.

Goldenberg, G., & Hagman, S. (1998). Therapy of activities of daily living in patients with apraxia. *Neuropsychological Rehabilitation, 8*, 123–141.

Gregory, C. A., & Lough, S. (in press). Practical issues in the management of early onset dementia. In J. R. Hodges (Ed.), *Early onset dementia: A multidisciplinary approach*. New York: Oxford University Press.

Institute of Medicine. (1997). *Enabling America: Assessing the role of rehabilitation science and engineering* (E. N. Brandt & A. M. Pope, Eds.). Washington, DC: National Academy Press.

Leopold, D. A., & Logothetis, N. K. (1996). Activity changes in early visual cortex reflect monkeys' percepts during binocular rivalry. *Nature, 379*, 549–553.

Levine, B., Robertson, I. H., Clare, L., Carter, G., Hong, J., Wilson, B. A., Duncan, J., & Stuss, D. T. (2000). Rehabilitation of executive functioning: An experimental–clinical validation of goal management training. *Journal of the International Neuropsychological Society, 6*, 299–312.

Luria, A. R. (1966). *Higher cortical functions in man*. New York: Basic Books.

Malec, J. F. (1999). Goal attainment scaling in rehabilitation. *Neuropsychological Rehabilitation, 9*, 253–276.

Motter, B. C. (1994). Neural correlates of attentive selection for color or luminance in extrastriate area V₄. *Journal of Neuroscience, 14*, 2190–2199.

Posner, M. I., & Petersen, S. E. (1990). The attention system of the human brain. *Annual Review of Neuroscience, 13*, 25–42.

Prigatano, G. P. (1999). *Principles of neuropsychological rehabilitation.* New York: Oxford University Press.

Saeki, S., Ogata, H., Okubo, T., Takahashi, K., & Hoshuyama, T. (1993). Factors influencing return to work after stroke in Japan. *Stroke, 24*, 1182–1185.

Shallice, T. (1981). Neurological impairments of cognitive processes. *British Medical Bulletin, 37*, 187–192.

Sundet, K., Finset, A., & Reinvang, I. R. (1988). Neuropsychological predictors in stroke rehabilitation. *Journal of Clinical and Experimental Neuropsychology, 10*, 363–379.

Taverni, J. P., Seliger, G., & Lichtman, S. W. (1998). Donepezil mediated memory improvement in traumatic brain injury during post acute rehabilitation. *Brain Injury, 12*, 77–80.

Teuber, H. L. (1964). The middle of frontal lobe function in man. In J. M. Warren & K. Akert (Eds.), *The frontal granular cortex and behavior* (pp. 410–444). New York: McGraw-Hill.

Treue, S., & Maunsell, J. H. (1996). Attentional modulation of visual motion processing in cortical areas MT and MST. *Nature, 382*, 539–541.

Van Essen, D. C., Anderson, C. H., & Fellerman, D. J. (1992). Information processing in the primate visual system: An integrated systems perspective. *Science, 255*, 419–423.

von Cramon, D. Y. Mathes-von Cramon, & Mai, N. (1991). Problem solving deficits in brain injured patients: A therapeutic approach. *Neuropsychological Rehabilitation, 1*, 45–64.

Weintraub, M. I. (Ed.). (2001). *Alternative and complementary treatment in neurologic illness.* New York: Churchill Livingstone.

World Health Organization. (2000). *The World Health Report 2000.* Geneva: Author.

Whyte, J., Hart, T., Schuster, K., Fleming, M., Polansky, M., & Coslett, B. (1997). Effects of methylphenidate on attentional function after traumatic brain injury: A randomized placebo-controlled trial. *American Journal of Physical Medicine and Rehabilitation, 76*, 440–450.

Zeki, S. (1992). The visual image in mind and brain. *Scientific American, 267*(3), 69–76.

Index